MW00980639

Pharmaceutics

Formulation and Processing of
Conventional Dosage Forms

Mrudula Bele

Assistant Professor in Pharmaceutics
MVP's College of Pharmacy,
Gangapur Road, Nashik,
Maharashtra

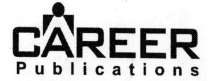

CAREER
Publications

Pharmaceutics
Formulation and Processing of Conventional Dosage Forms

First Edition : February 2012

ISBN:978-81-88739-91-2

© All rights reserved. No part of this book may be reproduced, stored in a retrieval system, or transmitted, in any form or by any means, electronic, mechanical, photocopying, recording, or otherwise, without the prior written permission of the publishers.

Published by :
Career Publications
Reg. Off. : 432/B, Deshmukh Bungalow ,
Vakil Wadi, Nashik - 422 001.
Maharashtra, India

Communication Address :
First Floor, Kaveri Smruti, Vakil Wadi,
Ashok Stambh, Nashik - 422001
Maharashtra, India.
Ph. : (0253) 2311210, 2310421, 2576175, 2311422
E-mail : info@careerandyou.com
        www.careerandyou.com

Pune Office :
First Floor, Gokhale
Classes Building, Tilak Road,
Pune - 411 030.
Maharashtra, India.
Ph. : (020) 24497602

Typesetting & Layout :
Satish More
Career Publications, Nashik.

Co-ordinating Editor :
Sudhanva Tipare
Hemlata Mali

Cover Design :
Kishor Pagare
Nishikant Wagh

Printer :
Replica Printers, Nashik

Price : ₹ 225.00

Pharmaceutics

Formulation and Processing of Conventional Dosage Forms

FOREWORD

It gave me immense pleasure to pen down my foreword about the upcoming book authored by Mrs. Mrudula Bele. The demand for an uncomplicated and standard book on conventional pharmaceutical dosage forms for undergraduate students has always been felt for long while teaching Pharmaceutics. The comprehensive treatise of the book seems most fascinating to me. The author has made enormous efforts to organise the updated content on the subject taken up in the book. The language and presentation technique of this book has been kept logical and simple for easy understanding of the subject theme. The author has tried hard for drawing figures in most simplified fashion for better understanding. The engorged content of this book would prove to be more useful to the concerned teachers and the readers.

Dr. S.K. Yadav

Principal,

Ravishankar College of Pharmacy, Bhopal

ACKNOWLEDGEMENT

It was some five years back, when Nishad had called me to ask if I would like to author a textbook on formulation of conventional dosage forms. I agreed!! However, I was always very lazy and it was only because of Nishad's and my colleague Dr. Milind Wagh's consistent perusal that I could finally do it. I am very happy that this book which I have been writing and writing and rewriting for last five years is now getting published. Eyes are misty though, that I cannot let Nishad know anymore that "I have finally done it". I could never thank Nishad, Sarika and Dr. Milind Wagh enough for being instrumental in publishing this book.

This book is an outcome of my teaching and learning experiments with the third year B.Pharm. students of my esteemed institute, MVP's College of Pharmacy, Nashik. My students taught me that teaching is the best way of learning. It was only because of the interactive lectures, and their demand for simplified notes that I thought of writing this book. My students made my notes popular in all over Maharashtra. One of my students told me one day that a 'xeroxwala' in Nashik is photocopying and selling my notes in the form of a 'book'!! So I thought why not write a book myself and take a credit of it !! I thank my students, faculty and Principal of MVP's College of Pharmacy for being a constant source of inspiration.

Thanks are due to my parents for consistently pushing me to finish this book. I am indebted to them for all the encouragement and motivation.

Spending time on writing this book was like snatching my time away from Hemant and Radha. I cannot thank you both enough for the patience and love...because without you my life would be meaningless!

Thanks are due to Dr. V.K. Maurya and Dr. S.K. Yadav who introduced me to the world of Pharmaceutics when I was their student. The foreword written by Dr. S.K. Yadav for my book is so special for me.

I would also like to thank Mr. Sudhanva Tipare, Ms. Hemlata Mali, Mr. Satish More, Mr. Sanjay Lolge and the entire Career team for their efforts in editing proof reading, typesetting and layouting this book.

- Mrudula Bele

To my aai and baba....
I am ......because you are!!

OUR EARLIER PUBLICATIONS

For B.Pharm

1)	Inorganic Pharmaceutical Chemistry (Theory)	: Dr. H.P. Tipnis & Dr. A.S. Dhake
2)	Inorganic Pharmaceutical Chemistry (Practical)	: Dr. D.P. Belsare & Dr. A.S. Dhake
3)	Anatomy Physiology and Health Education (Including Sports & Practical Physiology)	: Rahul P. Phate
4)	Modern Dispensing Pharmacy	: Dr. A.P. Pawar & Prof. R.S. Gaud
5)	Experimental Pharmaceutical Organic Chemistry: A Benchtop Manual	: Dr. K.S. Jain, P.B. Maniyar & Mrs. T.S. Chitre
6)	Biostatistics	: Dr. Sai Subramanian
7)	Pharmaceutical Analysis - I (Practical)	: Mrs. Sonali Sheorey & Ms. Meera Honrao
8)	Pharmacology (Part I) For Pharmacy	: Dr. Vivek Bele
9)	A Handbook of Experiments in Pre-clinical Pharmacology	: Dr. Sanjay Kasture
10)	Pharmacognosy & Phytochemistry (Volume - I)	: Dr. Vinod Rangari
11)	Pharmacognosy & Phytochemistry (Volume - II)	: Dr. Vinod Rangari
12)	Pharmaceutical Microbiology (Experiments and Techniques)	: Dr. C. R. Kokare
13)	Pathophysiology for Pharmacy	: Dr. Prakash Ghadi
14)	Introduction to Clinical Biochemistry	: Dr. S. P. Dandekar
15)	Principles and Applications of Biopharmaceutics and Pharmacokinetics	: Dr. H. P. Tipnis & Dr.Amrita Bajaj
16)	Business Accounting	: Dr. Mahesh Kulkarni
17)	Managerial Economics	: S. D. Geet, V. V. Morajkar & M. P. Wagh
18)	A Companion to Medicinal Chemistry	: N.N. Inamdar
19)	Practical Physical Pharmacy	: Dr.H.N. More & A.A Hajare
20)	Textbook of Pharmaceutical Analysis III (As per RGTU,Bhopal)	: Narendra Pratap,Sengar, Agarwal & Mrs. Singh
21)	Introduction to Pharmaceutics (For B.Pharm)	: Dr. Atmaram Pawar
22)	Clinical Pharmacy	: Dr. H. P. Tipnis & Dr. Amrita Bajaj
23)	Hospital Pharmacy	: Dr. H.P. Tipnis & Mrs. Amrita Bajaj
24)	A Textbook of Pharmacy Practice	: Dr.K.G.Revikumar & Dr. B.D.Miglani
25)	Vesicular & Particulate Drug Delivery Systems	: Edited by Prof.R.S.R.Murthy.
26)	Illustrated Glossary of Mycology	: Prof.Jitendra Vaidya
27)	Community Pharmacy	: Dr.H.P. Tipnis
28)	Spectroscopy	: Dr. D.P. Belsare, Prof. V.S. Kasture
29)	NIPER : A Companion	: N.N. Inamdar, A.H. Nathani

For D.Pharm

1)	Theory and Practice of Pharmaceutics - I	: Dr. A. P. Pawar
2)	Theory and Practice of Pharmaceutics - II	: Dr. A. P. Pawar
3)	Human Anatomy & Physiology	: Rahul Phate
4)	A Textbook of Biochemistry & Clinical Pathology	: Dr. Umekar, Lohiya & Kotagale
5)	Pharmaceutical Chemistry-II (for D.Pharm)	: Dr. A.S. Dhake, Dr. H.P.Tipnis
6)	Introduction to Pharmaceutical Chemistry	: S.K.Banerjee,Mashru & G. Banerjee
7)	Handbook for Community Pharmacists (Exclusively for Chemists & Druggists)	: Dr. Atmaram Pawar

For GPAT study...........

1)	GPAT : A Companion (For Pharmacy)	: N.N. Inamdar
2)	Pharmacy GATE Solved Question Papers	: N.N. Inamdar

Indian Reprints

1)	Managing Pharmaceuticals in International Health (Birkhauser)	: Anderson, Huss, Summers, Wiedenmayer
2)	Drug Metabolism (Springer)	: Caira, Mino R.; Ionescu, Corina (Eds.)
3)	Development and Manufacture of Protein Pharmaceuticals (Kluwer Academic/Plenum Publishers)	: Nail, Steve L.; Akers, Michael J. (Eds.)
4)	Liposomes Methods and Protocols (Humana Press)	: Basu, Subhash C.; Basu, Manju (Eds.)
5)	Drug Absorption Studies	: Carsten Ehrhardt
6)	Drug Delivery Systems	: Kewal Jain
7)	Polivinylpyrrolidone Excipients for Pharmaceuticals	: V.Buhler
8)	Chiral Separations	: G. Gobitz,Martin Schmid
9)	Optimization in Drug Discovery	: Zhengyin, Gary Caldwell
10)	Fundamentals of Clinical Research	: Bacchieri
11)	Modeling in Biopharmaceutics, Pharmacokinetics, and Pharmacodynamics	: Panos Macheras, Athanassios Iiiadis
12)	Biorelated Polymers	: Edited By: Emo Chiellini, Helena Gil, Gerhart Braunegg, Johanna Buchert, Paul Gatenholm and Maarten van der Zee
13)	Biopharmaceutical Drug Design and Development	: Edited By : Wu-Pong, Susanna, Rojanasakul, Yon
14)	New Approaches To Drug Development	: Edited By : P. Jolles

PREFACE

It is rightly said that one who has a 'Why' to live can get along with any 'how'!! Pharmaceutics is considered as an easier subject in the B.Pharm curriculum. However, I have experienced that students have many 'why's in their minds while learning pharmaceutics.

The whole idea behind writing this book was to address these 'whys' in formulation and manufacturing of conventional dosage forms. e.g. why a particular additive is chosen over the other? Why the USP limits have been set in a particular way? etc.

The dosage forms like tablets, hard and soft gelatin capsules, suppositories, dispersed systems and semisolids have been dealt with in this book. Topics like preformulation and tablet coating have also been discussed in depth.

The basic physicochemical principles involved in designing of any dosage form have been discussed in detail. The equipments used in manufacturing of the dosage forms and instruments used in their analysis have been discussed along with simplified diagrams. The principle behind every pharmacopeal method of evaluation have also been dealt with.

I hope all the undergraduate & postgraduate pharmacy students and teachers will find this book useful.

CONTENTS

Preformulation

INTRODUCTION:

When a new drug molecule shows considerable pharmacologic activity in animal trials, it is then to be subjected to evaluation in man. This evaluation includes testing of pharmacologic activity in humans and its correlation with the animal trials. Moreover it should also include evaluation of all those physicochemical properties of the new drug molecule that might affect its formulation into an effective dosage form. Preformulation commences when all these parameters are to be evaluated for a drug molecule after it has shown promising pharmacologic activity in animal trials. Preformulation encompasses activities ranging from supporting the discovery's identification of a new chemical ingredient to characterization of physical properties required for designing the dosage form.

Hundreds and thousands of compounds found in the chemical library are screened on animal models to find New Chemical Entities (NCEs) that have therapeutic potential. Although many initially promising NCEs are extremely

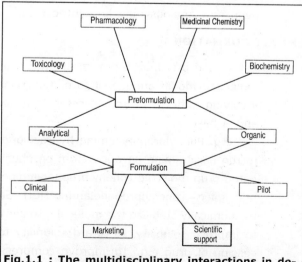

Fig.1.1 : The multidisciplinary interactions in development of a new drug candidate.

promising in *in vitro* studies, they are inactive in vivo because of their inadequate solubility and dissolution characteristics in the unfavorable aqueous environment of the body. This provides a demanding challenge for the preformulation scientist. The broad range of activities in preformulation requires a continuous interaction between scientists of different disciplines as shown in figure. 1.1

Almost all new drugs that are active orally are marketed as tablets, capsules or both. Only a few compounds are marketed as injections. Some other dosage forms may be required but they are usually drug specific.

Prior to development of a new drug into any of these three dosage forms, it is essential to study certain physicochemical properties; and other derived properties of the drug molecule. The preformulation studies often proceed in following order:

PRELIMINARY EVALUATION AND MOLECULAR OPTIMIZATION

Once a molecule is found pharmacologically active, a project team comprising of scientists from various disciplines as shown in the figure 1.1, have the responsibility of assuring that the molecule enters the development process in its optimum molecular form. For a physical pharmacist who has the responsibility to see how the product is going to be formulated and administered to the patient, solubility and stability are the two most important parameters which might adversely affect the drug performance.

Exhaustive experiments are to be carried out on the new drug to detect any problem areas. If any deficiency is found, a molecular modification is to be done which can improve drug properties. Salts, pro-drugs, solvates, polymorphs, or even new analogs may be synthesized.

i) SALT FORMATION :

Salt formation and pro drug approach are the two most commonly used approaches for molecular modification. Salt formation is one of the simplest chemical reactions, involving either a proton transfer or a neutralization reaction between an acid and a base.

e.g. Phenylpropanolamine hydrochloride is prepared by addition of a proton to the basic amine nitrogen atom on phenylpropanoplamine resulting in a protonated drug molecule (phenylpropanolamine-H$^{(+)}$) which is neutralized with a chloride anion (phenylpropanolamine-HCl). Salt forms of drugs are often prepared to chemically stabilize the molecule, to convert it to a less hygroscopic compound, to improve solubility, to retard solubility for sustaining release, to improve processing of drug e.g., to improve compressibility and flow properties and to improve bioavailability.

During synthesis, salts are usually formed in organic media to improve yield and purity.

Table 1.1: Property modification of drug molecules by salt formation.

Drug modified	Salt forming agent	Property modified
Ampicillin	N-alkylsulfamate	Absorption
Aspirin	Tromethamine	Oral absorption
Bephenium	Hydroxynaptholate	Toxicity
Cephalexin	Anthraquinone-1,5 disulphonic acid	Stability, absorption
Cephalosporins	Arginine	Toxicity
Dinoprost	Tromethamine	Physical state
Erythromycin	Aspartate	Solubility
	1 – Glutamine	Solubility, stability
Heptaminol	Decanoate	Sustained action
Kanamycin	Pamoic acid	Toxicity
Lincomycin	N-alkyl sulfamates	Oral absorption
Metformin	Carnitine	Toxicity
Propoxyphene	4-chloro-m-toluene sulphonic acid	Organoleptic properties
α-Sulphobenzene	Arginine	Stability
Penicillin		hygroscopicity, toxicity
Tetracycline	Betaine	Gastric absorption
Viracamine	Dioctyl Sulphosuccinate	Organoleptic properties

Table 1.2: Different types of salts used in marketed pharmaceutical products.

Anionic salts		
Acetate	Dihydrochloride	Phosphate
Benzoate	Edetate	Salicylate
Bicarbonate	Esylate	Stearate
Bitartrate	Estolate	Subacetate
Carbonate	Fumarate	Succinate
Chloride	Gluconate	Sulphate
Citrate	Calulamate	Tannate
	Hexylresorcinate	

Cationic salts (organic)
Benzalthine
Chloline
Diethanolamine
Ethylenediamine
Meglumine
Procaine

	Cationic salts (Metalic)
Hydrobromide	Aluminium
Hydrochloride	Calcium
Iodide	Lithium
Isothionate	Magnesium
Lactate	Potassium
Lactobionate	Sodium
Malate	Zinc
Maleate	
Mesylate	
Methyl sulphate	
Nitrate	
Pamoate	
Pantothenate	

II) PRODRUGS :

Salt formation is limited to molecules with ionizable groups. Prodrugs, however, may be formed with any organic molecule having a chemically reactive functional group.

A Drug substance, whose physicochemical properties are not optimum and hence limit its use, is chemically modified via the attachment of a premoiety in order to generate a new chemical entity called a prodrug. A prodrug is an inactive compound, formed by linking a drug to an inert chemical viz a premoiety, by a co-valent bond which should be broken *in vivo*. The co-valent bond may break spontaneously or enzymatically to yield the active drug. The pro-drugs are formed in order to optimize one or more of the following properties.

1. Physical properties: odor, taste, pain upon injection.
2. Physicochemical properties: lipophilicity, hydrophilicity, stability.
3. Pharmacokinetic properties: absorption through the epithelial membranes, passage through the blood-brain barrier, protection against presystemic metabolism or enzymatic degradation, onset of drug action, toxicity due to

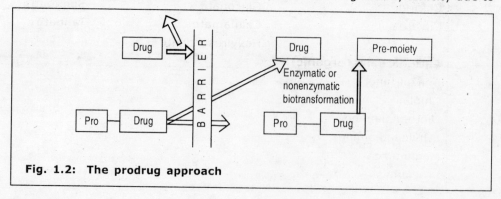

Fig. 1.2: The prodrug approach

local irritation or distribution in tissues other than target tissue, site specificity. e.g. Mesalamine (5-amino salicylic acid) is a drug useful in treatment of inflammatory bowel disease, since it is not absorbed into systemic circulation. Following oral administration, the drug is inactivated before reaching the lower intestine which is the site of action. Covalent bonding of this agent to sulfapyridine yields the prodrug sulfasalazine, an azo compound. This prodrug reaches the colon intact where cleavage by the bacterial enzyme azoreductase releases the active mesalamine for action.

Sulfasalazine

Colonic bacteria | Azoreductase

Mesalamine + Sulfapyridine

Table 1.3: Major areas of preformulation research.

Parent drug	Prodrug	Property modified
Chloramphenicol	Chloromphenicol palmitate	Taste
Clindamycin	Clindamycin palmitate	Taste
Sulfisoxazole	Acetyl ester	Taste
Trimcinolone	Diacetate ester	Taste
Ethyl mercaptan	Phthalate ester	Odor
Trichloroethanol	p-acetamido benzoate ester	Change of state
Salicylic acid	Acetyl salicylic acid	G.I. irritation
Kanamycin	Kanamycin pamoate	G.I. irritation
Nicotinic acid	Nicotinic acid hydrazide	G.I. irritation
Clindamycin	2-phosphate ester	reduced pain on injection
Chloramphenicol	Sodium succinate ester	Aqueous solubility
Tocopherols	Sodium succinate ester	Aqueous solubility
Corticosteroids	Phosphate ester	Aqueous solubility
Testosterone	Phosphate ester	Aqueous solubility
Menthol	β-glucoside	Aqueous solubility
Sulfanilamide	Glucosyl sulfanilamide	Aqueous solubility
Diazepam	L-lysine ester	Aqueous solubility
Metronidazole	Amino acid ester	Aqueous solubility
Azacytidine	Bisulfite prodrug	Stability
Ampicillin	Pivampicillin	Bioavailability
	Bacampicillin	Bioavailability
	Talampicillin	Bioavailability

Erythromcycin	Erythromycin estolate	Bioavailability
Naproxen	Dipalmitoyl glycerol ester	Bioavailability
Nadolol	Diacetate ester	Bioavailability
Epinephrine	Dipivalyl ester	Bioavailability
Triamcenolone	Triamcenolone acetonide	Prevention of presystemic metabolism
Propranolol	Hemisuccinate ester	Presystemic metabolism
Steroids	Propionate ester	Sustained release
Pilocarpine	Diester prodrug	sustained release
Timolol	Lipophilic ester prodrug	sustained release
Epinephrine	Diester ketone prodrug	Targetted delivery to eye
Acyclovir	Acyclovir monophosphate	Targetting to virally infected cells
Sulfasalazine	5-amino sulfasalazine	Targetting to colon
Formaldehyde	Hexamine	Targetting to urinary tract.

After choosing the optimum molecular form of a drug, its formulation development commences. In this phase, different physicochemical variables of the drug are quantified which assist in development of safe, effective and stable dosage form with maximum bioavailability.

Bulk Characterization: The synthetic process and the preformulation studies on an API are often conducted simultaneously. Therefore, comprehensive characterization of the bulk lots is essential to avoid misleading predictions of solubility and stability.

III) CRYSTALLINITY AND POLYMORPHISM :

A solid compound may be crystalline or amorphous. Crystals are characterized by repetitious spacing of constituents atoms or molecules in a 3-dimensional array. Whereas, amorphous solids have no such rhythmic patterns and atoms or molecules are randomly placed.

Crystal habit and internal structure of a drug affect several physicochemical

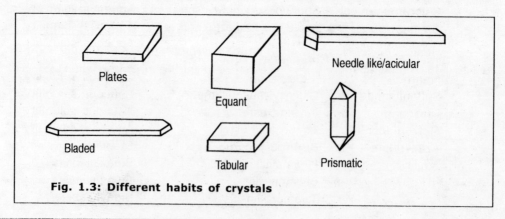

Fig. 1.3: Different habits of crystals

Plates

Equant

Needle like/acicular

Bladed

Tabular

Prismatic

properties. Crystal habit describes the outer appearance of crystals and the internal structure is described by the molecular arrangement. Different habits of crystals are shown in figure 1.3.

A compound having a single internal structure may have several crystal habits depending on the environment for growing crystals. Changes in the internal structure produce changes within the crystal habit, whereas chemical changes produce a change in both the internal structure and the crystal habit e.g. conversion of a salt to its free acid. Therefore the internal structure as well as crystal habit must be verified and described.

The internal structure may be classified in various ways :

Crystalline forms are thermodynamically more stable than amorphous forms and hence show greater solubilities and dissolution rates. Upon storage amorphous

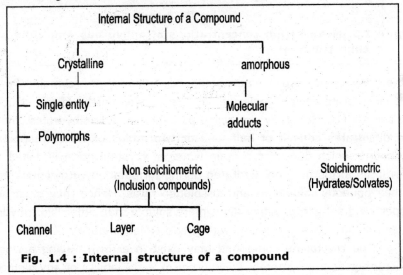

Fig. 1.4 : Internal structure of a compound

solids may revert to more stable forms; which is a major disadvantage

Table 1.4: Plasma levels of amorphous and crystalline Novobiocin in dogs following oral administration.

Hours after dose	Sodium Novo biocin (Crystalline) µg/ml, Plasma	Amorphous Novobiocin µg/ml, Plasma
0.5	0.5	5.0
1.0	0.5	40.6
2.0	14.6	29.5
3.0	22.2	22.3
4.0	16.9	23.7
5.0	10.4	20.2
6.0	6.4	17.5

Non-stoichiometric adducts consist of the solvent molecules entrapped in lattice structure. They are non-reproducible and hence are undesirable and should

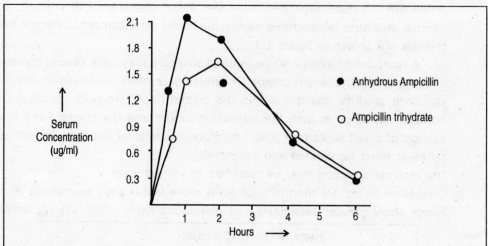

Figure 1.5: Mean serum concentrations of anhydrous Ampicillin and Ampicillin trihydrate.

not be developed. Stoichiometric adducts or solvates are molecular complexes that incorporate solvent molecules at specific sites in the lattice structure. When the solvent is water, they are called as hydrates. (Hemihydrates, monohydrates and dihydrates consist of half, one or two moles of water respectively). The compound which does not contain water of crystallization is called anhydrous. Anhydrous forms may get hydrated during formulation with remarkable increase in their aqueous solubilities and dissolution rates. Hence they must be identified properly e.g.anhydrous ampicillin is more soluble than ampicillin trihydrate, hence its dissolution rates are faster with greater bioavailability.

The crystalline compound may exist in a form having a single internal structure or as a polymorph. Polymorphism is the ability of any element or compound to crystallize as more than one distinct crystal species having entirely different internal structures e.g. carbon as cubic diamond or hexagonal graphite. Different polymorphs of a compound are, in general, different in structure and properties in the same manner as the crystals of two different compounds. Solubility, melting point, density, hardness and crystal forms may be different for the polymorphs and hence their performance as drug molecule differs. Metastable polymorphs often get transformed into stable polymorphs. Cimetidine exists in four polymorphic forms; A,B,C and D. Plasma concentrations of polymorphic forms; A,B and C were investigated and are summarised in figure 1.6. Form C is the more soluble polymorph and hence shows greater peak plasma concentration. Characterization of crystalline, solvated and polymorphic crystal forms can be done by several methods listed in Table 1.5.

Table 1.5 : Analytical methods for Characterisation of solid forms

- · Microscopy
- · Fusion methods
- · Differential scanning colorimetry (DSC/DTA)
- · Infrared Spectroscopy
- · X-ray diffraction
- · Scanning Electron Microscopy
- · Thermogravimetry
- · Dissolution/ solubility analysis

MICROSCOPY :

Differences in crystal morphology of polymorphic forms is sufficiently distinct if viewed microscopically. Hence microscopy is routinely used to describe polymorphic crystal habits.

Microscopes with crossed polarizing filters can distinguish between amorphous and crystalline forms. Amorphous substances and substances with cubic crystal lattices are isotropic i.e have single refractive index. Isotropic substances appear black with crossed polarized filters. Materials with more than one refractive index are anisotropic and appear bright with brilliant colours against black polarized background. The interference colour depends on crystal thickness and difference in refractive indices. Different polymorphs show different interference colours and can be distinguished by this technique. However, the technique is difficult and requires well trained optical crystallographers.

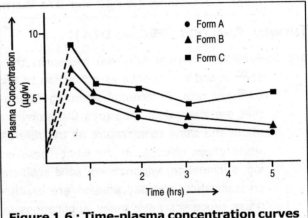

Figure 1.6 : Time-plasma concentration curves for three polymorphic forms of Cimetidine

FUSION METHODS (HOT STAGE MICROSCOPY) :

This involves use of a microscope equipped with a heated and lagged sample stage. This heating rate is controllable. It is a useful instrument for investigating polymorphism, melting points, transition temperatures and rates of transition.

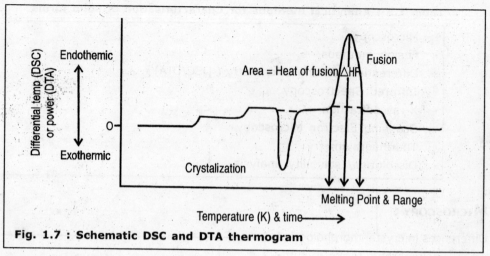

Fig. 1.7 : Schematic DSC and DTA thermogram

THERMAL ANALYSIS (DSC AND DTA):

DTA (Differential Thermal Analysis) measures the temperature difference between the sample and a reference as a function of temperature or time, while heating at a constant rate. Differential scanning calorimetry (DSC) is similar to DTA except that the instrument measures the amount of energy required to keep the sample at the same temperature as the reference i.e. it measures enthalpy of transition phase changes in the when there is a temperature change. Fusion, boiling, sublimation, vaporization, solid-solid transitions are often endothermic, while crystallization and degradation are exothermic. Quantitative measurements of these processes have many applications in preformulation studies.

For characterization of crystal forms, the heat of fusion (ΔHF) can be obtained from the area under the DSC-curve for the melting endotherm. Similarly, the heat of transition from one polymorph to another can be calculated. A sharp

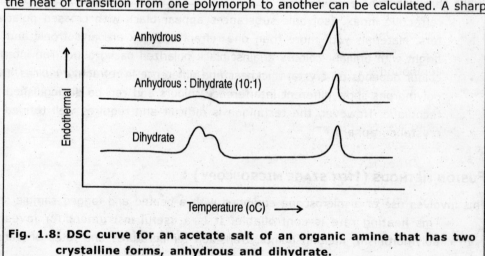

Fig. 1.8: DSC curve for an acetate salt of an organic amine that has two crystalline forms, anhydrous and dihydrate.

symmetric melting endotherm indicates good purity while a broad asymmetric peak suggest impurity.

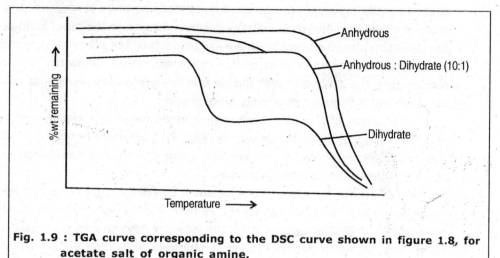

Fig. 1.9 : TGA curve corresponding to the DSC curve shown in figure 1.8, for acetate salt of organic amine.

THERMOGRAVIMETRIC ANALYSIS (TGA):

Thermogravimetric Analysis measures change in sample weight as a fuction of temperature or time. Comparing TGA and DSC data can aid in identification of thermal processes.

X-RAY DIFFRACTION:

X-rays are diffracted by crystals. This is because X-rays have wavelengths of about the same magnitude as the distance between the atoms or molecules of crystals. The X-ray diffraction pattern is photographed on a sensitive plate arranged behind the crystal and by such a method the structure of the crystal may be investigated. It provides a precise identification and description of a crystalline substance. Unit cell dimensions and angles conclusively establish the crystalline lattice system and provide specific differences between crystalline forms of a given compound.

Where whole crystals are unavailable for analysis, a powder of the substance may be investigated. The position and intensity of lines on such a diagram are compared with those on the photograph of a known sample and a qualitative and quantitative analysis is conducted.

Other methods such as Infrared diletometry, Proton Magnetic Resonance spectroscopy (PMR), Nuclear Magnetic Reasonance Spectroscopy (NMR) and Scanning Electron Microscopy (SEM) may be used for studying polymorphism and solvation.

POLYMORPHISM :

Polymorphs are either enantiotropic or monotropic. Enantiotropic polymorphs can be reversibly changed into another form by changing temperature or pressure. In monotropic polymorphism, one form is unstable at all temperatures and pressures. At a specified pressure, usually at 1 atmosphere, the temperature at which the two forms show identical free energies and may get transformed to the other form is called the transition temperature. They have identical solubilites in any solvent and identical vapor pressure and can co-exist at this temperature. Below the solid melting temperature, the polymorph with the low free energy, has lower solubility and vapor pressure and is thermodynamically more stable.

Identification of the polymorph that is more stable at room temperature, is important during preformulation studies. Also, it is important to determine whether polymorphic transformations are possible within the temperature range used for stability studies and during processing.

The difference in melting point between polymorphs (DMP) is a measure of the metastable polymorph stability. When DMP < 1^{0}C, then neither is significantly more stable. If DMP is 25-50^{0}C, then the lower melting species is difficult to crystallize and will revert rapidly. The closer the two m.p. DMP between 1 to 25^{0}C, then the unstable forms can be obtained easily before a solid –solid transformation occurs. Polymorphic compounds are best characterised by a complete pressure temperature phase diagram showing melt vapor, solid-vapor and solid-melt curves.

HYGROSCOPICITY:

Many drugs, particularly those that are water soluble salts, adsorb moisture from atmosphere. This moisture uptake may affect several properties of drugs viz. chemical stability, compressibility, flow properties.

Following procedure is used to test hygroscopicity: The drug substance is spread in a thin layer in several open containers to ensure maximum atmospheric exposure. These containers are then exposed to vanable relative humidity environments, obtained from several saturated salt solutions. Amount of moisture uptake is monitered for 0 to 12 weeks by any of the methods viz. gravimetry, TGA, Karl Fischer titration or gas chromatography. The data is represented as normalized (mg of water/gm of sample) or % of weight gain Vs time. Different storage conditions for the drug viz. storage in low humidity environment or special packaging with a dessicant may be assigned after examining this data.

FINE PARTICLE CHARACTERIZATION:

Certain physical and chemical properties of drug molecules are affected by the particle size distribution including drug dissolution rate, bioavailability, content uniformity, taste, texture, colour and stability. In addition properties such as flow characteristics and sedimentation rates are also important factors related to particle size. The way in which the particle size affects drug formulation should be found out. Particle size also significantly influences the oral absorption.

Particle size, shape and surface morphology may be determined by following methods:

i) ***Optical microscopy:*** A light microscope fitted with a calibrated grid may be used to find out size and shape. A slide is prepared by using a random sample. Several particles are sized and the resulting mean size and particle size range and frequency of particles falling in this range is found out and represented in the form of histograms. Photomicrographs of these slides may be taken using a Polaroid camera.

ii) ***Stream counting devices:*** Stream counting devices such as Coulter counter provide a convenient method for characterizing particle size distribution. The material is dispersed in a conducting medium like isotonic saline by sonication and by adding a few drops of surfactant. A small volume of this dispersion is then allowed to pass through an aperture on both sides of which a voltage is applied. Each particle while passing through the aperture, displaces the volume of the conducting medium equivalent to its own volume and develops a resistance. Other stream counters are based on principles of light blockage or laser light scattering.

iii) ***Gas adsorption:*** Dissolution and degradation of the drug may be more directly related to surface area rather than particle size. Gas adsorption method provides precise measurement of particle surface area. A layer of nitrogen molecules is adsorbed on sample surface at -196°C. Once the adsorption has reached maximum, the sample is reheated to room temperature. The nitrogen gas is then desorbed. Its volume is measured and converted to number of nitrogen gas molecules. A single nitrogen molecule occupies an area of 16 A^2. Weight specific surface area for the powder is calculated by multiplying no. of nitrogen molecules by cross sectional area of one molecule. Surface area may be determined for several partial pressures of nitrogen. (5 to 35% N_2 in He) and extrapolated to zero nitrogen partial pressure to yield true mono layer surface area.

SCANNING ELECTRON MICROSCOPY:

SEM is a useful tool to confirm physical observations related to surface area. The sample is exposed to high vacuum and coated with gold to make the sample conductive and then scanned with SEM which gives an idea of surface morphology.

BULK DENSITY:

Apparent bulk density is measured by pouring the pre-sieved drug sample in a graduated flask and measuring its weight and volume to give its bulk density (gm/ml). The tapped bulk density is found out by placing the graduated cylinder on a mechanical tapping apparatus till its volume is reduced to a minimum. This tapped volume is then used to find out the tapped bulk density.

The true densities and granular densities may be found out by liquid displacement methods.

The density determination is important in deciding the size of capsule in which is the drug is to be filled or to ensure homogeneity of a low dose tablet or capsule where there are large density differences between the drug and the excipients.

POWER FLOW PROPERTIES:

Determination of flow properties of a drug powder are important for several reasons. Flow property determinations help the formulation pharmacist determine in taking several decisions while designing a formulation. For example:

1. To choose among various methods of tablet compression viz. wet/dry granulation or direct compression.

2. To chose a proper feeding device e.g. auger or vibrating feeding hopper Angle of repose is an important property that can be determined for a powder to get an idea about its flow properties. It is the maximum angle that can be obtained between the free standing surface of a powder heap and the horizontal plane. There is a relationship between angle of repose (θ) and the ability of the powder to flow. Table 1.6 gives an idea about the type of flow one expects after determining the angle of repose.

Table 1.6: Angle of repose as an indication of powder flow properties.

Angle of repose (θ)	Type of flow
< 25	Excellent
25-30	Good
30 - 40	Passable
> 40	Very poor

Angle of repose determinations usually lack precision and hence are less important in determining powder flow rates. A useful emperical parameter is Carr's compressibility index.

CARR'S INDEX :

A simple test was developed by Carr and Neumann to evaluate flow properties of powders by comparing the poured (fluff/untapped) density and tapped density of a powder. Carr's compressibility index is defined as

$$\text{Carr's Index (\%)} = \frac{\text{Tapped density} - \text{Bulk density}}{\text{Tapped density}} \times 100$$

Table 1.7: Interpretation of carr's indices.

Carr's Index (%)	Type of flow
5 – 15	Excellent
12 – 16	Good
18 – 21	Fair to passable*
23 – 35	Poor*
33 – 38	Very poor
> 40	extremely poor

* May be improved by glidant

A similar index was developed by Hausner.

$$\text{Hausner ratio} = \frac{\text{Tapped density}}{\text{Bulk density}}$$

Hausner's index values of less than 1.25 indicate good flow (=20% Carr's index), while greater than 1.5 indicate poor flow (= 33% carr's index). Between 1.25 & 1.5, added glidant normally improves flow.

Carr's index and Hausner's ratio are one point determinations and do not always reflect the ease or speed with which the consolidation may occur.

A direct method of measurement is the flow through an orifice consisting of a metal tube from which drug flows through an orifice onto an electronic balance. A strip chart record directly gives the flow rate in grams/sec.

Flow rates (gm/sec) are determined for various orifices (1/8 to ½").

Following equation may be used to show the dependence of flow rate (W) on trece particle density (ρ), gravity (g) and orifice diameter (D_o)

$$D_o = A \left(\frac{4W}{60 \ \pi \rho \sqrt{g}} \right)^{1/n}$$

A and n are constants dependent upon the material and its particle size.

For cohesive powders tensile testing is done with the help of shear cells. The details of these tests are discussed in chapter 2.

SOLUBILITY ANALYSIS

Aqueous solubility of the drug dictates the ease with which it can be formulated as an aqueous solution for oral use and intravenous injections for preclinical studies. Preformulation solubility e.g. a drug for oral administration should be checked for solubility in media having isotonic chloride ion concentrations and acidic pH. The routes of administration may not be defined at this stage. But knowing the solubility of the drug and its solubilization mechanism can provide a basis of formulation work in the future.

Solubility analysis should include determination of aqueous, intrinsic, intrinoic solubility, pKa, temperature dependence, pH solubility profile, solubility products, solubilization mechanisms and rates of dissolution.

All the factors in solubility and dissolution experiments should be defined including pH, temperature, ionic strength and buffer concentrations.

AQUEOUS SOLUBILITY :

Aqueous solubility values that are important in early stage development are those in distilled water, 0.9% NaCl, 0.01 M HCl, 0.1m HCl and 0.1 m NaOH at room temperature as well as 37^{0}C. These early results are useful in developing suspensions and solutions for preclinical and toxicological studies.

A solubility of less than 1% or less than 1 mg/ml indicates a potential bioavailability problem and poor and erratic absorption from gastrointestinal tract. It often indicates a need for salt, particularly if the drug is to be formulated as a tablet or a capsule. In the range of 1-10 mg/ml serious consideration should be given to salt formation. If it is not possible to manipulate the solubility in this way, then liquid filling in soft gelatin capsules should be considered.

pk$_a$ DETERMINATIONS:

Solubility largely depends on pH. Therefore it is important to determine dissociation constant of a drug capable of ionizing in the pH range of 1 to 10. The concentration of ionized and unionized drug at a particular pH can be estimated by the use of Henderson – Hasselbalch equation.

For acidic compounds,

$$pH = pKa + log \frac{[\text{ionized drug}]}{[\text{unionized drug}]}$$

For basic compounds,

$$pH = pKa + log \frac{[\text{unionized drug}]}{[\text{ionized drug}]}$$

For weakly acidic drugs having pKa values more than 3, the unionized form is present in stomach in acidic pH. The drug is ionized predominantly in the neutral medium of the intestine.

pKa value can be most efficiently determined by detection of spectral shifts by UV or visible spectroscopy. Another method of potentiometric titrations is very sensitive for compounds having pKa values of 3 to 10. A suitable co-solvent such as methanol or dimethyl sulfoxide can be incorporated to avoid precipitation of unionized species.

The pH – dependence of solubility can also be used to obtain pKa value, in case of insoluble drugs. The pH of a solution where the equilibrium solubility is twice that of intrinsic solubility is the pKa.

EFFECT OF TEMPERATURE ON SOLUBILITY:

Most solution processes are endothermic, with positive heat of solution (ΔH_s). Therefore increasing the solution temperature increases the solubility.

Heat of solution is determined from solubility values of saturated solutions at 5°C, 25°C, 37°C and 50°C, ΔHs is determined using following equation:

$$\ln s = \frac{\Delta H_s}{R}\left(\frac{1}{T}\right) + C$$

S – Molar solubility at temperature T (°k)

R – Gas constant

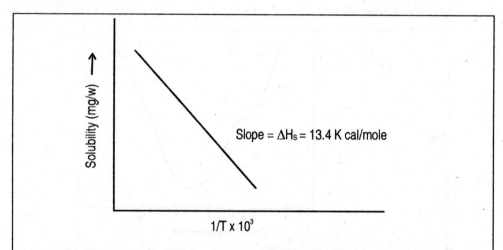

Fig. 1.10: A semi logarithmic plot of solubility against a reciprocal of temperature is linear over a limited temperature range and Hs can be obtained from slope.

SOLUBILIZATION :

The required drug may have poor or insufficient aqueous solubility. Sufficient experiments should be carried out in the preformulation studies for identifying possible mechanisms of solubilization.

The most frequently used approach for solubilization is co-solvency. Addition of co-solvents like ethanol, propylene glycol or glycerine significantly increases solubility. The extent of solubilization by addition of a co-solvent depends on polarity of the solute. More non-polar is the solute, greater is the extent of solubilization.

STABILITY ANALYSIS

The first quantitative assessment of stability of a new drug candidate occurs during preformulation. The drug candidate is tested under general conditions of handiling, processing and storage, both in solid state and solution state.

Solution state stability : The preformulation studies in solution state are carried out to identify the desired conditions for preparing stable solutions of the new drug candidate. The effect of pH, ionic strength, light, co- solvent, temperature and oxygen on the solution state stability of the candidate is studied in this phase.

i) pH : The drug samples in solution state are intentionally degraded at extreme pH and temperatures(0.1 N HCl/0.1 N NaOH/water at 90°C). This data gives idea on maximum rates of degradation. This study is followed by a generation of complete pH – degradation rate profile by using buffers of varying pH. The ionic strength, drug and co-solvent levels should be kept constant while studying the pH rate profile.

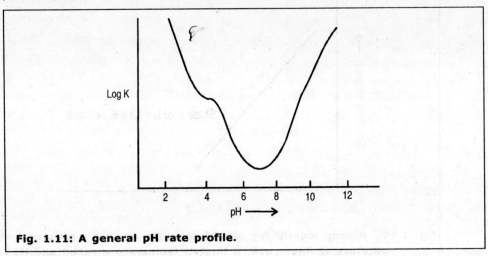

Fig. 1.11: A general pH rate profile.

ii) Ionic strength: The pH rate profile study should be carried out at constant ionic strength. Ionic strength for any new buffer solution can be found out from following equation:

$$\mu = \frac{1}{2} \varepsilon \, M_i Z_i^2$$

M_i – molar concentration of ion (all the ionic species in buffer plus drug should be considered.) Z_i –valency of ionic species.

iii) Co solvents : Co-solvents may be needed to produce drug concentration needed for analysis. If different co-solvents or the same co-solvent at different concentrations is added then the drug decay rates vary. They are found to vary linearly with the reciprocal of the dielectric constant of the solvent.

iv) Temperature : The stability solutions are placed in flame sealed ampoules and subjected to elevated temperatures not exceeding boiling points of solvent. Some ampoules are subjected to variable temperatures.

v) Light : The ampoules may be subjected to light stability by packaging in amber and yellow-green glass containers and protective samples in cardboard packages.

vi) Oxygen : To know the oxidation potential the ampoules are further tested with :

- excessive headspace for oxygen
- with a headspace of inert gas
- with an inorganic antioxidant
- with an organic antioxidant

Stability data generated in this way at each pH and temperature condition is used to find decay rate constants. The logarithm of decay rate constants are then plotted versus pH to generate the pH rate profile. The pH of maximum stability is the pH at which the graph shows the minimum.

The logarithm of decay rate constant is plotted versus absolute temperature for each buffer solution to generate the Arrhenius plot. A linear Arrhenius plot indicates a linear degradation mechanism and is useful for calculation of energy of activation. A broken Arrhenius plot is indicative of a change in decay mechanism.

EXCIPIENTS

Atmost all therapeutic products include excipients. In fact the total amount of excipients frequently used is greater than the active substances in the dosage form. All the therapeutic products must meet the following requirements to ensure safety, efficacy and quality :

- Convenience of administering
- Accuracy of dose
- Easy availability of drug in absorbable form
- Assurance of quality throughout shelf life
- Easy and reproducible process of manufacturing without compromising on performance.

It is impossible for any active pharmaceutical ingredient to have properties that allow incorporation in a therapeutic product that meets all above mentioned criteria. Therefore, it is desirable to add other materials to compensate any shortfalls. Therefore every therapeutic product is a combination of a drug and excipients.

An excipient (derived from words excipere to take out, receive) may be defined as a substances mixed with the active pharmaceutical ingredient to give it consistency or used as a vehicle for its administration.

CLASSIFICATION OF EXCIPIENTS :

There can be two ways of classifiying excipients:

- Depending on the type of dosage form in which they are used.
- Depending on the function they perform in the dosage form.

1. DEPENDING ON TYPE OF DOSAGE FORM IN WHICH THEY ARE USED:

This way of classifying excipients is based on the class of the dosage form in which they are being used. Fig. 1.12 indicates the classes in which they can be classified according to this system.

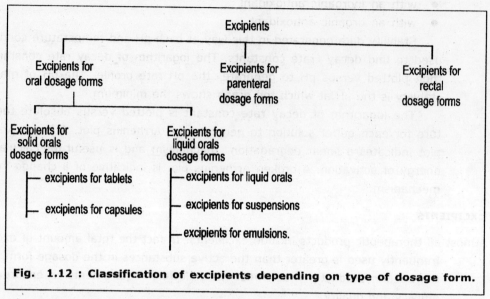

Fig. 1.12 : Classification of excipients depending on type of dosage form.

2. DEPENDING ON THE FUNCTION THEY PERFORM IN THE DOSAGE FORM:

As mentioned earlier, the excipients may perform different types of function in the dosage form and they may be classified accordingly as shown in figure 1.13.

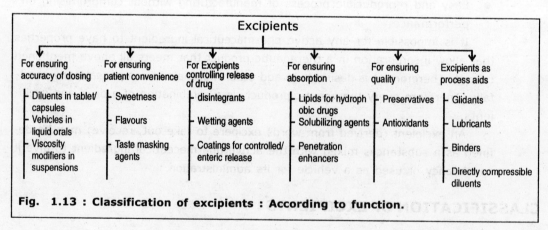

Fig. 1.13 : Classification of excipients : According to function.

Selection of excipients :

The selection of excipients for any particular active pharmaceutical ingredient is based on following criteria :

1. Nature and properties of active ingredient. e.g. stability, dose, compressibility etc.
2. Type of dosage form e.g. tablet, capsule, ointment etc.
3. The process by which it is going to be manufactured.
4. The target patient group e.g. adults, paediatrics, geriatrics.
5. The clinical condition of patients. e.g. diabetics, hypertensives

The excipient should be selected by considering all above parameters. The candidate excipients should then be evaluated for their functionality i.e. they function in the manner intended (do what they are meant to do).

Another important criteria in excipient selection is the regulatory status of the excipient and the country specific requirements for the same. The specifications for the excipients must comply with the pharmacopoeial standards of the particular country where the drug product is expected to be marketed. i.e. the United States Pharmacopoeia (USP) for the US, the European Pharmacopoeia (EP) for the Europe and the Japanese Pharmacopoeia (JP) for Japan. Unfortunately the specification tests for excipients are not the same in different pharmacopoeias. In some cases, the specifications are mutually exclusive i.e. for some excipients, it may be impossible to pass the specifications in all the three pharmacopoeias. e.g. the temperature specified for conducting the test for sulfated ash which is included as a specification for many excipients is 800+/- 25⁰C in the JP (refer Table 1.7).

The lack of harmonization for excipient standards between the different pharmacopoeias has been recognized by international regulatory agencies and a programme has been established to attempt to rationalise the difference. However, it will take more than a decade to alter this situation.

Table1.7 : Specifications for Sulfated ash/residue on ignition –according to different pharmacopoeias.

	EP II	USP XXII	JP XI
* First heating with Addition of H_2SO_4	Yes	No	Yes
* Temperature	600⁰C	800 ($\pm$) 25⁰C	450-550⁰C
* Final addition of ammonium carbonate	Yes	No	No
* Means of heating	Water bath Then flame	not specified	not specified

The desirability of harmonizing excipient standards has been recognized by the European, U.S and Japanese pharmacopoeas and an open conference sponsored by the USP, JP and EP in 1991 was the beginning of the harmonisation process. Table1.8 lists the excipients selected for harmonization.

Table 1.8: Excipients selected for harmonisation.

Excipient	Leading p'copoeia
Magnesium-stearate	USP
Microcrystalline cellulose	USP
Lactose	USP
Starch	USP
Cellulose derivatives	USP
Sucrose	EP
Povidone	JP
Stearic acid	EP
Dibasic Calcium phosphate	JP
Propylene glycol	Unassigved
Hydrochloric acid	USP
Alcohol	EP
Benzyl alcohol	EP
Talc	EP
Sodium chloride	EP
Sodium starch glycolate	USP
Sodium hydroxide	Unassigned
Polysorbate 80	JP
Calcium-disodium edetate	JP
Petrolatum	USP
Colloidal silicon dioxide	JP
Citric acid	EP
Methyl paraben	EP
Sodium sachharin	USP
Titanium dioxide	USP

Tablets

INTRODUCTION

Oral route of administration is the most preferred route. Parenteral route, and to some extent, transdermal route is used nowadays for systemic delivery of the drug. But parenteral route cannot be used for self-medication and is mainly preferred, during emergencies only, by healthcare workers, to treat comatose patients or for providing nutrition to hospitalised patients. The transdermal route has its own limitations in terms of eligibility of drug candidates for that purpose.

Hence, oral route of administration is most widely accepted route for providing systemic effects of drug. Therefore, for any newly discovered drug its eligibility for oral administration, is the most important factor which will decide its market value.

Solid oral dosage forms, i.e., tablets and capsules, represent the preferred class of oral dosage forms. This is because - a) They are unit dosage forms and deliver the dose of the drug accurately. Whereas, the liquid dosage forms are not unit dosage forms. The patient is required to measure the desired quantity of the medicine by using some measuring device; and such measurements typically show an error margin of 20-50 per cent; b) Transportation and handling of liquid oral dosage forms is much more costly than solid dosage forms. Also, breakage or leakage during shipment is a serious problem. Liquids are less portable and require more space on the pharmacists' counter; c) It is more difficult to mask the taste of drugs in liquid dosage forms.

Drugs are physically and chemically less stable in liquid dosage forms. The liquid dosage forms are still popular because - a) Public expects and prefers certain medicaments in liquid dosage forms, e.g. cough medicines; b) Some drugs are more effective in liquid dosage forms, e.g. antacids and adsorbents; c) Children and elderly patients have difficulty in swallowing tablets and capsules.

Tablets and capsules are the most preferred solid dosage forms. Tablets have two major advantages over solid dosage forms-

i) Tablet is a tamperproof dosage form. Capsules are mainly preferred for masking or hiding the contents, but they are more vulnerable to tampering. On the other hand, addition of any liquid, if aqueous, will cause disintegration, and if non-aqueous, will cause other visible changes. In tablets, addition of powder to a tablet is not feasible.

ii) Tablets are much cheaper than capsules. Capsules need an empty gelatin shell, the cost of which is much higher; and in addition to that, is the cost of filling. Also capsule-filling operation is much slower than tablet compression operation.

ADVANTAGES :

After considering all these points, following are the advantages of the tablet dosage form.

i) They are the unit dosage forms having greatest dose precision.

ii) Their cost is lowest.

iii) They are lightest and most compact.

iv) They are easier & cheap to transport and package.

v) They are the most economical of all the dosage forms

vi) The drugs show the best physical, chemical and microbiological stability in solid dosage forms.

vii) Product identification is easiest and cheapest using embossed punches.

viii) They are easier to swallow, with minimal tendency to float on the stomach fluid.

ix) They are best suited for large-scale production.

x) They can be formulated as certain special release products like enteric or sustained release dosage forms.

DISADVANTAGES :

i) Some drugs are difficult to compress into dense compacts due to their amorphous nature or flocculent, low density character.

ii) Some drugs are difficult or impossible to compress, like drugs having poor wetting properties and large dosage dissolution profiles.

iii) Some drugs need microencapsulation or tablets need coating, e.g. drugs having bitter taste, bad odour or drugs sensitive to moisture or oxidation.

UNIT PROCESSES OF TABLET MANUFACTURING :

The Process of tabletting involves following unit processes:
    i)   Solid-solid and solid-liquid mixing
    ii) Drying
    iii) Granulation
    iv) Fluidising
    v)   Pneumatic conveying
    vi) Compression

MIXING:

To mix is to put together in one mass or assemblage with more or less thorough diffusion
    of the constituent elements among one another. Mixing of solid particles is ac-
    complished through three principle mechanisms-

Diffusion: The redistribution of particles by the random movement of
particles relative to one another.

Convection: Movement of groups of adjacent particles from one place to
another within the mixture.

Shear : The change in the configuration of ingredients through formation of
slip planes in the mixture.

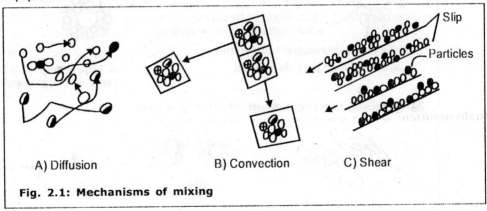

Fig. 2.1: Mechanisms of mixing

A. solid-solid mixing :

The unit operation of solid-solid mixing is separated into four principal steps-
1. Bed of solid particles expands
2. Application of 3-D shear force to the powder bed
3. Mix long enough to permit true randomisation of particles
4. Maintain randomisation after mixing has stopped

Initially, when dry materials or particles are loaded into a mixer, they form a
static bed. Before mixing can take place, this static bed must expand as a result
of mixing forces. There must be enough void spaces remaining in the mixer, after

it has been charged with the ingredients to be blended. Once particle movement is possible with the expansion of the powder bed, shear forces are necessary to produce movement between particles. Tension and compression forces merely change the bed volume. Induction of movement in all three directions requires adequate 3-D stress, resulting in turbulent particle movement. If these forces are inadequate, particles agglomerate in the powder bed and move together without mixing with adjacent particles, resulting in a poor mixture.

B. Liquid-solid mixing :

During tablet wet granulation, following blending events take place in sequence.

1. Pre-mixing of dry powders to be granulated called internal ingredients (solid-solid mixing).
2. Addition of liquids to solids to distribute the liquid uniformly throughout the pre-mixed powders. (solid-liquid mixing)
3. Mixing non-granulated or external ingredients with granules.

Fig. 2.2 indicate events that take place when a liquid is added to a powder bed being mixed.

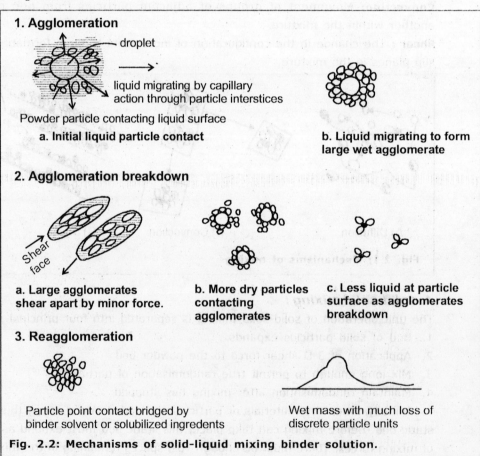

1. Agglomeration

droplet

liquid migrating by capillary action through particle interstices

Powder particle contacting liquid surface

a. Initial liquid particle contact

b. Liquid migrating to form large wet agglomerate

2. Agglomeration breakdown

Shear face

a. Large agglomerates shear apart by minor force.

b. More dry particles contacting agglomerates

c. Less liquid at particle surface as agglomerates breakdown

3. Reagglomeration

Particle point contact bridged by binder solvent or solubilized ingredients

Wet mass with much loss of discrete particle units

Fig. 2.2: Mechanisms of solid-liquid mixing binder solution.

Table 2.1: commonly used mixers for tabletting

Class	Examples
1. Rotation of entire mixer shell or body without agitator	Barrel blender double cone, blender V-blender, double cone blender, Cube blender.
2. Rotation of entire mixer shell or body with agitator	V-blender with agitator Double cone blender with agitator
3. Stationary shell with rotating blade	Ribbon mixer, Sigma blender, Planetary mixer, conical screw mixer
4. High speed granulators	Barrel type, bowl type
5. Air mixers	Fluidised Bed Dryer

Agglomeration: Droplets of solvent, such as water or solution, contact the moving powder particles that build up around the periphery of the droplet. As the powder is wetted by the liquid, the liquid migrates partly by capillary action into the particle interstices and forms large powder liquid agglomerates. It is assumed that the interfacial tension between the solid and liquid is low enough to cause satisfactory wetting of the powder. Otherwise, some surfactants may be added.

Agglomeration breakdown: After the initial large agglomerate formation, mixing, shear and tension forces break the large agglomerates down, such that the liquid is now carried throughout the mixture, via smaller agglomerates, which continue to diminish in size as the liquid is distributed over the powder particle surfaces. At this point, no hard agglomerates are detectable and the wet mass easily crumbles into powder if compacted by the grip of a hand.

Re-agglomeration: As the mixing proceeds and the liquid gets completely distributed throughout the mixture, the powder bed becomes a wet mass, acting similar to a highly viscous slurry. This slurry resists shear forces and begins to generally heat as particle-to-particle contact increases, requiring more mixer shear force for continued mixing. This is the result of the displacement of air by liquid at the particle surface, liquid viscosity and or partial solubilisation of some of the more soluble ingredients that may be present in the formula. Widely ranged sizes of agglomerates can be seen forming in the mixture as mixing proceeds. The end point of this is normally judged by how easily a wet compaction could be formed in the grip of a hand.

Paste formation: If mixing is continued beyond the normal granulating end point, a thick wet mass resembling a paste begins to form. This paste is difficult to break up for drying, will dry into extremely hard granules and usually form a poor compact in the tablet machine.

Mixing Equipment :

The mixing equipments can be classified following way:

i) Batch type mixers :

1. Rotation of the entire mixer shell or body with no agitator or mixer bed –
   a) Barrel b) Cube c) V-shaped d) Double cone

2. Rotation of the entire mixer shell or body with a rotating high shear agitator blade
   a) V-shaped b) Double cone c) Cube d) barrel

3. Stationary shell or body with rotating mixer blade
   a) Ribbon b) Sigma blade c) Planetary d) Conical screw

4. High speed granulators (Stationary shell or body with a rotating mixer blade and high speed agitator blade)
   a) Barrel b) Bowl

5. Air mixer (Stationary shell or body using air as an agitator)
   a) Fluidised bed dryer b) Fluidised bed granulator

ii) Continuous type mixers :
   a) Barrel b) Zigzag

The batch mixers are more frequently used.

A) Batch type mixers:-

I. Rotation of the entire mixer shell or body with no agitator or mixer blade-

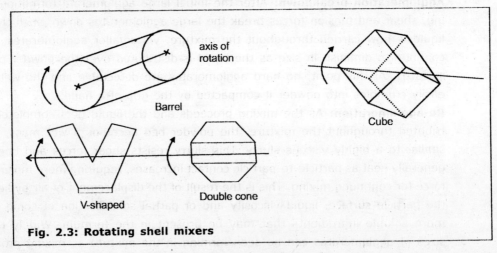

Fig. 2.3: Rotating shell mixers

The four types are shown schematically in the diagram. Cube and barrel mixers are not used very widely. But V-shaped and double cone blenders are used extensively for blending dry powders. Sometimes, baffles may be introduced to increase mixing shear.

Advantages:

1. Minimal attrition during blending of fragile granules
2. Large capacity

3. Easy loading and unloading
4. Easy cleaning
5. Minimal maintenance

Disadvantages:

1. High head space needed for installation
2. Segregation may take place with mixtures having wide particle size distribution.
3. Not suitable for fine particulate systems because there is not enough shear to decrease particle agglomeration.
4. If powders are free flowing, serial dilutions are required for addition of low dose ingredients.

Factors affecting the efficiency:

Following factors affect the efficiency of these blenders:

i) Fill Volume: Mixing efficiency is largely affected by the fill-volume. Adding material to approximately 50-60 per cent of the total blender's volume gives good degree of mixing.

ii) Blender speed: Slower the blender, lower the shear forces. Higher blending speeds provide more shear, but they also result in more dusting, causing segregation of fines. As the rpm increases, the centrifugal forces acting at the extreme ends of the mixing chamber exceed the gravitational forces needed for blending. Thus the powder will gravitate to the outer walls of the chamber.

The Double cone blender is usually charged and discharged through the same port : whereas, the V-shaped blender is charged and discharged through separate ports.

II. Rotation of the entire mixer shell or body with a rotating high shear blade:

This is a modification of the tumbling blenders with addition of a high speed (1200-3000 rpm) agitator mixing blades.

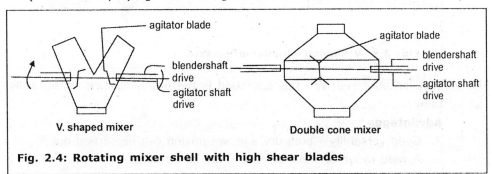

Fig. 2.4: Rotating mixer shell with high shear blades

The agitator blade gives added versatility to the tumbling blenders by virtue of the high shear attainable. Most mixers with agitator bars are also available with a separate liquid dispensing system, or incorporated into the agitator bar so that the solid-liquid blends can be easily blended without stopping the mixer for addition of granulating liquid. These units have a steam jacket around the shell for heating the wet granules and a vacuum system to remove the granulating liquid, the entire granulation and drying may be accomplished in one step in the following sequence -

1. Prepare the granulating solutions and adjust the feed rate through the pump.
2. Charge the blender with the ingredients to be granulated.
3. Pre-mix the dry solids and run the agitator mixer during blending.
4. Pump granulating solution into the processor and turn on full vacuum.
5. Mix until granulation is done.
6. Turn off vacuum, shut off agitator mixer and reduce blender shell revolution per minute to minimum.
7. Dry until the solvent collector contains specified amount of solvent.
8. Check LOD after drying is complete.

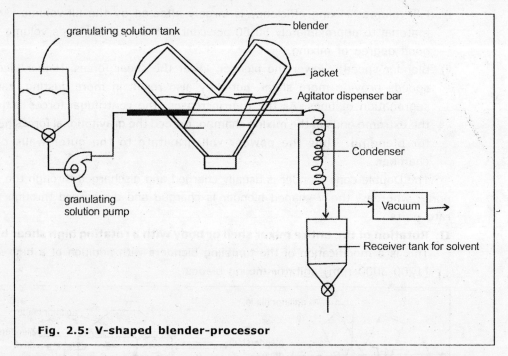

Fig. 2.5: V-shaped blender-processor

The problem encountered with this operation is the granules stick to the walls of container.

Advantages :

- Good versatility - both dry and wet mixing can be carried out.
- A wide range of shearing force may be obtained.

Disadvantages :

- Possible attrition of large, friable particles.
- Cleaning is a problem as the agitator assembly needs to be removed prior to cleaning.

III Stationary shell or body with rotating mixer blades -

The mechanical force for mixing is provided by moving blades in a fixed shell. The blades, which may be of various designs, are driven by motor-driven drive shaft.

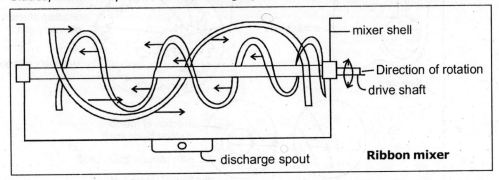

Ribbon mixer

Ribbon mixer : It consists of ribbon shaped blades that traverse the entire length of the U-trough and are attached to the drive shaft. It can be used for either solid-solid or solid-liquid mixing and gives less shearing action than the sigma or planetary mixer. The body of the mixer is usually covered to avoid dust explosion and evaporation of granulation liquid. It is an all purpose mixer, but has one major disadvantage - the possibility of dead spots at the end and in the corners of the mixer.

Sigma blade mixer : It gives high shear and kneading action, created by the intermeshing blades. It is an excellent choice for wet granulation, where heavy wettened powders require kneading for good liquid-solid distribution. It has close tolerance between the side walls and bottom of mixer shell. This creates a minimum of dead space during mixing. It is used primarily for liquid-solid blending.

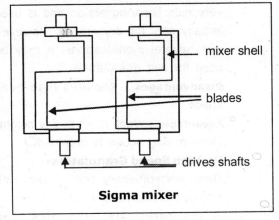

Sigma mixer

Planetary mixer : In this, the mixing shaft is driven by a planetary gear. As the planetary gear attached to the mixing blade, is driven in the indicated direction around the ring gear, it rotates the mixing blade. Both the mixer blades and mixer blade shaft positions are rotational. It is usually built with a variable speed drive so that slow speeds are used for dry mixing of powders and high speeds are used for kneading action during granulation. There are literally no dead spots in the mixing bowl and extra bowls may be used for mixing one batch after another without interruption. It is better suited for mixing of smaller batches.

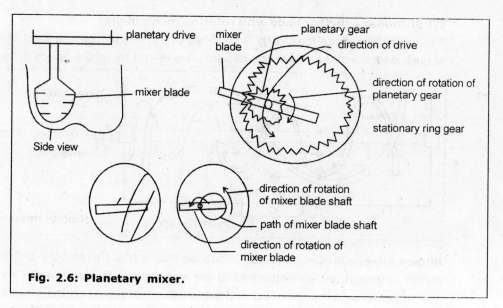

Fig. 2.6: Planetary mixer.

Conical screw mixer : The screw shaft rotates round the periphery of the cone and the screw turns so that the pitch transfers the material from the bottom of the mixer to the top. It provides a very mild shearing action and is used initially only for dry mixing. However, with several modifications, it may be used for wet granulation.

Disadvantages : Requires high head space.

Advantages : When filled to any height, same mixing action is obtained.

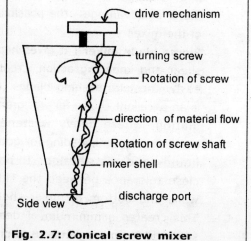

Fig. 2.7: Conical screw mixer

IV. High Speed Granulators-

These are stationary shell mixers with a large mixer scraper blade which mixes the ingredients, eliminates dead spots and presents the mixer contents to a high speed chopper blade that intimately mixes the ingredients. The high speed chopper is driven by a separate motor driving the larger mixer-scraper blades.   **Advantages :**

i) Extremely rapid ii) Intimate solid-solid and solid-liquid mixing
iii) Product has fairly uniform wet granule size.

Disadvantages :

i) Product contamination from the packing gland where the shaft passes through the mixer shell.
ii) Limited batch size, as the larger equipments are very costly.

ii) Limited batch size, as the larger equipments are very costly.

The barrel type mixers are top loading with bottom discharge doors. Care must be taken during mixing, as too long a mixing time may cause unwanted particle size reduction.

V. Air mixers (stationary shell using moving air as agitator)-

The example of this class is Fluidized bed dryer which performs

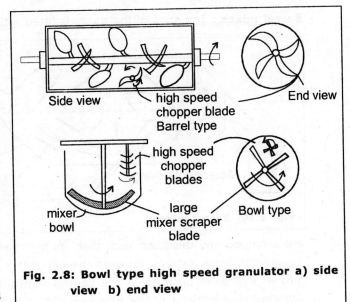

Fig. 2.8: Bowl type high speed granulator a) side view b) end view

mixing very intimately and efficiently. By fluidizing the powder bed, enough shear is developed to mix beds of some of the smallest particles. By introducing a spray system for granulating liquid, the same equipment may be used for mixing, granulating as well as drying.

B) Continuous mixers:

They are used in pharmaceutical industries and are reserved for mass production that requires 8-24 hrs/day of mixing year-round to meet the market's demands. Ingredients to be mixed are accurately metered into the mixer at one end and are discharged at the other end as a homogenous mixture ready for further processing.

Disadvantages-

- Auxiliary equipments like storage hoppers, automatic weighing units, conveying methods and metering equipments should be selected properly.

- There must be enough flexibility to enable production to be increased or reduced.

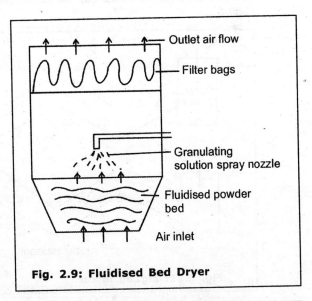

Fig. 2.9: Fluidised Bed Dryer

Barrel mixer : The shell of the mixer is fitted with baffles internally. The baffles

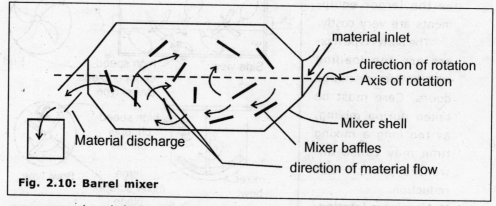

Fig. 2.10: Barrel mixer

are arranged and designed such that, as the mixer shell rotates, the incoming ingredients begin moving towards the opposite end of the blender. Mixing begins at this point because of the baffle's tumbling action. As the material approaches the midpoint of the tumbling shell, the baffles are so positioned as to cause the folding back of the granulation mixture over itself in the direction of the inlet end. This action continues up to the discharge end, where, in addition to another set of baffles designed to move the material out of the discharge port, overflow also causes the blended dry solids to discharge. After set up, equilibrium blending is reached and the process becomes continuous.

Zigzag blender : It is also a rotating shell type mixer. But in this mixer, the shell takes the shape of several V-shaped blenders in series. As the material is metered into the rotating mixer, the throughput rate is determined in part by the angle of the axis of rotation, which can be varied (as the angle increases the throughput also increases).

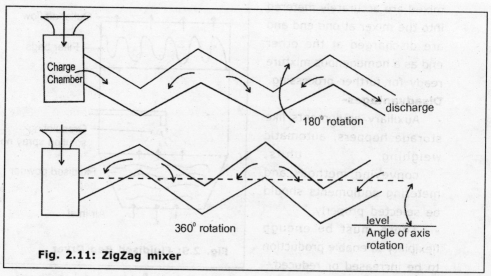

Fig. 2.11: ZigZag mixer

A single pre-weighed charge can be dumped into a charge chamber and portions of it enter into the V-shaped tubular sections by gravity as the shell rotates. With each rotation, one half of the blend in each downward V recycles back to the preceding chamber and one half moves forward to the next arm of the blender. Because of the inclined axis of rotation towards the discharge, material movement is always forward. As the first charge clears the mixer, the next charge is added.

DRYING :

Drying plays an important role in wet granulation method of tabletting. Different types of dryers that can be used for drying granules are as follows:

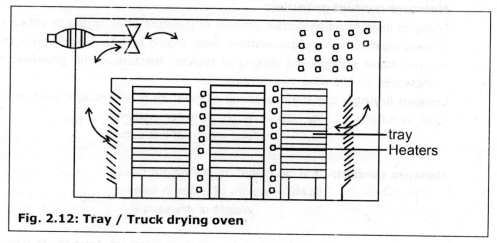

Fig. 2.12: Tray / Truck drying oven

Truck Dryer/Tray Dryer :

This dryer consists of trucks on which trays are placed. In a tray dryer, material to be dried is placed on tiers of trays in a cabinet. Truck dryer is more convenient than tray dryer, because it offers greater convenience of loading and unloading. Drying in these two dryers is a batch process.

Tray dryers are either direct or indirect type. In direct type, heating is accomplished by forced circulation of large volumes of hot air. Indirect dryers use heated shelves or radiant heat sources inside the drying chamber to evaporate moisture, which is then removed by either a vacuum pump or small amounts of circulating gas.

Trays have solid, perforated or meshed bottoms. Temperature and airflow must be constantly maintained to achieve uniform drying. Fans and heating coils are integral part of the oven. The coils are electrically heated or steam heated.

Tunnel Dryers :

This is a modification of tray dryers for continuous operation. Trucks are continuously moved through drying tunnels by a moving chain. Trucks are loaded on one side of the dryer, allowed to remain in the chamber for a sufficiently long time and then discharged at the exit. This is a semi-continuous process.

Conveyor dryers are more advantageous over tunnel dryers because they are truly continuous. The trucks here are replaced with a conveyor belt or screen.

Air is heated with the help of electrically heated or steam heated coils and circulated by fans. Additionally, the tunnel walls may be heated for improving drying rates.

Fluidised Bed Dryers:

Fluidised bed dryers are the most widely used equipments in tablet manufacturing. With certain modifications, fluidised bed dryers can also be used for mixing wet granulation, coating and spheronisation processes in tabletting. They are discussed in detail elsewhere in this chapter.

Moisture content granules:

Granules need to retain certain amount of moisture after drying to obtain tablets of good quality. Too dry granulations yield friable tablets. Granulations that are too wet cause sticking and picking of tablets. Moisture in the granules may be represented in following two ways-

Loss on drying:- It is the expression of moisture on wet weight basis and calculated as follows,

$$\% \text{ LOD} = \frac{\text{Weight of water in sample}}{\text{Total weight of wet sample}} \times 100$$

Moisture content:- It is calculated on dry weight basis.

$$\% \text{ MC} = \frac{\text{Weight of water in sample}}{\text{Weight of dry sample}} \times 100$$

These values can be determined by using a moisture balance. It has a heat source for rapid heating and a scale calibrated in percentage LOD or percentage MC. A weighed sample is placed on the balance and allowed to dry till constant weight is reached.

For example, if exactly 10g of moist solid is brought to a constant dry weight of 6g:

$$MC = \frac{10-6}{6} \times 100 = 66.7\%$$

Whereas,

$$LOD = \frac{10-6}{10} \times 100 = 40\%$$

GRANULATION

Granulation is the process in which powder particles are made to adhere to form larger particles called granules. Granulation is done after mixing the necessary powdered ingredients, so that a uniform distribution of each ingredient throughout the mixture is achieved.

Reasons for granulation:

i) To prevent segregation of the constituents in the powder mixture-

Segregation occurs due to differences in the size or density of the components, the smaller particles concentrating at the base of a container while the larger ones above them. An ideal granulation will contain all the constituents of the mixture in each granule and segregation of the ingredients will not occur.

It is also important to control the particle size distribution of the granules because, although the individual particles may not segregate, if there is a wide variation in size distribution, the granules themselves may segregate. If this occurs in the hopper of a tablet compression machine, it will result in products having large weight variations. These machines fill by volume rather than weight and if the different regions in the hopper contain granules of different sizes, a given volume in each region will contain a different weight of granules. This will lead to unacceptable distribution of active ingredient within the batch.

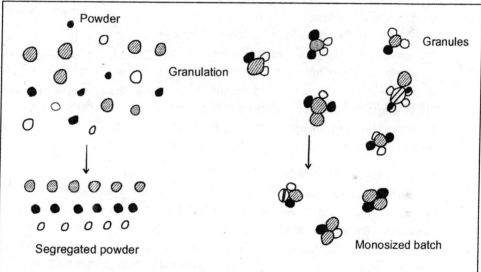

Fig. 2.13: Schematic representation depicting how granulation eliminates segregation

ii) To improve flow properties of the mixture-

Many Powders are cohesive due to their small size or surface characteristics, and do not flow well. Poor flow results in weight variation within the final product due to nonuniform filling of tablet dies. Granules of such powders are larger and more uniform in size and hence have good flow property.

iii) To improve compression characteristics of the mixture-

Some powders are difficult to compress even after addition of binder. But granules of the same formulation are easily compressed, and produce stronger tablets.

iv) Other reasons-

1. Granulation of toxic materials reduces hazards of generating toxic dust.
2. Slightly hygroscopic materials adhere and form cakes. Granulation may reduce this hazard because, even if granules absorb some moisture, they still retain their flowability.

Summary of reasons for Granulation-

- To avoid segregation
- To improve flow properties
- To improve compressibility
- To avoid dusting
- To avoid static charge build-up and dust explosion

Characterisation of granules :

i) Angle of repose - Granules begin to slide when the angle of inclination is large enough to overcome frictional forces. This balance of forces cause powders poured from a container, onto a horizontal surface, to form a heap. The sides of the heap formed in this way make an angle with the horizontal which is called angle of repose. It is defined as the maximum angle that can be obtained between the free standing surface of a powder heap and the horizontal plane as shown in the figure

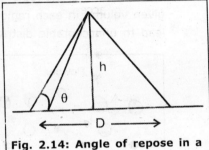

Fig. 2.14: Angle of repose in a powder heap

Angle of repose is defined by the equation, $\theta = \dfrac{2h}{D}$

Angles of repose measurement has been used as an indirect methods of quantifying powder flowability because of its relationship with interparticulate cohesion. There are different methods of determining angle of repose and they are shown in the table below. As a general guide, granules having angle of repose between 20° and 40° indicate reasonable flow properties. Above 50° however, powders show poor flowability.

Table 2.2: Methods of measuring angle of repose.

	Apparatus	Method	Angle defined
1.		Fixed static height cone	angle of repose
2.		Fixed static base cone	angle of repose

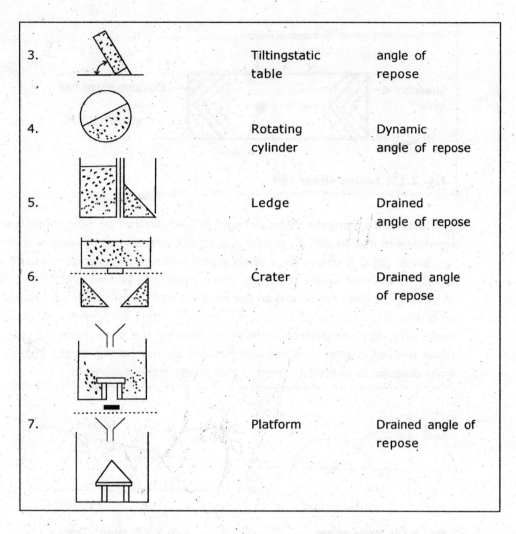

3.		Tiltingstatic table	angle of repose
4.		Rotating cylinder	Dynamic angle of repose
5.		Ledge	Drained angle of repose
6.		Crater	Drained angle of repose
7.		Platform	Drained angle of repose

There are two main types of angles of repose- the poured angle and the drained angle. The poured angle is the angle measured on a pile poured freely onto a flat surface.

The drained angle is the angle measured on the conical surface of the powder in a flat-bottomed container, if the powder is discharged through an orifice in the base.

Table 2.3: Angles of repose and corresponding type of flow

Angle of repose (°)	Type of flow
< 25	Excellent
25-30	Good
30-40	Passable (may improve with glidants)
> 40	Very poor

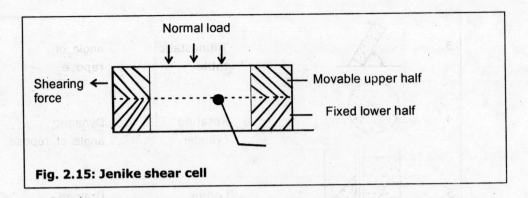

Fig. 2.15: Jenike shear cell

ii) Shear cell strength: Shear strength of granules can be determined from the resistance to flow caused by cohesion and can be measured by using a shear cell.

Shear cell is a simple piece of apparatus which is designed to measure shear stress, at different values of normal stress. Powder is packed into the two halves of the cell. Weights are placed on the lid of the cell. A cord is connected from the lid of the cell, by a pulley, to weights, so as to apply shearing stress across the two halves. The shear stress is found by dividing the shear force by cross sectional area of powder bed and will increase as the normal stress increases. A Mohr diagram is plotted to present this stress interrelationship.

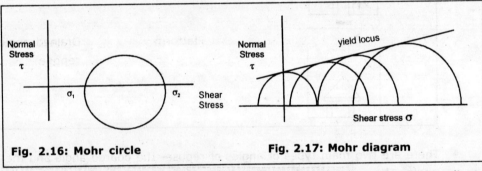

Fig. 2.16: Mohr circle   **Fig. 2.17: Mohr diagram**

A Mohr diagram is constructed by plotting the normal stress, τ, as ordinate and shear stress, s, as abscissa. For two values of shear stress on abscissa at which failure occurs and the cell is sheared, σ_1, and σ_2 are used as the diameter of a Mohr circle with radium $r_1 + r_2$. A series of Mohr semicircles is constructed in this way, with different pairs of shear stresses causing failure. A line is constructed to touch all the Mohr semicircles and is called the yield locus. It is characteristic of a powder under given conditions.

A flow factor, f.f., can be obtained by determining the reciprocal slope of a curve or tangent to a curve of unconfined yield stress s_u, plotted against the maximum normal on a yield locus (Figure 2.18).

The relationship between flow factor and powder flowability is shown in the table below.

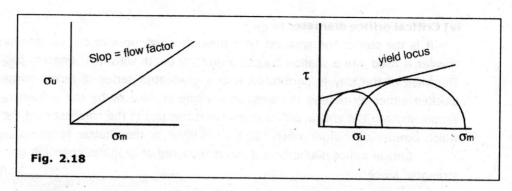

Fig. 2.18

Table 2.4: Relationship between flow factor and powder flowability

Flow Factor value	Flow description
> 10	Free flowing
4-10	Easy flowing
1.6.4	Cohesive
< 1.6	Very cohesive

iii) Tensile Strength : Tensile strength is characteristic of the internal friction or cohesion. The powder is packed into a split plate, one half of which is fixed and the other half free to move by means of wheels. It runs on tracks on a table.

The table is then tilted towards the vertical, until the angle is reached at which powder cohesion is overcome and the mobile half plate breaks away from the static half plate. The tensile strength s, of powder can be found out as -

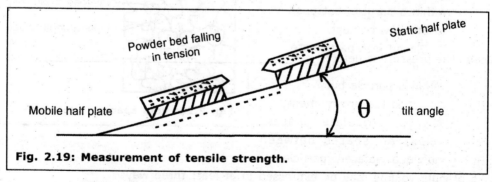

Fig. 2.19: Measurement of tensile strength.

$$\sigma_\tau = \frac{M \sin \theta}{A} \times 10^5 \ P_a$$

Where,

M - Mass of mobile half plate + powder

θ - Angle of tilted table to the horizontal

A - Cross Sectional area of powder bed

iv) Critical orifice diameter :

It is the size of the smallest hole through which powder can be discharged. Powder is filled into a shallow tray to a uniform depth with near-uniform packing. The base of the tray is perforated with a graduated series of holes, which are blocked either by resting the tray on a plane surface or by the presence of a simple shutter. The critical orifice diameter is the size of the smallest hole through which powder discharges when the tray is lifted or the shutter removed.

Critical orifice diameter is a direct measure of granules cohesion and arch strength, since:

$$\tan \alpha = \frac{r}{x}$$

Where,

r - particle radius

x - radius

$$\text{and } \tan F' = \frac{\tan \phi}{1 - \tan \phi \, r/x - r^2/x^2}$$

Where,

F' - angle of form which is obtuse angle between the contracting powder dome and the horizontal

$\tan \phi$ - the co-efficient of friction.

v) Volume : It is difficult to measure true volume of granules because they contain three types of air spaces or voids-

1. Open intraparticulate spaces/voids: Present within a particle, but open to the environment.

2. Closed intraparticulate spaces/voids: Present within a particle but closed to the environment.

3. Interparticulate spaces/ voids: Air spaces between individual adjacent particles.

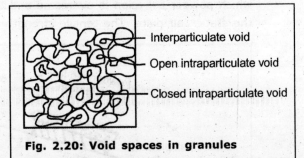

- Interparticulate void
- Open intraparticulate void
- Closed intraparticulate void

Fig. 2.20: Void spaces in granules

The granule volume may be expressed in at least three ways-

1. True volume (V_t): Total volume of the solid particles excluding all the voids. This has got a characteristic value for each particle.

2. Granular volume (V_g) : The cumulative volume of all the particles including the volume of intraparticulate voids and excluding interparticulate voids.

3. Bulk Volume (V_b) : Total volume of the powder including both the intra and inter granular spaces.

Under experimental conditions, it is advisable to consider volume V of the sample, relative to the true volume V_t. A useful dimensionless quantity relative volume (V_r) may be defined as-

$$V_r = \frac{V}{V_t}$$

When almost all air spaces are removed, $V_r \to 1$. This occurs during tabletting.

vi) Porosity - In some cases, voids present in the powder mass are more significant than the solid component.

Therefore, another term, porosity (ε) is introduced. It is defined as:

$$\varepsilon = \frac{V_v}{V_b}$$

Where,

V_v - total volume of voids

Therefore, $V_v = V_b - V_t$

Therefore, $\varepsilon = \dfrac{V_b - V_t}{V_b}$

$$= 1 - \frac{V_t}{V_b}$$

It is frequently expressed in percentage as, $\%\varepsilon = 100 \times \left(1 - \dfrac{V_t}{V_b}\right)$

True Volume can be measured by a helium pycnometer. This works on the principle that, within a sealed system containing helium (a non-adsorbing gas), the change in pressure caused by a finite change in volume of the system is a function of its total volume. The instrument is schematically shown in the diagram. The volume of the system is varied by means of a piston, until a preset constant pressure is produced. The pressure is detected on a pressure detector. The piston movement (U) necessary to achieve this pressure is read from scale. The pycnometer is calibrated first by using a sample of known volume, V_c. The operating equation for the instrument is-

Where,

$$V_t = \frac{V_c}{U_1 - U_2}(U_1 - U_s)$$

U_1, U_2 and U_s - variable volume scale readings for an empty cell, with standard volume and with test material respectively.

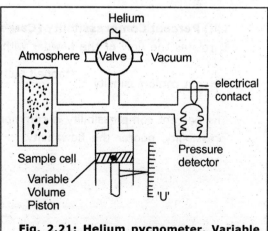

Fig. 2.21: Helium pycnometer. Variable volume positions are read from scale.

Granule volume (V_g) can be measured by measuring liquid displacement by a powder pycnometer (specific gravity bottle method). Liquids that do not readily wet the powder are used, e.g. inert organic liquids, mercury.

Bulk volumes (V_b) can be measured in a number of ways, ranging from simple pouring of known weight into a graduated vessel or using standard tapping or vibrating procedures. Depending on that, the bulk volume may be tapped bulk volume or untapped bulk volume.

vii) Density

Three different densities can be determined for granules, based on the three volumes.

$$\text{The true density } (\rho_t) = \frac{\text{Mass (M)}}{\text{True Volume } (V_t)}$$

$$\text{The granular density } (\rho_g) = \frac{\text{Mass (M)}}{\text{Granular Volume } (V_g)}$$

$$\text{The bulk density } (\rho_b) = \frac{\text{Mass (M)}}{\text{Bulk Volume } (V_b)}$$

Depending upon the method used for determining bulk volume, the bulk density can be tapped or untapped.

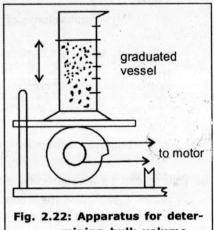

Fig. 2.22: Apparatus for determining bulk volume

graduated vessel

to motor

viii) Percent Compressibility (Carr's index)

It relates the flow of the powder with its compressibility. It is defined as-

$$\text{Percent compressibility} = \frac{(\text{tapped bulk density - untapped bulk density})}{\text{tapped bulk density}} \times 100$$

The percent compressibility is commonly known as Carr's index. Higher the compressibility, poorer the flowability.

Table 2.5: Relationship between flowability and Carr's index.

Carr's index (% compressibility)	Type of flow
5-15	Excellent (free flowing granule)
12-16	Good (free flowing powdered granules)
18-21	Fair (powdered granules)
23-28	Poor (very fluid powders)
28-35	Poor (fluid cohesive powders)
35-38	Very poor (fluid cohesive powders)
> 40	Extremely poor (Cohesive powders)

Another value, that may be defined by Hausner's ratio, is given as-

$$\text{Hausner's ratio} = \frac{\text{tapped bulk density}}{\text{untapped bulk density}}$$

Table 2.6 : Relationship between Hausner ratio and Carr's index.

Hausner's ratio	Type of flow	Equivalent Carr's index (%)
< 1.25	Good	20
> 1.25	Poor	30

ix) Granule Morphology: Granule morphology can be assessed with the help of optical microscopy. Samples may be sorted using a device in which the granulation is fed onto a triangular metal deck and vibrated. Particles of different shape segregate on this deck and are collected for microscopic analysis.

x) Particle size analysis: Particle size of granules affects tablet weight, weight variation, disintegration time, granule friability, granule flowability and drying rate kinetics. Particle size and size distribution may be determined by microscopy, sieving, sedimentation, adsorption and electrical conductivity measurement, i.e., Coulter-counter.

xi) Surface area: Determination of the surface area of finely milled drug powders may be useful for drugs that have limited water solubility. In this case, particle size and surface area largely affect the dissolution rate. In general, inverse relationship exists between particle size and particle surface area of the particles. However, granules may have convoluted structure with considerable internal surface area. Gas absorption and air permeability are the two methods used for particle surface area determination. In the former one, amount of gas adsorbed onto the granules to form a monolayer is measured and used to calculate surface area. In air permeability method, the amount of air that permeates a bed of granules used to calculate surface area of sample.

Table 2.7: Evaluation parameter in granule characterisation.

Evaluation parameter	Method/equipment used
1. Angle of repose	Fixed height cone
	Fixed base cone
	Tilting table
2. Dynamic angle of repose	Rotating cylinder
3. Drained angle of repose	Ledge
	Crater
	Platform
4. Shear Strength	Jenike shear cell
5. Tensile Strength	Split plate apparatus
6. Critical orifice diameter	Tray with graduated, perforated base
7. True Volume/density	Helium pycnometer
8. Granular volume/density	Liquid displacement (mercury)
9. Bulk volume/density	Bulk density apparatus
10. Granule morphology	Optical microscopy
11. Granule size/size distribution	microscopy, sieve analysis, sedimentation, coulter-counter
12. Granule surface area	gas adsorption, air permeability

xii) Hopper flow rates: Instruments to obtain hopper flow rates continuously monitor the flow of material out of conical hoppers onto a recording balance device.

xiii) Compaction: Process of compressing granules into a tablet is complex. Instrumented tablet presses are used to measure the forces applied during compression.

Granulation methods:

Table: 1.8: Granulation methods utilised in pharma industry.

Method	Process
Agitation	Agglomeration of powders by mechanical agitation in the presence of the required proportion of liquid (wet granulation).
Compaction	Compression of powders into a solid mass which is broken down into smaller fragments (dry granulation).
Globulation	Drop formation of solutions, slurries or melts, followed by a solidification stage, e.g. spray drying, spray congealing.
Heat bonding	Action of heat to give a sintered mass.

Except for heat bonding, all other methods are used for pharmaceutical wet granulation. Granulation by low shear or high shear mixers or fluidised bed granulators is preferred. Dry granulation methods using sluggers or roller compactors are not used extensively. Granulation by globulation or extrusion is used only for specialised products like pellets or controlled release dosage forms. Alternatively, tablets may also be prepared by direct compression of the free flowing mixture of drug substances along with excipients. This decreases number of production steps, but has the disadvantage of segregation and dust formation associated with dry granulation.

i) Direct compression: Some crystalline substances such as sodium chloride, sodium bromide and potassium chloride may be compressed directly. But very few substances are easily compressible. In some cases, although the drug substance is easily compressible, the addition of other excipients may make it difficult. Most materials possess relatively weak forces of intermolecular attraction or are covered with films of adsorbed gases that tend to hinder compression. Directly compressible diluents are to be added in large quantities in order to make these drugs compressible. Therefore, this method cannot be used for large dose drugs, as it will produce tablet of large size & weight. In case of small dose drugs, uniform blending of the drug with coarser, directly compressible diluents, cannot be achieved. Thus, this method can be used only for moderate dose drugs with directly compressible diluents.

A directly compressible diluent is a diluent that can be compacted with little difficulty and may be compressed even with large quantities of drugs and other additives mixed with it. Directly compressible materials, in addition to possessing good flow and compressibility, must be inert, tasteless, re-workable, easy to disintegrate and inexpensive.

Disadvantages :

i) The difference in particle size and bulk density of the drug and other diluents leads to stratification and segregation of ingredients, which further leads to poor content uniformity in the tablet. This is of special concern especially in case of low-dose drugs.

ii) A large-dose drug, may present problems if it is not easily compressible by itself. To facilitate compression, a large amount of directly compressible diluent must be added. This leads to a tablet which is too large to swallow and is expensive.

iii) Sometimes, the directly compressible diluent may interact with the drug, e.g. reaction of spray dried lactose with amine compounds that leads to yellow discolouration called as Millard reaction.

iv) Because of the dry nature of directly compressible drug, static charges may build up during screening, mixing which may prevent uniform distribution of the drug.

v) Dust explosion may pose a problem.

The equipment and procedures used are basically sieving, milling, mixing and compression.

Table: 2.9: Advantages and disadvantages of dry granulation.

Advantages	Disadvantgages
1. Less number of steps	1. Requires specialized machines
2. Low equipment and labour cost	2. Non-uniform colour distribution
3. Less time consuming	3. More dusting
4. Useful for moisture & heat sensitive materials	
5. Improved disintegration time due to absence of binder.	

Directly compressible diluents

The most important requirements for filler/ binders are -

1. It should have high compaction to ensure that the compacted mass will re main after the release of the pressure.
2. It should have good flowability to ensure that the powder blend flows homogenously and rapidly.
3. It should have good blending properties to avoid segregation.
4. It should be less sensitive to lubricant.
5. It should be stable.
6. It should be inert.
7. It should be compatible with all substances.
8. It should promote tablet disintegration.
9. It should have batch to batch reproducibility
10. It should be cost effective

Celluloses

i) Microcrystalline cellulose (MCC):

It is the most widely used direct compression filler. This diluent has the function of a disintegrating agent, and chemically it is identical to natural cellulose. Only the physical form is changed from fiber to particle form. It has high dilution capacity, low lubricant requirements, high compressibility and fast disintegration.

MCC has very low coefficient of friction and therefore does not require lubricant for itself. It has highest compressibility. It transforms many materials that are normally non-compressible into highly compressible powders. Although not primarily a disintegrant, it does absorb moisture and acts as an auxiliary to other disintegrants.

Disadvantages of MCC as a filter are:

i)   Flow properties are not at par with the other directly compressible diluent.

ii) High cost

MCC is available in two grades- PH 101 (powder) and PH 102 (granular). It is most popularly available under the brand name of Avicel. Some other popular brands are Emcocel and Medicel.

ii) Powdered Cellulose:

It is purified, mechanically disintegrated cellulose prepared by processing cellulose obtained as a pulp from fibrous plant materials. It is also known as microfine cellulose or cellulose flocs. It is available in several grades under the trade names Elcema and Solka Floc.

When it is not in agglomerated form, it has poor flow properties, so it is an unsuitable direct compression excipient when used alone. It has poor compressibility. Tablets formed with powdered cellulose require almost three times the compression force as compared with MCC. The diluting potential is low and binding properties are poor. But it has some inherent lubricating property, which minimises the ejection force and is inexpensive.

Sugars and sugar alcohols:

i) Lactose:

It is a disaccharide obtained from milk and yields D-glucose and D-galactose on hydrolysis. It contains either one molecule of water (a monohydrate termed as hydrous lactose) or is anhydrous. The third variety of lactose is the one prepared by spray drying and is called spray dried lactose.

Lactose is inexpensive and therefore frequently used as main excipient. Its flowability and compressibility is poor and cannot be used as directly compressible diluent. Lactose is first placed in solution. Partial crystallisation is allowed to take place before spray drying the slurry. The final product contains mixture of large crystals of lactose monohydrate and spherical aggregates of crystals held together. The fluidity is improved by virtue of large particle size and intermixing of spherical aggregates.

Spray dried lactose requires high compression pressure to produce hard tablets. It has high dilution capacity. It shows good flow properties and does not affect the release rate of the drug. A major problem with spray dried lactose is a change in colour, or browning, when formulated with amines. The reaction is called Maillard reaction and it is catalysed by presence of moisture and alkaline stearate lubricants. The tablets are formulated with stearic acid rather than stearates if they are likely to undergo Maillard reaction. Spray dried lactose available commercially includes Pharmatose and Zeparox.

Anhydrous lactose may also be used as directly compressible diluent. Its flow properties are poor and it may pickup moisture from the surrounding, causing a change in tablet dimensions. Anhydrous lactose is less likely to undergo Maillard reaction as it is free from moisture.

Modified spray dried lactose (fast flow lactose) consists mainly of spherical aggregates of microcrystals held together by a higher concentration of glassy structure than in normal spray dried lactose. During manufacturing process, crystals, are never allowed to grow, but are agglomerated into spheres by spray drying. It is much more compressible and has better flow properties than spray dried lactose. It is available commercially under the names 'Fast Flow Lactose' and 'Tablettose'.

ii) Sucrose-based diluents:

Sucrose is a disaccharide of dextrose and Levulose obtained from sugarcane or sugar beat, as a white to colourless crystalline material, soluble in water.

Compressible sugars are modifications of sucrose resulting from processing or combination with other materials to convert sucrose to a direct compression vehicle. Sucrose is allowed to undergo spontaneous crystallisation from a strongly agitated supersaturated solution containing a second ingredient. The result is micro-sized crystal agglomerates, in which the second ingredient is uniformly incorporated into the latticework. Examples of such co-crystallised products of sucrose are:

i) Di-Pac : Sucrose (87%) is modified by co-crystallisation with maltodextrins (3%).

ii) Nu-Tab : Consists of processed sucrose, 4% invert sugar and 0.1 to 0.2% each of cornstarch and magnesium stearate.

iii) Sugartab : 90-93% processed sucrose and 7-10% invert sugar.

The compressible sucrose-based diluents are excellent fillers for chewable tablets made by direct compression, due to their sweet taste. They are highly compressible and free flowing; non-hygroscopic and soluble. They are inexpensive and available commercially in various colours.

The main disadvantage of sucrose-based diluents is, they are not acceptable for diabetic patients, they are calorie contributors and cariogenic.

iii) Mannitol and sorbitol:

It is the most useful diluent for lozenges and chewable tablets. Mannitol and its isomer, sorbitol, have negative heat of solution and a sweet taste. Mannitol has advantages over sorbitol due to its less hygroscopicity. Mannitol is highly expensive.

Modified mannitol, prepared by spray congealing of the hot melt, shows better compressibility and flow properties and therefore is used for direct compression. It is also available as granulated mannitol.

iv) Starches :

Unlubricated native starches have good compression characteristics, but poor flow properties. They are therefore, less suitable as directly compressible diluents.

Table 2.8: Commonly used direct compression diluents

Class	Chemical name	Trade name	Composition
A. Celluloses	1. Microcrystalline cellulose	Avicel Emcocel Medicel	Cellulose modified physically in particle form
	2. Powdered cellulose	Elcema Solka floc	Powdered cellulose NF Powdered cellulose NF
	Lactose		
B. Sugars and Sugar alcohols	1. Anhydrous lactose		Lactose NF, anhydrous
	2. Spray dried lactose	Pharmatose Zeparox	Lactose in porous spheres
	3. Modified fast flow lactose	Tablettose	Agglomerated spray dried lactose
	Sucrose		
	Compressible sucrose	1 - Di Pac	97% sucrose +3% dextrin
		2 - Nu Tab	Sucrose+invert sugar+ Corn starch + Mg. stearate
		3 - Sugartab	90-93% sucrose + 10-7% invert sugar
	Mannitol		
	Sorbitol	Sorbitol 1162,834 Neosorb-60	Sorbitol-NF (Crystalline for direct compression)
	Dextrose	Ceralose	Dextrose, anhydrous
Starches	Pre-gelatinised Starch	StaRX 1500	
	Dextrins	Emdex Celutab	93-99% dextrose 93-99% dextrose
Inorganic Salts	Dicalcium phosphate dihydrate	Emcompress Di-Tab, DICAFOS	Dibasic calcium phosphate U.S.P.
	Tricalcium phosphate	Tri-Tab, TRICAFOS	Tricalcium phosphate anhydrous (for direct compression)
	Calcium sulphate dihydrate	Compactroll/ Delaflor	Direct Compression calcium sulphate.

Pre-gelatinised starch is starch that has been chemically or mechanically processed to rupture all or part of its granules in presence of water, and subsequently dried.

A special pre-gelatinised starch for direct compression is available as STA - RX 1500. It does not differ from starch U.S.P. chemically.

Dextrates are purified mixtures resulting from the controlled enzymatic hydrolysis of starch. It contains between 93 and 99% dextrose. Two such directly compressible modified starches are Emdex and Celutab. They consist of porous spheres that have excellent flow properties. They are sweet to taste and can be used as direct compression diluents for chewable tablets.

v) Dextrose:

Dextrose is available commercially by the name Ceralose. It is available both, as a monohydrate and as anhydrous dextrose. It has poor compressibility.

Inorganic salts:

1. Dicalcium phosphate, dihydrate: It is available in the free flowing form as Emcompress, Di-Tab and DICAFOS.
2. Tricalcium phosphate: Available as Tri-Tab and TRICAFOS
3. Calcium sulphate dihydrate: Available as Compactroll

Table 2.9: Advantages and disadvantages of direct compression.

Advantages	Disadvantages
1. Reduced Processing time	1. Chances of non-uniformity of contents are more for low dose drugs due to segregation of powder particle.
2. Reduced labour cost	2. High dose drugs cannot be compressed due to requirement of diluents in high amounts that increases tablet weight.
3. Fewer manufacturing steps and less number of equipments	3. More precision required during blending
4. Less process validation and lower consumption of power	4. Chances of toxicity to personnel are more in case of potent drugs due to dusting
5. Suitable for moisture and Heat-sensitive drugs	5. Chances of static charge build up and dust explosion
6. Reduced disintegration time as each primary particle is directly disintegrated rather than granules	

Dry Granulation (Compression Granulation):

Compression granulation is a valuable technique for granulation of large dose drugs where direct compression is not possible and the drug is sensitive to moisture or heat or both, e.g. many aspirin and vitamin formulations.

In dry granulation methods, powder particles are aggregated under high pressure. All particulate matter can be aggregated when compacted at high pressure because bonding forces are established by direct contact between solid surfaces.

Two methods are used for dry granulation-

i) Slugging: In this components of a tablet formulation are compacted by means of a tablet press or specially designed machine, followed by milling and screening, prior to final compression into a tablet. Powders are first compressed into large tablets or slugs which are milled to make granules. Conventional slugging machines produce slugs upto 25 mm in diameter or larger. When an initial blend of powders is forced into dies of a large capacity tablet press, and pressed using flat faced punches, the compacted masses are called slugs. Slugs are then milled and screened to produce granular form of tabletting material which can flow more easily. When a single slugging process is insufficient, slugs are sometimes screened and slugged again. When slugging is done twice, it strengthens the bonds that hold the tablet together.

ii) Roller Compaction: This method is used for dry granulation on large scale on a specially designed machine called roller compactor with a capacity of as much as 500 kg per hour.

Two cylindrical rolls rotate in opposite directions to draw the powder feed into the gap between the rolls. The feed is compressed into sheets or large ribbon-like pieces called as briquets. By means of hydraulic pressure, one roller is forced against the other. Powdered material is fed between rollers by a screw conveyor system. The ribbon shaped pieces are then milled and compressed.

The roller compaction is affected by- hydraulic pressure exerted on com-

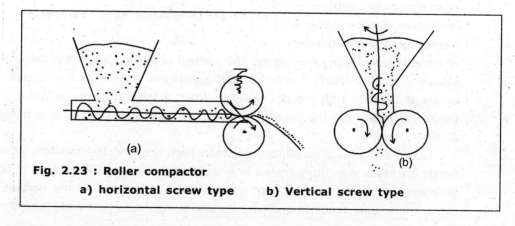

Fig. 2.23 : Roller compactor
   a) horizontal screw type   b) Vertical screw type

paction roll, rotational speed of rolls and rotational speed of feed screws. The feed screw usually consists of a variable speed vertical and horizontal screw. Horizontal screw packs up the powder from hopper and maintains continuous flow to vertical screw. Vertical screw delivers powder to compaction rolls. It delivers the powder and maintains a continuous flow on rolls. Vertical screw is usually set so that it delivers more material than the compaction rolls accept, assuring constant loading during compaction.

Many modifications in roll designs, shapes and sizes of screw feeder are available. Sometimes the machine is provided with liquid cooled rolls.

Advantages :

i) increased production capacity

ii) greater control of compaction pressure

iii) no need for excessive lubrication .

iii) Wet Granulation:

Wet granulation methods also involve unit operations of milling and mixing like the other two methods. But the unique operations are wet massing of the powders, wet milling and drying. In this method, the granules are formed by binding powders together with an adhesive. A solution, suspension or slurry of the binder is added to the powder mixture, or sometimes, the dry binder is incorporated in the powder

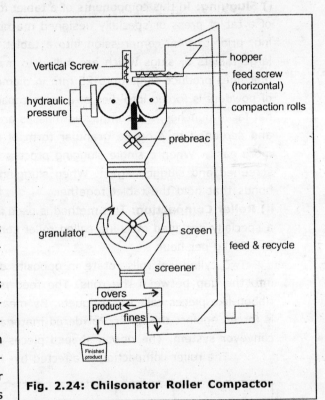

Fig. 2.24: Chilsonator Roller Compactor

mix and liquid is added separately. The method of introducing binder depends on solubility of the binder. If only a small quantity of solvent is permissible, the binder is blended with the dry powder. When a large quantity is desired, the binder is dissolved in the liquid. The binder solution should be fluid in nature to disperse readily.

Liquid bridges are developed between particles, and the strength of these bonds increases with the increase in amount of the liquid. The amount of liquid. Whenever a powder is mixed with a liquid which is able to wet the particle surfaces, the system tends to decrease its free surface energy, by the formation of

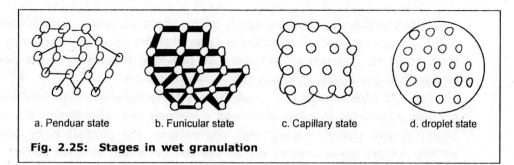

a. Penduar state   b. Funicular state   c. Capillary state   d. droplet state

Fig. 2.25: Stages in wet granulation

liquid bridges between particles. If the amount of wetting liquid is increased, the liquid bridges coalesce and change gradually into the liquid state as depicted in the feed.

At low liquid levels, discrete lens shaped rings are formed at the points of contact of the particles. This is the pendular state which persists until the liquid rings begin to coalesce. Relative amount of liquid phase in the agglomerate is conveniently described by the liquid saturation, S, that is, the ratio of the volume of liquid phase to the total volume of pores. For pendular state, S is upto 25 per cent, for funicular state, S is 25-80 percent and when S is greater than 80per-cent, liquid is in capillary state.

Size enlargement by agglomeration proceeds by one or more of the following mechanisms-

*   Nucleation of primary particles because of formation of liquid bridge bonding
*   Coalescence between colliding agglomerates and nuclei
*   Layering of particles from degradation of established agglomerates.

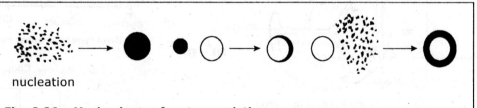

nucleation

Fig. 2.26: Mechanisms of wet granulation

Once the granulating liquid has been added, mixing continues until a uniform dispersion is attained and all the binder has been activated.

Wet granulation involves following steps-

*   Deagglomeration of starting materials by milling
*   Dry mixing
*   Liquid addition and wet massing
*   Wet sieving to remove large lumps
*   Drying
*   Milling or sieving to achieve desired size distribution

After addition of granulating agent, mixing continues until a uniform distribution has been attained. Granulation in large blenders requires 15 minutes to 1 hour. The time depends on wettability of powders, proportion of the powder mixture and granulating fluid and efficiency of the mixer.

The wet screening process involves converting the moist mass into coarse, granular aggregates by passage through a hammer mill or oscillating granulator, equipped with screens having large perforations. The purpose is to increase particle contact points, further consolidate the mass and increase surface area to facilitate drying. Overlying wet material dries slowly and forms hard aggregates which tend to turn to powder during milling.

A drying process is required to remove all the solvent that was used and also to decrease the moisture content to an optimum level of concentration within the granules. During drying, interparticulate bonds result from fusion or recrystallisation and curing of the binding agent.

After drying, granulation is screened again. Size of screen depends upon the equipment used and size of tablet to be made.

Use of inflammable or explosive solvents for wet granulation may cause explosion and pollution hazards.

Equipments for wet granulation :

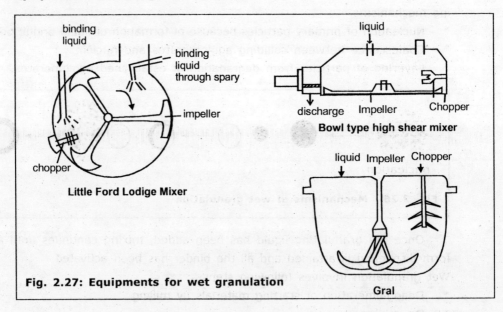

Fig. 2.27: Equipments for wet granulation

1) Low shear mixers- Twin arm kneader, sigma blender, Nauta mixer (Conical screw), changeable bowl planatory mixer.

2) High shear mixers: They employ a rotating agitator and a high speed chopper.

Traditional equipment : If each step of wet granulation is carried out in separate equipment, following equipments are used.

Table 2.10: Equipments in traditional wet granulation process.

Step	Equipments
Dry blending	V-blender, Double cone blender
Wet massing	Sigma blade mixer, planetary mixer
	Granulation Oscillating granulator
	Drying Tray dryer, truck dryer, Fluidised bed dryer

The Lodige mixer is a horizontal cylinder equiped with a central shaft and plough shaped blades rotating at relatively high speeds.

The Diosna, Little ford MG2 mixers are vertical bowl type high shear mixers

The Gral mixer is a modification of industrial planetary mixer containing two mixing devices.

Advantages of Wet Granulation:

1. Cohesiveness and compressibility of powders is improved due to added binder which coats the powder particles, causing them to adhere to each other so that they can be formed into granules. Thus properties of formulation components are improved to overcome their tabletting deficiencies. During the compaction process, granules are fractured, exposing fresh, clean powder surfaces, which improves compressibility. Lower pressures are needed to compress tablets, resulting in improvement in tooling life.

2. High-dosage drugs having poor flow and compressibility properties must be prepared by wet granulation to obtain suitable flow and cohesion for compression. Proportion of binder required in this case is quite low as compared to proportion of dry blender needed in direct compression.

3. Good distribution and uniform content for soluble low dosage drugs is obtained if these are in binder solution of the wet granulation. This is direct advantage over direct compression, where content uniformity of drugs and colour distribution can be a problem.

4. Wet granulation prevents segregation of components of a homogenous powder mixture during processing, transferring and handling; therefore composition of each granule becomes fixed.

Limitations:-

1. It is an expensive process because of the time, labour, equipment, energy and space requirements. However, a number of improvements have been made in the method that helps reduce the cost, e.g. high shear mixers, fluidized bed dryer, V-blender processor.

2. It is difficult to carry out wet granulation of moisture-sensitive drugs. It can

be done using anhydrous solvents. But in that case, special precautions are needed to avoid explosion and protect the environment. This increases cost of processing.

3. Some soluble dyes in wet granulation often cause migration of the dye during drying (mottling). This can be prevented by use of insoluble lakes.

4. An inherent limitation of wet granulation is that any incompatibility between formulation components will be aggravated by the granulating solvent bringing them in close contact.

Table 2.11: Advantages and Disadvantages of wet granulation

Advantages	Disadvantages
1. Excellent cohesiveness and compressibility due to added binder	1. High labour and equipment cost
2. Excellent flow properties	2. High space and time requirements
3. Good distribution and uniform content for low dose drugs	3. Large number of steps
4. Prevention of segregation	4. Migration of soluble dyes
5. Improved dissolution rates for hydrophobic drugs	5. Aggravation of incompatibilities between formulation components
	6. Aqueous granulations not suitable for moisture-sensitive drugs
	7. Not suitable for heat-sensitive drugs.

Table 2.12: Steps in tablet production via wet Granulation, dry Granulation and direct compression, respectively.

Wet granulation	Dry Granulation	Direct Compression
1. Weighing	1. Weighing	1. Weighing
2. Milling	2. Milling	2. Milling
3. Dry blending	3. Dry blending	3. Dry blending
4. Wet mixing	4. Slugging/Roller compaction	4. Blending of lubricant & disintegrant
5. Granulation	5. Sizing	5. Compression
6. Drying	6. Blending of lubricant and disintegrant	
7. Sizing	7. Compression	
8. Blending of lubricant and disintegrant		
9. Compression		

Novel methods of granulation: Several advanced methods are being used for granulation. These methods produce agglomerates that are very close to the spherical shape and are called as pelletisation techniques. Pellets can be compressed as tablets, filled in capsules or administered as loose powders. Apart from having excellent flow properties, pellets possess following advantages-

1. They can be divided into desired dose strengths without formulation or process variable.
2. They can be blended to deliver incompatible drugs.
3. They can be used for sustained release of drugs
4. Pellets disperse freely in gastrointestinal tract after taking orally and maximise absorption of the drug, while minimising local irritation of the mucosa caused by irritant drugs, as only a little amount of the drug is available in a single pellet.

Variety of techniques are available for pelletisation, namely, extrusion-spheronisation, solution, suspension and powder layering using fluidised bed dryer, granulation, balling, spherical crystallisation, melt solidification.

Extrusion-spheronisation:

Extrusion-spheronisation is basically a shaping and forming technique and involves several unit processes like sifting, blending, wet massing and drying. But the two steps that dictate the outcome of the process are extrusion and spheronisation. Process: Fig. 2.28 shows the steps involved in the process of extrusion-spheronisation.

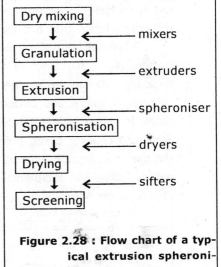

Figure 2.28 : Flow chart of a typical extrusion spheronisation process

The process is a multistep procedure involving dry mixing, wet granulation, extrusion, spheronisation, drying and if necessary screening.

1. Dry mixing: The drug and excipients are mixed in suitable blenders.
2. Wet granulation: The powders are converted to plastic mass by addition of binder solution using suitable granulating equipments.
3. Extrusion: The plastic mass is converted into cylindrical extrudates, like noodles, by using extruders.

A Variety of extruders are available and can be classified as screw extruders, gravity fed or roll extruders and ram extruders.

Screw extruders have screws that rotate along the horizontal axis and hence transport the material. They force the material through an aperture plate. Two types of screw extruders are available : Axial screw extruders and radial

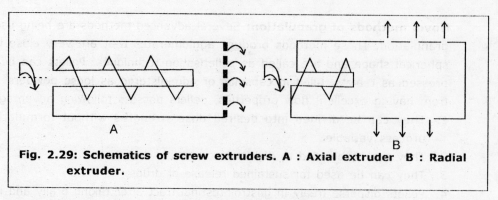

Fig. 2.29: Schematics of screw extruders. A : Axial extruder   B : Radial extruder.

screw extruders (fig 2.29). In axial extruders, the aperture plate is positioned axially.

It consists of a feeding zone, a compression zone and an extrusion zone. In radial extruder, transport zone is short and the material is extruded radially through screens that are mounted around the horizontal axis of the screws.

Gravityfed extruders include rotary gear extruders and rotary cylinder extruders (fig 2.30). Both of them consist of two counter rotating cylinders, but basically differ in the design of these cylinders. In rotary cylinder extruder, one cylinder is hollow and perforated and the other is solid and acts as a pressure roller. In rotary gear extruder, there are two hollow counter rotating gear cylinders with counter bored holes. In ram extruders, a piston displaces and forces the material through a die at the end (fig 2.31). The extruder converts the plastic mass of drug and excipients into cylindrical noodle-like extrudates. These extru-

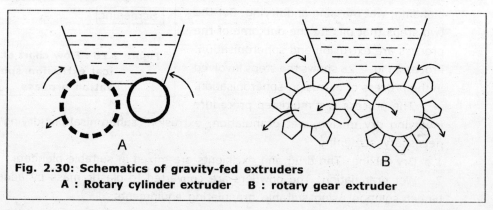

Fig. 2.30: Schematics of gravity-fed extruders
A : Rotary cylinder extruder   B : rotary gear extruder

dates are then fed to a spheroniser.

Spheronisation: A spheroniser, also called a marumeriser, consists of a static cylinder or stator and a rotating friction plate at the base. The friction plate is a rotating disk with a characteristically grooved surface. Fig. 2.32 shows a standard friction plate with a cross-hatch pattern, where the grooves intersect at 90°.

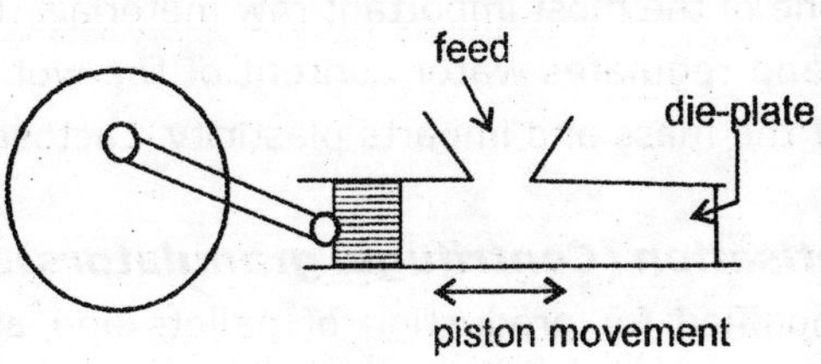

Fig. 2.31: Schematics of a ram extruder

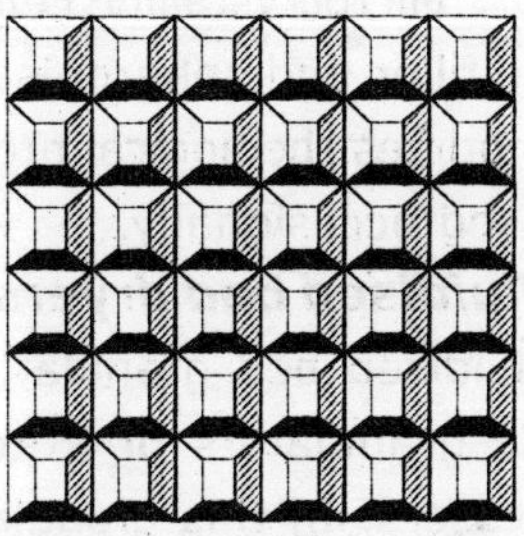

Fig. 2.32: Spheroniser friction plate with a cross-hatch pattern.

The width of grooves is selected according to the pellet diameter, and is in general one and a half to two times the target pellet diameter. The rotational speed is variable and ranges from 100-2000 rpm and depends on the diameter of the unit.

The defined quantity of extrudate is fed into spheroniser from top and the spheronised particles are discharged by centrifugal force via a discharge chute positioned in the vertical wall of the cylinder. The extrudates are rapidly chopped into lengths of approximately twice their diameter by the action of the plate. These cylinders are then spheronised by interparticulate collisions and frictional forces between the particles and walls. The cylinders are first compressed along their length and their ends get rounded, eventually producing dumbells which are further compressed along their length to provide spherical pellets. Fig. 2.33 depicts various stages of spheronisation process.

5. Drying: Since relatively high amounts of water or solvents are incorporated in the formulation, the final pellets contain significant quantities of residual moisture. They are dried either on trays or in a fluid bed dryer.

6. Sizing: Sizing may be necessary to separate the various fractions if the particle size distribution is wider than required.

Formulation : The excipients play an important role in extrusion and spheronisation technique because the granulated mass should be plastic and sufficiently cohesive and self-lubricating during extrusion step.

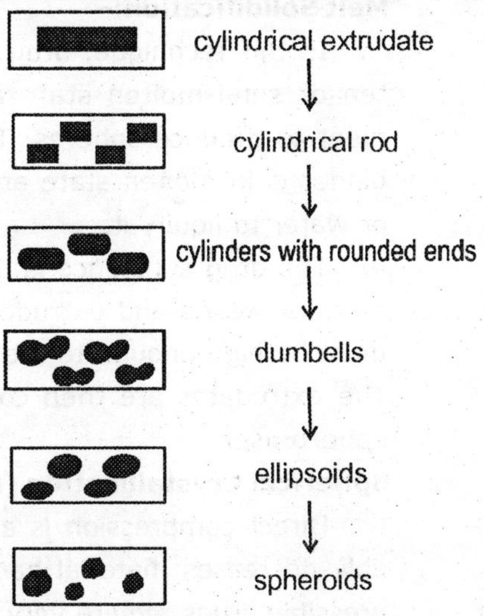

Fig. 2.33: Shape transitions during a spheronisation process

Microcrystalline cellulose is one of the most important raw materials. It is used as filler and spheronisation aid and regulates water content of the wet mass. It modifies rheological properties of the mass and imparts plasticity. Lactose may be used occasionally.

Fluidised bed dryers in pelletisation (Centrifugal granulators).

Fluidised bed granulators are modified for production of pellets and are called CF-granulators or Roto-processors. In this granulator, a disc rotates at the bottom of the fluidised bed granulator (fig. 2.34). Binder solution is admitted through a nozzle tangentially. The rotating disc pushes the particles towards the vertical wall. Fluidising air is admitted through a slit between the disc and the wall. It generates a strong force

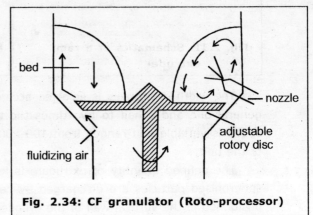

Fig. 2.34: CF granulator (Roto-processor)

and carries the particles vertically along the wall of the container. The particles lose their momentum and cascade down toward the center of the rotating disc. At the same time, they receive the binder solution through the nozzle. A combination of centrifugal force, fluidising air velocity and gravitational force, along with the application of binder solution, converts the powder mass into pellets.

Melt Solidification:-

In this technique, drug substances and excipients are converted into a molten or semi-molten state and subsequently shaped using appropriate equipment to produce spheres. The process is similar to wet granulation, except the binder is in molten state and therefore does not require addition of any solvent or water to liquify it.

The drug substance is first blended with appropriate additives, such as polymers or waxes and extruded at a predetermined temperature. The temperature must be high enough to melt at least one or more of the formulation component. The extrudates are then converted to spheroids by using any type of jacketed spheroniser.

Spherical Crystallisation (Balling):-

Direct compression is a revolutionary technique of tabletting as it considerably decreases material handling and processing time. But high dose non-compressible drugs require very high amount of directly compressible vehicles. Tabletting of high dose, non-compressible drug by direct compression, therefore, still remains a challenge. The compressibility of non-compressible active ingredients can be improved by modification of physical form. A modified crystallisation technique, called spherical crystallisation is devised for this purpose.

Spherical crystallisation is a novel particle design technique, by which crystallisation and agglomeration can be carried out simultaneously, in one step. When a particulate solid is suspended in one liquid, and a second liquid which preferentially wets the solid and is immiscible with the first liquid, is added. The mixture is shaken in an appropriate vessel that agglomerates the solid. By appropriately controlling several parameters, spherically agglomerated crystals are obtained. These agglomerates have good flowability and compressibility.

The technique transforms fine crystals into spherical, dense agglomerates. In this process, as a crystallisation solvent, a mixture of three partially miscible solvents is used, e.g. ethanol-water-chloroform. When the composition of the mixture is correctly chosen, a small amount of solvent, termed, 'bridging liquid' is liberated from the system. This liquid collects crystals produced during crystallisation and transforms them into a spherical form.

Methods :- The simple spherical crystallisation method involves following steps:

i) The substance is dissolved in a 'good solvent'.

ii) Solution is poured into a poor solvent under controlled conditions, so that crystallisation is favoured.

iii) The fine crystals that are formed are agitated in liquid suspension.

iv) A bridging liquid that preferentially wets the crystal surfaces is added, which causes bridging.

v) The agglomerates are spherical if amount of the bridging liquid and rate of agitation is controlled.

Some other methods of spherical crystallisation-

Quasi Emulsion solvent diffusion method : When a bridging liquid (or plus a good solvent) solution of the drug is poured into a poor solvent under agitation, quasi emulsion droplets of bridging liquid or good solvent are formed in poor solvent, which induce crystallisation followed by agglomeration.

Neutralisation method :- An antidiabetic drug, tolbutamide, is dissolved in sodium hydroxide solution, hydroxyl propyl ethyl cellulose aqueous solution and hydrochloric acid are added to neutralise NaOH solution. This crystallises out tolbutamide. A bridging liquid (ether) is added, which causes agglomeration.

The evaluation parameters for agglomerates formed by spherical crystallisation method are particle size and particle size distribution, density measurements, angle of repose, shape and surface topography by use of Scanning Electron Microscopy, crystalline form of agglomerates by X-ray diffraction, strength and friability and wettability.

Cryopelletisation :- In cryopelletisation, droplets of a liquid formulation are converted into solid spherical particles by using liquid nitrogen as a fixing medium. Droplets of solution or suspension of a drug are allowed to come in contact with liquid nitrogen at -160°C. The material instantaneously and evenly freezes due to rapid heat transfer.

The equipment consists of a container equipped with perforated plates at the bottom. Immediately below the plates, at a predetermined distance is a reservoir of liquid nitrogen in which a conveyor belt with transport baffles is immersed. The conveyor belt has a variable speed. The frozen pellets are transported out of the nitrogen bath into a storage container at -60°C prior to drying.

Spray drying and spray congealing :- In spray drying, drug entities in solution or suspension are sprayed into a hot air stream to generate dried, highly spherical particles.

During spray congealing, drug is allowed to melt, dissolve or disperse in hot melts of waxes or fatty acids and sprayed into an air chamber where the temperature is below melting temperature of the waxes. The droplets congeal in the form of perfect spheres.

Table 2.13: Novel methods of granulation

Method	Description
1. Extrusion spheronisation	Wet mass is first extruded into cylindrical shapes, chopped and converted to spheres
2. Fluid bed granulation	Modified fluidised bed dryers are used to prepare Spherical agglomerates with the aid of centrifugal force
3. Melt solidification	Drug and excipients are converted into semi-molten state and then shaped into spheres
4. Spherical crystallisation	It is a particle design technique where crystallisation and agglomeration takes place simultaneously
5. Cryopelletisation	Solution or suspension is rapidly congealed at 160°C by using liquid nitrogen
6. Spray drying	Drug is suspended or dissolved in a solvent, sprayed and dried rapidly to produce spherical agglomerates.
7. Spray congealing	Drug is suspended or dissolved in hot melt of low melting waxes, which is then sprayed in cool air current where droplets congeal to spherical agglomerates.

COMPRESSIBILITY AND COMPACTABILITY OF POWDERS

The compressibility of powders is defined as its ability when held within a confined space, to reduce in volume upon application of pressure.

The compactability of powders is defined as the ability to gain strength of the formed assemblage of particles, upon application of pressure.

EVALUATION OF COMPRESSION BEHAVIOUR

The compression and volume reduction may be studied by two ways :
- by characterization of ejected tablets
- by characterization of compression events.

The tablets may be characterized in following ways :

Tablet inspection :

The changes in physical properties of particles may be studied by scanning electron microscopy and profilometry. The inspection of tablets with the help of the above mentioned techniques reveals the fragmentation pattern, permanent shape changes due to deformation and formation of cracks within tablets.

Pore structure of tablets :

The mean pore size, pore volume and pore size distribution in tablets may be studied by mercury intrusion porosimetry.

Specific surface area :

The measurement of surface area of powders before and after compression gives an idea about fragmentation. The techniques like gas adsorption (BET surface area analysis) and air permeability may be useful in determining surface area of powders. The compression and decompression events during tabletting may be characterized by following ways:

Force displacement profiles - The force displacement profile is the relationship between upper punch force and upper punch displacement during compression. Force displacement profiles are an important means of characterizing compression behavior of powders.

The force displacement curve may be divided into three different regions

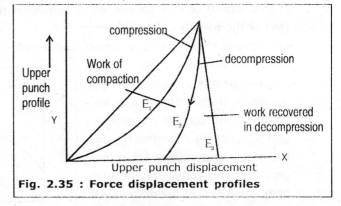

Fig. 2.35 : Force displacement profiles

Viz. E1, E2 and E3. The areas E1 and E3 should be small for a powder to perform well in tabletting. The profiles are useful as indicators of tablettability of powders. Following are other useful parameters to decribe compression & decompression.

1. Upper punch force versus die wall force
2. Tablet porosity versus upper punch pressure.
3. Upper punch force / pressure versus compression time.
4. Lower punch force / pressure versus compression time.
5. Upper punch force/pressure versus lower punch force / pressure.
6. Punch force versus punch displacement.
7. Tablet relative volume versus upper punch pressure force.

TABLET VOLUME / APPLIED PRESSURE PROFILES

The relationship between volume & applied pressure is the most important approach in deriving a mathematical expression for compression. A large number of volume-pressure relationships have been established. However, the two important ones are : Heckel equation and Kawakita equation

Heckel equation :

Tablet porosity is measured on an ejected tablet (out of die) or on a powder column (in die)

The compression of a powder can be described in terms of a first order reaction, where the pores are the reactant & the densification is the product. Following expression is derived :

$$\ln(1/e) = KP + A$$

Where,

e - tablet porosity

P - applied pressure

A - constant suggested to reflect particle rearrangement & fragmentation

K - slope of the linear part of the relationship. It reflects the deformation of particles during compression.

The reciprocal of K is considered to represent the yield stress or yield pressure (py) of the particles. $\ln(1/e) = \dfrac{P}{py} + A$

Yield stress is the stress at which plastic deformation starts. The typical Heckel plot is shown in fig. 2.36.

The profile shows an initial curvature (region I) which is associated with particle fragmentation & repacking. After this region, the relationship become linear (region II). This region of the plot obeys the heckel expression. In this region, it is believed that particle deformation controls the compression process. The recip-

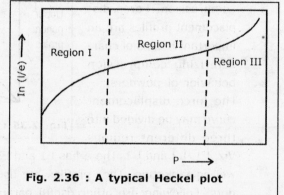

Fig. 2.36 : A typical Heckel plot

rocal of the slope of this region is the yield pressure. After this region, profile again deviates from the linear relationship (Region III). The curvature reflects elastic deformation of the whole tablet.

Kawakita equation

The equation assumes that during powder compression in a confined space, the system is at equilibrium so that the product of a pressure term & volume term is constant. The equation is written in following linear form :

$$P/C = (1/ab) + (p/a)$$

P - applied pressure

C - degree of volume reduction

a, b - constant

The degree of volume reduction relates the initial height of the powder column (h_o) to the height of the powder compact at an applied pressure p (h_p) as:

$$C = (h_o - h_p) / h_o$$

Mechanism of compaction :

The assemblage of particles in the form of a tablet gains strength as a result of interparticlate bonding. The bonding is of following five types. (Rumpt classification):

1. Bonding due to addition of liquid
2. Bonding due to addition of binders
3. Solid bridges
4. Intermolecular and electrostatic forces.
5. Mechanical interlocking.

Evaluation of compactability :

As defined earlier, compactability is the ability of a powder to form a coherent tablet. The compactability i.e. the ability to form a coherent tablet is understood in a broader sense. A powder with a high strength broader sense. A powder with a high strength forms a tablet with a higher fracture resistance. Thus measurement of fracture resistance i.e. tensile strength of a tablet, is an indirect measure of tablet compactability. Compactability is often evaluated by studying the effect of compaction pressure on the strength of resulting tablet. This often exhibits a linear relationship.

Leuenberger & Aldeborn developed equations to model

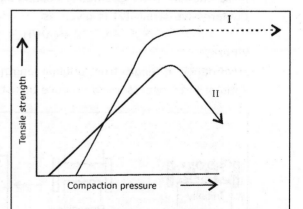

Fig. 2.37 : Relationship between compaction pressure & tensile strength. (I) tablets showing no lamination (II) tablets showing lamination

compactability. In both equations bond structure is related to an endpoint representing maximum tensile strength (Tmax). It assumes that over a cross section of tablet, number of bonding & non bonding sites exist. This number depends on applied pressure (p), tablet relative density (r=1-porosity, e). A term compression susceptibiity (v) was introduced in the expression, It describes compressibility of powder and has a unit of 1/ pressure.

$$T = T_{max} (1 - e [v p_p])$$

As seen from the compactability profile (fig 2.37), the tensile strength initially increases with increase in pressure and finally, levels off.

TABLET COMPRESSION:

Physics of tablet compression (Ref. Encyclopaedia vol. 18)

The applied forces may have various effects on powders as follows:

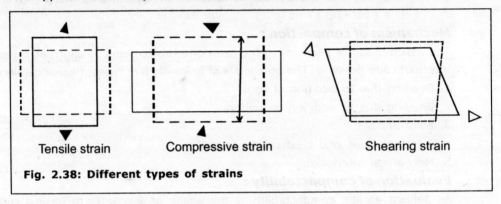

Fig. 2.38: Different types of strains

i) **Deformation:** When a solid body is subjected to opposing forces, there is a finite change in its geometry, depending upon the nature of the applied load. Compressive strain (z) is given as

$$Z = \Delta H/H_o$$

Where,

ΔH -Change in length from original length H_o

Ratio of force necessary to produce this strain to area, A is called stress $S = F/ A$.

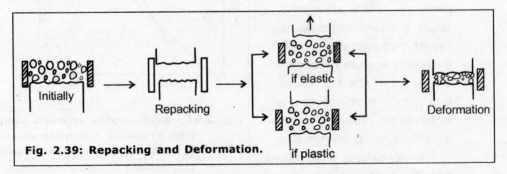

Fig. 2.39: Repacking and Deformation.

ii) Compression :

When external mechanical forces are applied to a powder mass, there is normally a reduction in bulk volume as a result of one or more of the following effects -

a) **Repacking** : With application of external load, the particles rearrange themselves in the void spaces and repack. This is the major cause of volume reduction in initial stages of application of load. As the load increases the rearrangement becomes more difficult and further compression involves particle deformation. Some types of particle deformations-

b) **Elastic deformation** : If on removal of load, the powder mass spontaneously reverts back to its original form, it is called as elastic deformation to some extent, e.g. aspirin.

c) **Plastic deformation** : After exceeding the elastic limit of the material (yield value), the deformation may become plastic, i.e., the particles undergo viscous flow. This is a predominant mechanism when the shear strength is less than tensile or breaking strength.

d) **Brittle Fracture** : Upon exceeding the elastic limit of the material (yield value), the particles undergo brittle fracture if the shear strength is greater than the tensile or breaking strength. Under these conditions the larger particles are sheared and broken into smaller particles which fill the voids.

e) **Micro-squashing** : Irrespective of the behaviour of larger particles, smaller particles may deform plastically, a process known as micro-squashing. The proportion of the fine powder in the sample may therefore be significant.

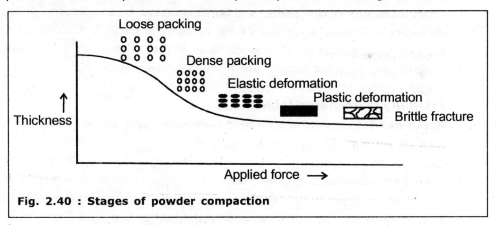

Fig. 2.40 : Stages of powder compaction

Consolidation / Compaction :

i) When surfaces of two particles approach each other, closely enough, their free surface energies result in a strong attractive force, a process known as cold welding. This force is mainly of Van der Waals attractive force. This increases mechanical strength of the powder bed when compressed.

ii) Most particles have irregular shape, so that there are many points of contact in a bed of powder. Applied compression load is transmitted through these particle contacts. When the force is appreciable, this transmission may result in generation of frictional heat. There is local rise in temperature, which causes melting of the contact area of the particles, which re-

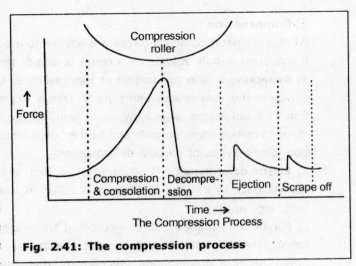

Fig. 2.41: The compression process

lieves the stress in that particular region. In that case, the melt solidifies, giving rise to fusion bonding. This further increases mechanical strength.

During tablet formation, load is applied to the powder mass. Plastic deformation and brittle fracture creates clean surfaces which bond together. Plastic deformation is believed to create maximum number of clean surfaces and it is known to be time-dependant. Therefore, higher rate of force application results in formulation of lesser number of clean surfaces resulting in weaker tablets. Also, higher concentration of materials that form weak bonds may lead to weak tablets. Creation of new surfaces of bonding occurs simultaneously. A high quality tablet is formed when the extent of bonding exceeds fragmentation, with increase in temperature of powder mass due to friction, stress relaxation increases and stronger tablets are formed. Under certain conditions, pre-compression helps to remove entrapped air, thereby increasing stress relaxation.

Friability of uncoated tablet - I.P.

Apparatus : It consists of a drum of transparent synthetic polymer with polished internal surfaces and subject to minimum static build up. It has a diameter of 283-291 mm & a depth of 36-40 mm. One side of the drum is removable. A curved projection with an inner radius of 75.5 to 85.5 mm & extending from the middle of the drum to the outer wall enables the tumbling of the tablets at each turn of the drum. The outer diameter of the central ring is 24.5 mm to 25.5 mm. The drum is attached to the horizontal axis of a device that rotates at 25 ± 1 rpm. It should be ensured that with every turn of the drum the tablets roll or slide and fall onto the drum wall or onto each other.

Method : For tablets with an average weight of 0.65g or less, take a sample of whole tablets corresponding to about 6.5g and for tablets with an average weight of more than 0.65g, take a sample of 10 whole tablets.

Dedust & weigh the required number of tablets. Place the tablets in the drum & rotate it 100 times. Remove the tablets, remove any loose dust from them and weigh them accurately. The test is run only once. If the results are difficult to interpret or if the weight loss is greater than the targeted value, the test is repeated twice & the mean of the three tests is determined. A maximum loss of weight, not more than 1.0% is acceptable for most tablets. If obviously cracked, chipped or broken tablets are present in the sample, the sample fails the test.

iii) Decompression : After compression and consolidation, the formed compact must be capable of withstanding the stresses encountered during decompression and tablet ejection. The same deformation characteristics that come into play during compression play a role during decompression. After application of maximum compression force, the tablet undergoes elastic recovery. Because the tablet is constrained in the die, elastic recovery occurs only in the axial direction. If the rate of elastic recovery is high the tablet may cap or laminate in the die due to rapid expansion in radial direction only. If tablet undergoes brittle fracture during decompression, compact may form failure plains due to fracturing of surfaces. Tablets that do not cap are capable of recovering by plastic deformation. Since plastic deformation is time dependent, stress relaxation is also time dependent. Therefore higher rates of decompression, i.e., faster machine speed, results in weaker tablets.

iv) Ejection: It occurs in 3 stages-
1. Initial ejection peak force required to break the tablet adhesion to the die wall. That is the highest force encountered during ejection.
2. Forces required for pushing the tablet up in the die wall, which are typically lower than at the ejection peak. Inadequate lubrication or damaged dies, where tablet continues to adhere to the die walls resulting in tablet failure.
3. Declining forces as the tablet emerges from the die.

v) Scrape off : Tablet scrape off occurs immediately after ejection when tablet rests on the lower punch. Higher scrape off forces may result in tablets sticking to lower punches, or under extreme conditions shearing the bottom of the tablet.

Equipments :

i) Eccentric or Single punch tablet press

The single punch tablet machine is also called as eccentric tablet machine, because the movement of the upper punch and application of force is produced by an eccentric wheel that rotates. They produce one tablet at a stroke and their capacity is quite low. The tablet press consists of – i) hopper for holding and feeding granulation, ii) dies that define the size and shape of the tablet and iii) punches for compressing granulation into dies.

The press consists of - a i) upper punch connected to the main shaft which is connected to the eccentric, ii) lower punch held by the lower shaft, iii) die held in place by the die table and iv) powder feeder moving back and forth on the die

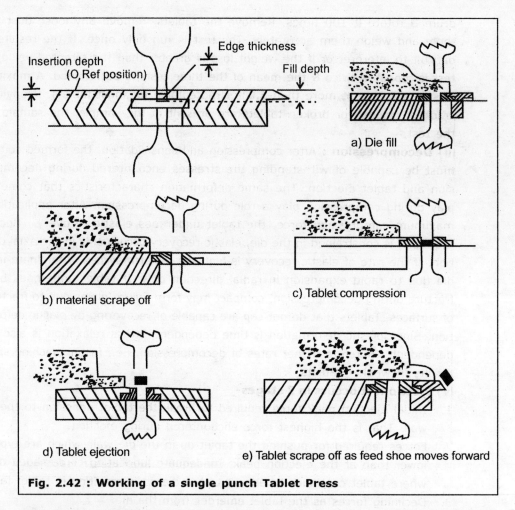

Fig. 2.42 : Working of a single punch Tablet Press

table. The punch reference position of zero is located at the top of the die. Sequence of tablet compression is shown in the Fig. 2.42.

a.   The feeder moves over the die and lower punch. The lower punch drops to a preset height which is the fill depth. As the lower punch drops, the powder fills the die cavity.

b.   The feeder begins to recede. As it clears the die cavity, it scrapes off the excess material. Many times, the feeder incorporates the agitator bar, which helps the material to flow into the die cavity.

c.   Upper punch descends into the die cavity and material is compressed. Lower punch remains stationary. Maximum depth at which upper punch enters into die is called as insertion depth. The difference between fit depth and insertion depth determines the tablet edge thickness.

d.   Upper punch is pulled from the die and away from compact, lower punch begins to move upward and ejects the tablet.

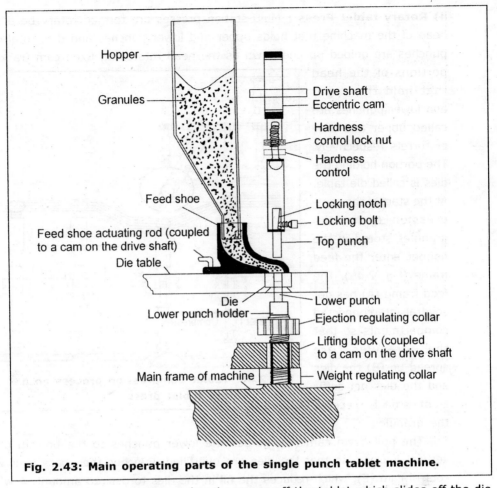

Fig. 2.43: Main operating parts of the single punch tablet machine.

Labels in figure:
- Hopper
- Granules
- Feed shoe
- Feed shoe actuating rod (coupled to a cam on the drive shaft)
- Die table
- Die
- Lower punch holder
- Main frame of machine
- Drive shaft
- Eccentric cam
- Hardness control lock nut
- Hardness control
- Locking notch
- Locking bolt
- Top punch
- Lower punch
- Ejection regulating collar
- Lifting block (coupled to a cam on the drive shaft
- Weight regulating collar

e. The feeder moves forward and scrapes off the tablet which slides off the die cavity, refer figure 2.44 and 2.45.

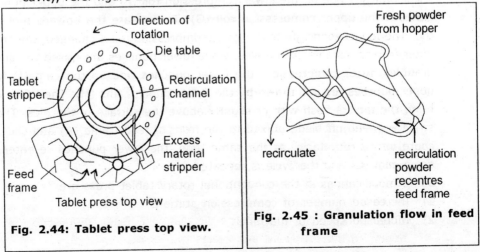

Labels in figure 2.44:
- Direction of rotation
- Die table
- Tablet stripper
- Recirculation channel
- Excess material stripper
- Feed frame
- Tablet press top view

Fig. 2.44: Tablet press top view.

Labels in figure 2.45:
- Fresh powder from hopper
- recirculate
- recirculation powder recentres feed frame

Fig. 2.45 : Granulation flow in feed frame

ii) Rotary tablet Press : Multi-station presses are termed rotary because the head of the machine that holds upper and lower punches and dies rotates. The punches are guided up and down as the head rotates on fixed cam tracks. The portions of the head that hold the upper and lower punches are called upper and lower turrets respectively. The portion holding the dies is called die table. At the start of the compression cycle, the granules stored in the hopper enter the feed frame (Fig. 2.46). The feed frame (A) has got several interconnected compartments so that the granules are spread on (B) the dies and the dies get sufficient time to receive the granules.

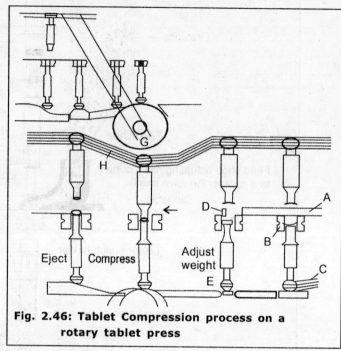

Fig. 2.46: Tablet Compression process on a rotary tablet press

The pull down cam (C), guides the lower punches to the bottom of their vertical journey, so that the dies are overfilled. Punches then pass over weight control cam (E), which reduces the fill in the dies to desired amount. A wipe off blade (D) at the end of the feed frame removes the excess granules. Then the lower punches ride on the lower compression roll (F) and the upper punches ride beneath the upper compression roll (G). To regulate the upward movement of the lower punches, height of the lower compression roll is changed. Upper punches enter a fixed distance in the dies, while lower punches are raised to squeeze the granules. After compression, the lower punches ride up the cam (I) while the upper punches are withdrawn by the upper punch cams (H). The lower cams (I) bring the tablets flush with or slightly above the surface of the dies. The tablets strike a sweep off blade affixed to the front of feed frame (A) and slide down a chute into a receptacle. At the same time, the lower punches re-enter the pull down cam (C) and the cycle is repeated.

Some modifications in the conventional rotary tablet press are :

1) Increased number of compression stations
2) Increased speed of machine

3) Use of hydraulic or pneumatic pressure to control pressure rolls in place of older spring type pressure rolls.

4) Pre-compression stations to allow compression of difficult granulations.

5) Chilling of compression components to allow compression of low melting point substances such as waxes.

iii) Double rotary machine: A double rotary machine is the one which consists of two hoppers, two sets of compression rolls. Compression takes place at compression stations and one compression cycle is complete with half rotation of the die table and upper and lower turrets.

Compression machine tooling : The basic mechanical unit in all tablet compression equipment includes a lower punch that fills into a die from the bottom and an upper punch, with a head of the same shape and dimensions that enters the die cavity from the top, after the tabletting material fills the die cavity. The tablets assume the size and shape of punches and die used. See Fig. 2.43 Spherical Shallow Standard Deep

Generally, round tablets are used more. Oval, capsule-shaped (caplets), square, triangular, or other irregular shapes may be used. The curvature of the faces of punches determines the curvature of the tablets.

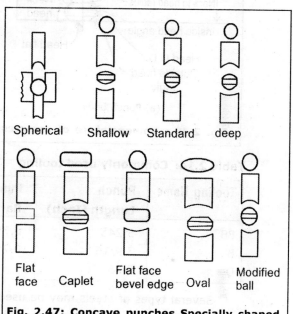

Fig. 2.47: Concave punches Specially shaped punches.

The dies and punches are called compression machine tooling. Each tooling set consists of a die and upper and lower punches Fig. 2.48 illustrates the terminology used to describe the compression tooling. The most commonly used tooling is BB tooling. It is 5.25" long, and has nominal barrel diameter of 0.75" and head diameter of 1". B tooling is similar to BB tooling except that the lower punch is shorter, having the length of 3 9/16". D tooling is used for larger tablets. It has 1" barrel diameter, 1.25" head diameter and 5.25" length. The dies used with above punches are either a 0.945" outer diameter (outer diameter) die capable of making a 7/16" round tablet or 1 3/16" outer diameter die capable of making a 9/16" round tablet.

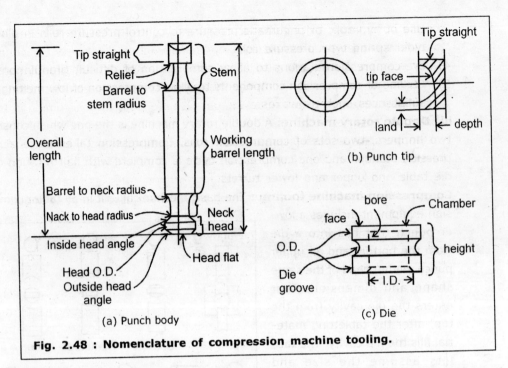

Fig. 2.48 : Nomenclature of compression machine tooling.

Table 2.14: Commonly used tooling

Tooling Name	Punch Length (Inch)	Punch Diameter Barrel (Inch)	Punch Diameter Head (Inch)
BB	5.245	0.75	1
B	3 9/16	0.75	1
D	5.25	1	11/4

Several types of steels may be used to manufacture tooling. These steels differ in toughness and wear strength. Tablets having various sizes, shapes and contours may be produced by using different types of tooling. Visibly unique tablets may be produced by using tooling carrying certain other information like company names or symbols, trade names or dosage strength. These numbers or letters may be engraved or embossed on the punch faces. Even though tablets having a variety of shapes may be produced, some practical aspects limit the implementation of different designs. The upper punches may turn around during the compression process. This

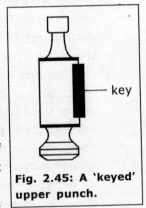

Fig. 2.45: A 'keyed' upper punch.

movement does not create any problem while compressing round tablets. But when the punch tip is not round, i.e., a tablet having some novel shape is being produced, the upper punch must not rotate, otherwise it will strike the edge of the die bore, while it descends for compression. 'Keying' of the punches is done to avoid this problem. A slot is cut longitudinally into the barrel of the punch and a key is inserted. This key, also called as 'anti-turning device', slightly protrudes and engages a similar slot, cut into the upper punch guides on the tablet press. Lower punches do not require keying because their tips always remain in the die and do not rotate.

In order to produce physically perfect compressed tablets, a regular maintenance schedule for the tooling should be set up. They must be highly polished and must be kept free from rust and imperfections. In cases where the tooling is likely to get abraded, chromium plated toolings are used. Punches should never be dropped on hard surfaces. When the punches are in the machine, the upper and lower punches should not be allowed to contact each other, as this may cause flattening of edges of curved punches. When the punches are removed from the machine, they should be washed thoroughly with soapy warm water and dried well. The dies and punches should be coated thoroughly with some oil or grease to prevent rusting. They should be stored in boxes or paper tubes.

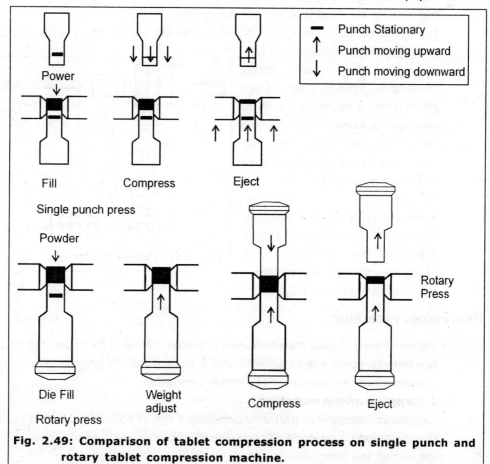

Fig. 2.49: Comparison of tablet compression process on single punch and rotary tablet compression machine.

Auxiliary Equipments:

1. **Forced feeders:** If the dwell time of the die under the feed frame is too short or the flow properties of granules are too poor, the die fill is incomplete, which results in weight variation and unsatisfactory content uniformity of the tablets. To overcome this problem, mechanised feeders may be used to force the granulations into the die. (Fig. 2.51)

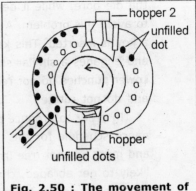

Fig. 2.50 : The movement of tablets on the die table of a double rotary press.

2. **Granulation level sensors:** If the granulation hopper is not refilled after adequate time, the tabletting machine runs dry, giving rise to a series of unacceptable events, viz., production of low weight tablets, inability to compress the granules into tablets and degeneration of tooling. Granulation level sensors are used to stop the press automatically when the granulation level drops to a critical level.

3. **Compression force monitors:** They monitor the force at each compression station, which correlates with tablet weight. They are also capable of initiating corrective actions like altering the amount of die fill to maintain a fixed force, ejecting tablets that are out of specification, counting and documenting the machine operation.

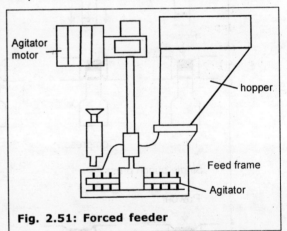

Fig. 2.51: Forced feeder

4. **Tablet dedusters:** They remove traces of loose powder adhering to tablets following compression. The tablets are conveyed directly from the tabletting machine to a tablet deduster

PROCESSING PROBLEMS:

Various problems occur during manufacturing of tablets. Some of them are due to formulation defects, some due to the equipment, while some are combinations of the two. Following are the reasons of capping & lamination.

1. Capping and lamination :

Capping is complete or partial separation of top or bottom crowns of tablet from the main body. Lamination is separation of tablet into two or more distinct layers.

• During compression, sufficient die wall pressure in produced on the tablets due to plastic deformation. This pressure cannot be relieved by elastic recovery when punch pressure is removed. In some tablets, this die-wall pressure produces enough stress to initiate a crack in the tablet. The tablet is confined in the die and can expand only in axial direction during decompression. This may cause separation of top or bottom portion of the crown of the tablet. The stress relaxation is time-dependent. Therefore, initiation of fracture is also time-dependent. Tablets that do not fracture are able to release the stress during decompression by plastic deformation. Pre-compression, slowing down the tabletting rate and decreasing final compression pressure, are the remedies to this problem.

• Often deep concave punches produce tablets that cap. Curved portion of the tablet expands radially, while the body cannot and the tablet caps. Use of flat punches can eliminate this problem.

• A granulation that is too dry lacks cohesion and the tablets tend to cap. Addition of hygroscopic substances, like sorbitol and PEG 4000, can help to maintain proper moisture level.

• In direct compression, some powders may have poor compressibility and may cause capping.

• Concave edges of punches gradually turn inward with use and form a claw that can pull off crowns of tablets. This can be eliminated by avoiding use of concave punches.

• Dies develop a wear 'ring' in the area of compression. As the ring enlarges, tablets that are compressed have a diameter that is too large to pass easily through the narrower portion of die above the ring. This causes the tablet to cap or laminate. A simple solution is to turn the die so that compression occurs above the ring. Coating the die walls with inert material like tungsten carbide also protects the die.

• Another cause of lamination may be sweep-off blade. During ejection, the lower punch must raise flush, which protrudes slightly above the die, so that the whole tablet strikes the sweep-off blade. If punch remains below the die, the sweep-off blade cuts the tablet.

2. Picking and sticking:

Picking is a term used to describe the sticking of the surface material from the tablet to a punch and being removed by it. These are usually small fragments from the tablet face at first. But the condition becomes progressively worse with time. Tablets may chip or break if picking occurs on the lower punch or may get pulled apart if it occurs on the upper punch.

• This is usually due to incompletely dried or incompletely lubricated granulations. The remedy is to control the moisture in the granulation.

• On rotary machines, increasing the pressure, decreasing the speed and/or increasing the proportion of binder, helps to overcome these defects.

- Use of light mineral oil as lubricant is also effective.
- Another remedy is to use highly polished punches or chromium plated punches.
- In some cases colloidal silica added to the formula acts as polishing agent and makes the punch edges smooth. On the other hand, frictional nature of this material may require addition of extra lubricating agent to facilitate release of tablet from the die.
- Low melting point substances, either active ingredients or the additives, such as stearic acid or PEG, may soften sufficiently due to heat of compression and cause sticking. Dilution of the active ingredient with a high melting point material may help. The low melting point additive should be replaced with a suitable high melting point additive.
- Sticking refers to the tablet material being removed by the die wall. When sticking occurs, additional force is required to overcome the friction between the tablet and the die wall during ejection. Serious sticking during ejection may cause chipping of the tablet's edges, thus producing a rough edge. Sticking does not allow lower punches to move freely and may exert unusual pressures on cam tracks and punch heads.
- Picking is of particular concern when the tips of punches have engraving or embossing on them. Small enclosed areas such as those found in the letters A, B and O are difficult to manufacture clearly. To avoid this, letterings should be kept as big as possible or the tablet should be re-formulated to a larger size.
- Filming is a slow build-up of a thin film of the material on the punches when pressure is applied. This is mainly due to loss of polish on the punch faces, high humidity or high temperature. If this build up is allowed to progress, tablets from bevelled edge or concave punches fill in punch concavities and become flat, while tablets from flat faced punches become concave because of build up of granulation around the edges of the punch faces.

Remedies are:

i)   Decreasing moisture content
ii)   Changing lubricant
iii) Increasing proportion of binder
iv)   Increasing clean punch faces with 5 per cent light mineral oil.
v)   Polishing punch faces

3. Chipping and Cracking : Chipping is a defect in which pieces are broken or chipped out of the tablet. This may occur on the faces, but usually occurs on the edges. This may be due to sticking, or damaged punches.

- Cracking refers to tablets that are cracked anywhere, but often in the centre of the top. Cracking is due to expansion. Chipping or cracking problems may be solved by replacing the chipped punches or by increasing the binder or polishing punch tips.

4. Mottling : Mottling is unequal distribution of colour on a tablet with light or dark areas on a uniform surface. Mottling may be because of the drug whose colour differs from the tablet excipients or a drug whose degradation product is coloured. Use of a colouring agent may solve this problem. But a soluble dye can cause mottling by migrating to the surface of the granulation during drying. This can be solved by changing the solvent system, binder system, reduce the drying temperature or grind to a smaller particle size.

• Certain coloured binder solutions may not be distributed well because they must be hot when added to much cooler powder mixtures. The adhesive then precipitates from solution and carries most of the colour with it. Further wetting or over-wetting is needed to disperse the binder and colour. But additional mixing may result in tablets with increased Disintegration time. A better remedy is to incorporate finely powdered binders into product before adding granulating fluid or to disperse colour additive during powder blending step.

5. Weight Variation : The weight of the tablet is decided by the amount of granules in the die cavity. All the factors that affect die-filling process also affect the weight of the tablet.

• Granule size and size distribution before compression : The ratio of the smaller sized granules to larger sized granules and the difference between the granule size affects the tablet weight. Although the volume in the die is same, different proportions of small and large particles may change the weight of fill in each die. If large granules are being used to fill a small die cavity, relatively few granules are required and the difference of only a few granules around the average may represent a high percentage weight variation. If a large number of granules are required for die-fill, a variation of few granules around the average would produce a minor weight variation.

• Poor flow : The granules should flow continuously and uniformly from the hopper thorough the feed frame. If the granules do not flow readily, some dies are filled incompletely. Incomplete filling takes place also when the speed of the machine is too high, so that it is in excess of the granulation's flow capabilities. Remedies to solve this problem would be - i) Addition of a glidant like talc or increasing the amount of the glidant. ii) Induced die feeders which mechanically force the granules into the die cavity.

• As particulate solids move due to gravity through smaller openings, they experience uneven pressure due to the granules above and alongside. Depending on the geometry of the hopper, this may give rise to either of the two causes of poor flow - arching/bridging or rat holing. Problems of poor hopper flow can be handled by

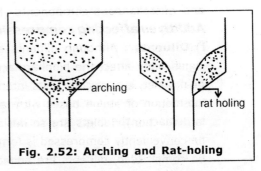

Fig. 2.52: Arching and Rat-holing

duce segregation and stratification of the particles. This classification of the particles not only causes weight variation, but also leads to poor content uniformity. Many times, poor particulate flow is caused not by any defect in granulation, but because of the poor design of the hopper. Weight variation is also caused by excessive flow through hopper. Restricting the flow out of hopper often corrects the problem.

• **Poor mixing** : Sometimes lubricants and glidants are not thoroughly mixed because of which flow of particles is impaired.

• **Punch variation** : When lower punches are of unequal length the fill in each die varies.

6. Hardness variation : The causes of hardness variation and weight variation are always same. Hardness depends on weight of material and space between the upper and lower punches at the moment of compression. If the volume of the material or space varies, hardness is inconsistent.

7. Double Impression: This problem occurs with punches which have a monogram or other engraving on them. During compression, the tablet receives imprint of the punch. In some machines the lower punch is free to drop. and then travel uncontrolled till point of ejection. At this point the punch can make a new lighter impression on the bottom of the tablet resulting in a double impression.

• Similarly, when compression is carried out at two stages, i.e., pre-compression and compression, the engraved upper punches may give rise to this problem. During pre-compression, the tablet receives a lighter impression. If the upper punch is uncontrolled, it can rotate during the short travel in between the pre-compression and compression rolls and create a double impression. To solve this problem, newer punches have anti-turning devices as an integral part of their construction.

FORMULATION OF TABLETS:

The excipients added to the tablets can be classified based on their function. They include those which affect compressional characteristics of the tablets, i.e., diluents, binders and adhesives, lubricants, anti-adherents and glidants, those which affect the biopharmaceutics, chemical and physical stability and marketing considerations of the tablet like disintegrants, colours, flavours and sweeteners and miscellaneous components (buffers/adsorbents).

Additives affecting compressional characteristics

i) Diluents : Although diluents are thought of as inert ingredients, they can significantly affect the biopharmaceutics, chemical and physical properties of the final tablet, e.g. calcium salts interfering with absorption of tetracycline from GIT, interaction of amine bases with lactose in presence of alkaline lubricants (Maillard reaction). Tablets are so designed that the smallest sized tablet, which can be conveniently compressed is formed. But when dose of the drug is too small to be compressed, diluents are added to make up the volume.

Table 2.15: Problems in Tabletting:

Problem	Reason	Remedy
Capping and Lamination	i) Plastic deformation of tablet	Slow down the speed Use pre-compression
	ii) Too dry granulation	Addition of hygroscopic substances
	iii) Claw formation in concave punch	Avoid use of concave punch
	iv) Wear ring in die	Turn the die
	v) Collision with sweepoff blade	Adjusting the punch height
Picking and Sticking	i) Incompletely dried granules	Control moisture in granules
	ii) Incompletely lubricated granules	Use of proper lubricant Use of highly polished punches
	iii) Melting of low melting point additives	Replace with high melting point additive
Mottling	i) Colour of drug differs from excipient	Use of colouring agent
	ii) Degradation product of drug is coloured Migration of soluble dye	Changing solvent, reducing drying temp., replacing dye with insoluble lake
	iii) Precipitation of colour with binder solution	Use of powdered binders rather than solution
Weight variation	i) Larger granule size/wider with narrow size distribution	Use small sized granules
	ii) Poor flow -arching/rat-holing	i) Use of glidants ii) Use of induced feeders
	iii) Poor mixing of glidant	Increase in mixing time
	iv) Unequal length of punches	Replace the punchcs.
Hardness variation	Reasons and remedies are same as of weight variation	
Double impression	Uncontrolled rotation of punch	Use of anti-turning devices for punch

ii) Ideal properties of a diluent are -

i) It should be physiologically inert ii) It should be non-toxic iii) It should be economical iv) It should be readily available v) It should be should not be contraindicated by itself (e.g. sucrose based diluents in diabetics) vi) It should be physically and chemically stable with the drug vii) It must be free of any unacceptable microbiological load viii) It must be colour compatible ix) If the drug product is also a food item, e.g. vitamin preparations, it must be an approved food additive. x) Should not adversely affect bioavailability of the production.

The moisture content of the diluent is an important factor to consider. Many diluents exist as hydrates and contain appreciable bound water as water of crystallisation. Such diluents can very well be used for moisture-sensitive drugs, provided the bound moisture is not released under any exaggerated conditions of temperature during storage. Some diluents, although contain some quantities of unbound moisture, have little affinity for atmospheric moisture. Such diluents should be preferred over anhydrous diluents, which although contain no unbound moisture, have high affinity for atmospheric moisture. Some popularly used diluents:

1. **Lactose U.S.P.:** It is the most widely used diluent and exhibits good stability with most drugs. Hydrous form is used for systems that are wet granulated. Two grades – 60-80 # (coarse) and less than 80-100 # (regular) are available. Lactose formulations show good drug release and the granulations are easily dried. It is a low cost diluent, but may discolour in presence of amine salts and alkaline lubricants.

2. **Lactose U.S.P., anhydrous:** exhibits all properties of hydrous lactose & does not show Maillard reaction. Tablets show fast disintegration and low weight variation with absence of sticking, picking and capping. It has a greater tendency to pick up moisture and therefore should be packaged properly.

3. **Lactose U.S.P., spray dried:** It has improved flow properties and due to general spherical form, it is commonly combined with microcrystalline cellulose and is used as direct compression vehicle. It can accommodate 20-25 per cent of the drug and should be used at 40-50 per cent of tablet weight for its direct compaction properties. Its flow properties are adversely affected if it losses its 3 per cent moisture content. It undergoes Maillard reaction with amine containing drugs.

4. **Starch U.S.P.:** It is obtained from corn, wheat or potatoes. It has poor flow and compression characteristics and possesses high moisture content between 11-14 per cent. Specially dried grades of starch with moisture content of 2-4 per cent are available but at high prices. Various directly compressible starches are available, e.g. Sta-RX 1500 may be used as diluent/binder/disintegrant.

It is self-lubricating and may be compressed alone. But when combined with drug, it requires the addition of lubricant. Sta-Rx contains 10 per cent moisture and is prone to softening when combined with excessive amounts of magnesium stearate.

Two hydrolysed starches are Emdex and Celutab, which contain 90- 92 per cent dextrose and 3-5 per cent maltose. They are free-flowing and directly compressible. They can be used in place of mannitol in chewable tablets because of their sweetness and smooth feel in mouth.

5. Dextrose, commercially available as cerelose, is also used as diluent. It is available in two forms, hydrous and anhydrous.

Sometimes, it may be used to replace some of the spray-dried lactose, which may reduce tendency of tablets to darken.

6. Mannitol is the most expensive diluent, but it is still used for chewable tablets because of its negative heat of solution and sweetness. It produces cooling sensation in mouth. It is non-hygroscopic and used in vitamin preparations, where moisture sensitivity is a problem.

7. Sorbitol is an optical isomer of mannitol. It is sometimes combined with mannitol to decrease diluent cost, but it is hygroscopic.

8. Sucrose-based diluents - Sugartab (90-93 per cent sucrose plus 7-10 per cent invert sugar) DiPac (97 percent sucrose plus 3 per cent modified dextrins), Nu Tab (95 per cent sucrose, 4 percent invert sugar and cornstarch and magnesium stearate).

They are used as direct compression vehicles in regular as well as chewable tablets. They minimise the need of artificial sweeteners. They have a tendency to pick up moisture.

9. Microcrystalline Cellulose (Avicel): It is direct compression vehicle. Available in two grades - pH101(powder) and pH102 (granules).

It is a unique material as it can also act as disintegrant. It is expensive and typically combined with other materials to reduce the cost.

Some other materials are dibasic calcium phosphate dihydrate NF (Emcompress), Calcium sulfate dihydrate, Calcium lactate trihydrate, inositol and amylose.

Binders and Adhesives :

Binders are added either in dry or in liquid form during wet granulation.

Acacia and tragacanth are natural gums and are used as aqueous solution of 10-25 per cent concentration. They are effective as solutions rather than dry powders. They are of natural origin and vary in composition. They are usually heavily contaminated. Granules should be dried quickly at higher temperature to avoid microbial proliferation.

Gelatin is a good binder and forms tablets as hard as acacia and tragacanth.

It also has the advantage of being easier to prepare and handle. Solutions must be used warm.

Starch paste is the most common granulating agent. It is prepared by dispersing starch in water and then heating it for some time. During heating, starch undergoes hydrolysis to dextrin and glucose. A properly made paste is translucent, indicating complete conversion to glucose. It produces cohesive tablets that readily disintegrate readily.

50 per cent glucose solution in water is also a common wet granulating agent. Properties are similar to sucrose solution, which are used in 50-75 percent concentration. These are low cost adhesives. Unless sugar solutions are highly concentrated, bacterial proliferation may be a problem.

Modified natural polymers such as cellulose derivatives; methylethyl cellulose, Sodium carboxy methyl cellulose, Hydroxypropyl methyl cellulose are common binders and adhesives. They can also be used dry for direct compression, but are more effective in aqueous solutions. Hydroxy propyl cellulose may also be used as an alcoholic solution to provide anhydrous adhesive. Ethyl cellulose can only be used as an alcoholic solution. Polyvinyl pyrrolidone is also an alcohol soluble binder used in concentration of 3-15 per cent. Granules dry rapidly and compress extremely well. Polyvingl pyrrolidone is specially used for multivitamin chewable tablets, where moisture sensitivity can pose a problem.

Non-aqueous binders are compatible with moisture sensitive drugs. Most non-aqueous vehicle binders have, as their main disadvantage, the possible need of explosion-proof drying facilities and solvent recovery systems. Usually, granulations are partially air-dried and then dried in oven below the explosive limit of alcohol in air.

Pre-gelatinised starch can also be used by blending dry with various components of a tablet formula.

ADDITIVES AFFECTING BIOPHARMACEUTICAL CHARACTERISTICS

A) Disintegrants:

The purpose of disintegrant is to facilitate break up of tablet after administration. Disintegrant may be added prior to granulation or prior to compression or at both the stages.

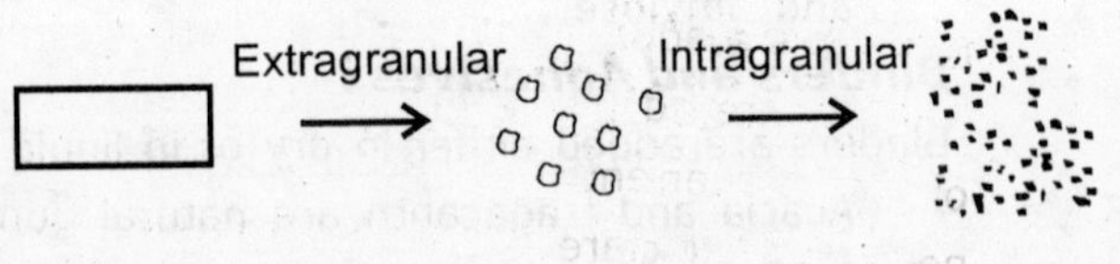

The disintegrants, depending upon the step at which they are added can be extragranular or intragranular.

Fig. 2.53: **Process of disintegration**

Extragranular formulations disintegrate more rapidly. Most effective lubricants are hydrophobic and impair wetting of the tablet particles and thus retard disintegration and dissolution. To avoid this, disintegrants are often combined with lubricants to aid extragranular disintegration. Usually both extra and intra granular disintegrants are added in combination.

Table 2.17: Commonly used binders for wet granulation.

Binder	Concentration in granulating liquid (% w/v)	Granulating solvent
Starch	5-10	Water
Pre-gelatinised starch	2-10	Water
Gelatin	2-10	Water
Acacia, tragacanth	5-20	Water
Sugars (Glucose, sucrose)	upto 50	Water
Polyvinyl pyrrolidone	2-20	Water or alcohol
Methyl cellulose	2-10	Water
Sodium-carboxymethyl cellulose	2-10	Water
Ethyl cellulose	5-10	Alcohol or Alcoholic water
Polyacrylamides	2-8	Water
Polyvinyl oxazolidones	5-10	Water or water+ alcohol
Polyvinyl alcohols	5-20	

Six different categories of disintegrants are starches, clays, cellulose, algins, gums and miscellaneous.

Starches are the most common disintegrating agents. They show a great affinity for water through capillary action, resulting in expansion and disintegration of tablets. Higher levels of starches result in rapid disintegration, but loss of bonding cohesiveness and hardness. Starch contains absorbed water and should be dried at 80-90°C. They should be stored properly when not in use.

Kaolin and Bentonite are clays that swell in contact with water. They are off-white in colour and show batch to batch variations. They are, therefore, used for coated tablets (to offset their colour).

Veegum is highly refined isomorphous silicate. It is superior to kaolin and can be obtained as a pure white powder.

Celluloses such as purified cellulose, methyl cellulose, Na-CMC + CMC are evaluated as disintegrants, but are not used widely. Solka-Floc is a name applied to several grades of purified cellulose. They are white, fibrous, inert, neutral materials which can be used as disintegrants in combination with starch for pH and moisture sensitive drugs like aspirin and penicillin. Microcrystalline cellulose is available in two grades. Avicel PH 101 & PH 102 in formulation. It can perform as disintegrant, binder, glidant and filler, making it an extremely versatile excipient. It absorbs water by fast capillary action. Avicel and starch make excellent disintegrant combination.

Alginates are extracted from natural algae. They are available as alginic acid or its sodium salt and are effective in 5-10 per cent quantity. They have great affinity for water, starch and Avicel. They do not retard flow.

Gums can absorb water and swell and hence can be used as disintegrants. But they also exhibit good bonding properties and their exact concentration as disintegrants should be decided, e.g. agar, karaya gum, locust bean gum, pectin and tragacanth. Guar gum is marketed under the trade name of Jaguar. It is available in various particle size ranges and is not sensitive to pH or moisture content of tablet. It is an excellent disintegrant, but has the disadvantage of being buff coloured which tends to discolour on aging due to the alkaline nature of tablets.

Miscellaneous disintegrants include effervescent mixtures, surfactants, hydrous aluminium silicates and super-disintegrants.

Superdisintegrants : Effervescent mixtures of citric/fumaric/tartaric acids with sodium carbonate and sodium bicarbonate, if added to granules, generate carbon dioxide in contact with water. This causes disintegration of tablet by disruption. It is essential to maintain dehumidified conditions while processing tablets containing effervescent mixtures.

The new generation disintegrants, called as super-disintegrants, substantially reduce the disintegration time. They absorb water several times their own volume and swell causing fast disruption of tablets. They are particularly useful in tablets containing highly water insoluble drugs and in dispersible tablets. Croscarmellose sodium, available by the trade name Ac-di-sol, is cross-linked sodium carboxymethyl cellulose. It is water-insoluble anionic cellulose. It shows good water uptake, high capillary action and rapid swelling properties. It is required in low concentrations.

Sodium starch glycolate, available by brand names of Primogel and Explotab are modified starches. They are low substituted carboxymethyl starches. They swell upto 200-300 per cent of their volume, as compared to 10-25 per cent in case of natural starches.

Soya polysachharides available by trade names of Emcosyl are all natural super-disintegrants. Being a dietary fibre, it is extremely important as disintegrant in nutritional products.

Polyplasdone is cross-linked polyvinyl pyrrolidone. It has porous morphology which rapidly takes in liquids into the particle to speed swelling. It also has very good flow properties and compressibility.

Cation exchange resins have been investigated as super-disintegrants. e.g.

Polacrilin Potassium. It is a potassium salt of weak acid, based on a methacrylic acid divinylbenzene copolymer.

B) Lubricants, antiadherants and glidants

Lubricants decrease friction between granules and die walls during compression and ejection.

Antiadherants decrease sticking to punch and to some extent to die walls. Glidants improve flow characteristics of granules.

Table 2.16: Commonly used disintegrants

Commonly used disintegrants Disintegrant	Concentration in granulation (% w/w)
Starch U.S.P.	5-20
Modified starch (Sta-Rx)	5-15
Microcrystalline cellulose (Avicel)	5-20
Purified cellulose (Solka-Floc)	5-15
Alginic acid	5-10
Guar gum	5-10
Kaolin	5-15
Bentonite	5-15
Veegum	5-15
Effervescent mixtures	5-15
Super-disintegrants	
Sodium-starch glycolate (Explotab/Primogel)	1-8
Croscarmellose sodium (Ac-di-sol)	5-10
Crospovidone (Polyplasdone)	0.5-5

Lubrication occurs by two mechanisms, fluid lubrication and boundary lubrication. In fluid lubrication, two moving surfaces are separated by a continuous layer of lubricant, e.g. mineral oil. It should be used when finely atomised as it otherwise produces oily spots. Boundary lubrication occurs due to adherence of polar portions of molecules with long carbon chain to the metal surfaces of die wall.

When lubricants are added, they form a coat around granules. But because the best lubricants are hydrophobic, they retard disintegration and require addition of an extragranular disintegrant. Such mixtures of a lubricant and extra disintegrant mixed with the granulations is called as running powder.

Lubricants : Lubricants are divided into water soluble and water insoluble categories. Water insoluble lubricants are hydrophobic and can harm drug bioavailability, disintegration and dissolution times and tablet strength. They are subgrouped into fluid lubricants and boundary lubricants. Water-insoluble fluid lubricants include stearic acid ,mineral oils, hydrogenated vegetable oils, paraffins and waxes. Boundary lubricants include a series of metallic stearates, talc, starch and sodium stearyl fumarate.

Salts of fatty acids are the most widely used lubricants and magnesium stearate is the most common amongst them. Metal soaps form dense, high melting films between the substrate and die wall surfaces to reduce friction and aid tablet ejection. Magnesium stearate is highly effective in this respect. It is an excellent lubricant and acceptable antiadherent, but has relatively poor glidant properties.

Table 2.17 : Commonly used lubricants

Lubricant	Suggested Percentage(%)
Water insoluble - fluid	
Light mineral oil	1-3
Stearic acid	1-2
Hydrogenated vegetable oils	1-2
Glyceryl behenate	0.5-4
Water insoluble- boundary layer	
Magnesium stearate	0.5-2
Calcium stearate	0.5-2
Zinc stearate	0.5-2
Talc	5-10
Starch	5-10
Sodium stearyl fumarate	0.5-2
Calcium stearate, sodium stearate	
Lauryl sulfate mixture	
(Stearowet C)	
Water soluble	
Polythylene glycols	2-10
Sodium acetate	5-10
Sodium benzoate	2-5
Sodium chloride	5-20
DL-leucine	1-5
Sodium lauryl sulphate	1-3
Magnesium lauryl sulphate	1-3

Fatty acids are better lubricants than fatty alcohols and hydrocarbons. The most commonly used fatty acid, is stearic acid which is a poorer lubricant than magnesium stearate.

Glyceryl, sorbitan and sucrose fatty acid esters can be used, but their lubricity is poor than magnesium stearate.

Talc is a water-insoluble boundary lubricant with some glidant properties. It is best utilised in combination with magnesium stearate.

Starch is not a very effective lubricant, but can be used as an auxiliary lubricant in combination with others. It acts as disintegrant, as well as an auxiliary lubricant.

Water-soluble lubricants are preferable for complete dissolution of tablets, i.e., soluble and effervescent tablets.

Use of boric acid is questionable because of its toxicity. Sodium benzoate and sodium chloride find little use. Generally, PEG 4000 and 6000 are used in soluble tablets. They are non-reactive and can be used with pH sensitive drugs. PEG solutions are sprayed onto powders.

Magnesium and sodium lauryl sulphates are water-soluble lubricants with high HLB values. They are often used with stearates to overcome their hydrophobicity. Calcium stearate and SLS is commercially available as stearowet-C.

Glidants : Poor flow of powders in compression results in several defects like weight variation, arching and rat holing. Glidants improve flow characteristics of granules and powders. They reduce the angle of repose of powder blend in turn increasing their flow properties. Efficiency of a glidant in improving flow properties can be determined out by finding its glidant index.

$$\text{Glidant index} = \frac{\text{Powder flowability with glidant}}{\text{Powder flowability without glidant}}$$

Commonly used glidant excipients are given in Table - 2.18.

Many of them also possess lubricant properties and blend with lubricants and antiadherents and can be used to provide both properties.

Table 2.18

Glidant	Suggested percentage
Talc	1-5
Silica aerogels	
Cab-o-sil	0.1-0.5
Syloid	0.1-0.5
Calcium silicate	0.5-2
Magnesium-stearate	0.2-2
Calcium-stearate	0.2-2
Zinc-stearate	0.2-7
Calcium-stearate Sodium-stearatet	0.2-2
Sodium lauryl sulphate (stearowet-C)	1-10
Starch	0.2-2
Magnesium- lauryl sulphate	0.2-2
Magnesium- oxide	1-3
Magnesium-carbonate	1-3

Talc is a widely used glidant with excellent antiadherent properties. Excessive amounts cause wetting problems. Starches are excellent glidants and have additional disintegrant properties.

Various forms of silica can be used successfully. It is the best glidant currently. Pyrogenic silicas have small particle size, are spherical in shape and are available in hydrophobic and hydrophilic forms. They are available by commercial names of Cab-o-sil and Aerosils. Magnesium oxide is considered to be an auxiliary glidant with silica. Magnesium stearate and talc also additionally reduce static electricity charges in powders.

Antiadherents : Some solids have significant adhesive properties and can adhere to tooling surfaces, causing sticking and picking. Antiadherents have polishing effects on these surfaces for release of such particles. Most lubricants have certain antiadherent properties. Talc is an excellent antiadherent. Starches and microcrystalline cellulose have some antiadherent properties.

Table 2.19 : Commonly used antiadherents

Antiadherent	Suggested percentage (%)
Talc	1-5
Cornstarch	1-5
Metallic stearates	0.25-1
Micro crystalline cellulose	5-10

Lubricants must be added in very fine particle size (200). Smaller the particle size, better is the lubricating action, because of larger surface area available.

Table: 2.20 : List of FDA certified colour additives

FDA certified colour additives
FD & C Red No. 3 (erythrosine)
FD & C Red No. 40 (Allura red)
FD & C yellow No. 5 (tartrazine)
FD & C Yellow No. 6 (sunset yellow)
FD & C Blue No. 1 (brilliant blue)
FD & C Blue No. 2 (indigotine)
FD & C Green No. 3 (fast green)
D & C Blue No. 6 (indigo)
D & C Green No. 5 (alizarin cyanine green f)
D & C Green No. 6 (quinazarin green)
D & C Red No. 19 (rhodamine B)
D & C Red No. 22 (eosin Y)
D & C Red No. 33 (acid fuschin D)
D & C Red No. 37 (rhodamine B stearate)
D & C yellow No. 10 (quinoline yellow ws)
Ext. D &C green No. 1 (napthol green B)
Ext. D & C orange No. 4 (orange II)
Ext. D & C yellow No. 1 (metanil yellow)

Table 2.21: Commercially available natural colours

Colorant	Colour	Source
Carmine	Red	Dried female cochineal insects
Grape-skin extracts	Purple	Grapes
Annatto	Yellow	Extract of seeds of *Fixa orellana*
Beet juice, dried	Red	Beets
Cranberry juice, dried	Red	Cranberries
Caramel	Brown	Sugar
Turmeric	Yellow	Turmeric

C) *Flavours and Sweeteners:-*

Flavours are rarely used as liquids because of their moisture sensitivity and tendency to volatilise when heated. Aqueous flavours are little accepted due to their poor stability upon aging, therefore flavours are incorporated as solids in the form of spray-dried beadlets and usually at the lubrication step.

To avoid oxidation, oils are emulsified with acacia and spray dried. Dry flavours are usually easier to handle and more stable. Oils, if at all used, are diluted with alcohol and sprayed onto granules. They may also be adsorbed onto granules, or on excipients, and added. Usually flavours are incorporated at concentration not more than 0.75% w/w.

Sweeteners are usually added to chewable tablets, when commonly used diluents like mannitol, sucrose and dextrose are unable to mask the taste of components. The only FDA approved sweetener is saccharin (500 times sweeter than sucrose). But it has a disadvantage of bitter aftertaste which can be minimised by incorporating 1% NaCl.

Aspartame is a non-drug approved sweetener, 180 times sweeter than sucrose. It shows discolouration with ascorbic and tartaric acid. Because of possible carcinogenicity of pharmaceutical sweeteners (cyclamate, saccharin), formulators tend to design products without such agents.

D) *Adsorbents :*

Adsorbents, such as Silicon dioxide (Cab-o-sil, Syloid, Aerosil), adsorb large amounts of liquids without getting wet. This allows incorporation of many oils, eutectic melts and fluid extracts into tablets. Silicon dioxide adsorbed systems can hold upto 50 per cent by its weight of water. Other potential adsorbents are bentonite, kaolin, magnesium silicate, tricalcium phosphate, magnesium carbonate and magnesium oxide.

Organoleptic additives

I) Colorants -
Colorants are incorporated in the tablet for three reasons-
i)   Identification of similar looking products.
ii) Colours can help to minimise mix-ups during manufacture
iii) The product has an aesthetic value because of colours.

Many dyes are banned due to some reason or the other and the manufacturer has to depend on product shape, size and engraving for product identification. The colorants are chosen from the limited number of dyes and lakes and small number of natural and derived colours that fall under the FD&C and D&C Act. Dyes are water-soluble materials, while lakes are formed by adsorption of water soluble dye on an inert adsorbent, e.g. $Al(OH)_3$ which yields the dye insoluble.

Photosensitivity of the colorants may be affected by the drug, excipients and methods of manufacturing and storage. UV absorbing chemicals have been added to tablets to minimize their photosensitivity. Postal shades are usually chosen as they show least amount of mottling. Colours near the midrange of visible spectrum (yellow /green) show less mottling than those at either extremes (blue/red).

Method of incorporation:
Water-soluble dyes are usually incorporated in the granulating solution, but this may lead to mottling during drying. Colours may also be adsorbed on carriers (starch, lactose, Calcium sulphate aqueous, sugar), from aqueous or alcoholic solutions. Resultant mixtures are dried and used as stock systems for many lots. Water-soluble dyes may also be dry blended with an excipient, prior to final mixing. Lakes are almost always blended with other dry excipients, because they are insoluble. Usually tablets made by direct compression use lakes as no granulation step is used.

TYPES OF TABLETS

Table 2.22: Describes different types and classes of tablets ad their brief description

Class	Description
Oral tablets for ingestion Compressed tablets	These are the standard compressed tablets made either by wet, or dry granulation, or by direct compression.
Multiple compressed tablets a) Compression coated tablets	These are either tablet within a tablet or tablet within a tablet within a tablet. They are compressed either to separate physically or chemically incompatible ingredients or to produce repeat action products.
b) Layered tablets	They are two or three layered tablets devised for the above two reasons
Repeat action tablets	Core tablet is usually coated with shellac and releases its contents in the intestine. Second dose is added in coating, which is released in the stomach.
Delayed action and enteric coated tablets	Delayed action tablets release the drug after some time lag. Enteric coated tablet is an example of delayed action tablet that releases the drug only after reaching the intestine.
Sugar + Chocolate coated tablets	Chocolate-coated tablets are obsolete as they are too easily mistaken for candy by children. Sugar-coated tablets are coated with sugar syrup to produce elegant glossy tablets. The main aim is to mask the taste of the drug and sometimes to separate incompatible drugs.
Film coated tablets	The purpose of the film coating is same as that of sugar coating, but the process is simple and less time consuming.
Chewable tablets	These tablets are intended to be chewed prior to swallowing. The purpose is ease of administration of drugs having large doses, and quick reduction in particle size of drug leading to quick action, e.g. antacid tablets.
Tablets used in the oral cavity	
Buccal and sublingual tablets	They are intended to be held in the mouth

	where they slowly release active ingredients which are absorbed through buccal or sublingual mucosa. The major advantage is quick onset of action with no first pass effect, e.g. isosorbide dinitrate tablets.
Troches and lozenges	They are to be slowly dissolved in the oral cavity to exert their local soothing effect in mouth or throat, in case of common cold. They are formulated as demulcents, astringents and antitussives.
Dental cones	They are to be placed in the empty socket after tooth extraction. Their purpose is to exert antibacterial effect in the socket and they usually contain antibacterials or astringents to retard bleeding.
Tablets used by other routes	
Implantable tablets	They are implanted subcutaneously in animals or man. The purpose is to provide prolonged drug effect, up to one year. They are implanted surgically. They are particularly implanted to deliver growth hormones in food producing animals.
Vaginal tablets	They undergo slow dissolution and release the drug in vaginal cavity. They are used to deliver antibacterial agents, antiseptics or astringents.
Tablets used to prepare solutions	
Effervescent tablets	They contain organic acids and bases along with active ingredients. They react in presence of water-producing carbon dioxide and thus make flavoured carbonated drink.
Dispensing tablets	They are to be dissolved in given quantity of water to produce solutions that are to be used topically. They usually contain mild silver proteinate, mercury bichloride and quaternary compounds. They are now obsolete.
Hypodermic tablets	They are to be dissolved in sterile water for injection, to make an extemporaneous injectable solution. They are rarely used.
Tablet triturates	They were prepared extemporaneously by the pharmacists by moulding. They are only of historic importance.

COMPRESSION-COATED TABLETS

Compression coating was a technique developed after the invention of sugar coating, but prior to film coating. It has some advantages over sugar coating and some disadvantages as compared to film coating.

Advantages over sugar coating

- Elimination of water or other solvents in the coating procedure eliminates the need of barrier coating to prevent water from penetrating the core.
- Incompatible substances can be separated by placing one in the core and the other in the coating.
- It the drug discolours or tends to give mottled appearance, it can very well be incorporated in the core. Compression coating be can used to make sustained release tablets.

Disadvantages over film coating:

- Process of compression coating is much slower than film coating and requires very complex equipments.
- The increase in tablet weight because of compression coating is much large compared to film coating. Therefore, compression coating cannot be used for large dose drugs.

EQUIPMENTS FOR COMPRESSION COATING:

Two different types of equipments are used for making compression coated tablets.

i) Some machines are used for putting coatings on cores that were compressed on other machines.

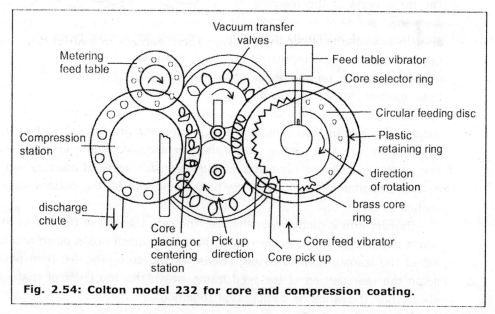

Fig. 2.54: Colton model 232 for core and compression coating.

ii) In some machines, compression of cores takes place on one side of the machine with almost immediate transfer to other side for application of coating.

Following are some of the equipments for compression coating :

1) Colton model 232 : Previously compressed cores are fed by vibrating feeder unit onto a circular feeding disc which is rotated clockwise or counter-clockwise (fig 2.54). The disc is tapered slightly downward from its center to its edge. A vibrator gently agitates the disc so that the core tablets separate into a single layer. Around the periphery of the disc is a plastic ring which prevents the tablets from piling up or escaping from the core selector ring immediately below. The selector ring has 33 V-shaped slots around its inner edge which engages the cores. The cores are picked out of the slots by transfer cups connected to a vacuum system through flexible tubing. The spring loaded cups are guided into contact with the cores. The core centering ring and the transfer cups are synchronised with the speed of the die table.

Bottom layer of the coating enters the die from hopper feed frame. At the same time core is picked up by a transfer cup, which is guided into the die. Vacuum is interrupted and the core rests on the bed of coating. A metering feed plate passes under a hopper and feed frame and over the die into which is deposited the top layer of granulation. The whole is then compressed in the usual manner by passing punches between compression rolls.

2) Manesty drycota : It consists of two heavy duty presses with a transfer device in between. The three parts of the machine are joined and kept in synchronisation by a common drive shaft. Cores of tablets are compressed in normal manner on one press. Upon ejection, they are brought

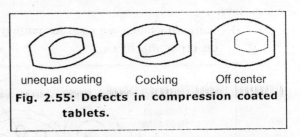

unequal coating   Cocking   Off center

Fig. 2.55: Defects in compression coated tablets.

up flush with the surface of the die adjustment, to the other side of the feed frame. They rise up into cups on transfer arms and are carried across the bridge to the other side, i.e., coating side of the machine. The feed frame on the coating side of the machine is narrowed to allow transfer arms to pass. Granules flow from the hopper the in front of the feed frame and fill the bottom layer of the coating in die.

Transfer arm is guided over this die. The core falls out of the cup as the lower punch is pulled down to make room. The upper punch drops down and taps the top of the transfer cup to assure release of the core. The die then passes beneath the rear portion of the feed frame where the top layer of coating is applied. Then the whole is compressed together.

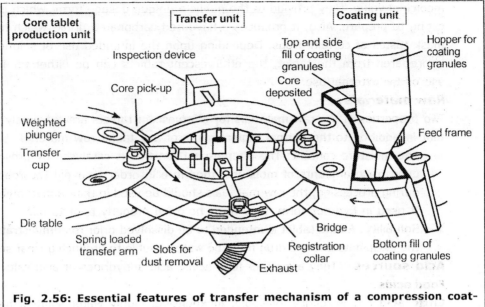

Fig. 2.56: Essential features of transfer mechanism of a compression coating machine.

Formulation :

Almost any formula that will produce a firm tablet is satisfactory for producing the core granules. The coating granules should have excellent cohesiveness and ability to adhere tightly to the core. They should be plastic enough to expand slightly with slight expansion of the core after extrusion of entire tablet from the die. The maximum size of the granules must be less than the space between the deposited core and walls of the die so that the granules will readily fill the space.

Centering of the core is extremely important; especially for special types of coatings like enteric coating. Speed of the machine tends to centrifuge the core towards the periphery of the die table and opposite to the direction of rotation. Reducing the speed of the press is a solution to this problem, but it is not economical. The coating granules should be formulated in such a way that they should be soft, somewhat like lactose. Such granules prevent the core from sliding on the bottom layer of the coating. Plastic materials, such as gelatin, PEG, can be included. Edges of compression coated tablets are thicker and therefore large amount of lubricant is needed to facilitate easy extrusion from die. Usually similar materials are used in coating and cores, based on the theory that like substances will bond together better than unlike ones.

EFFERVESCENT TABLETS

Effervescence is defined as evolution of bubbles of gas from a liquid as a result of some chemical reaction. Effervescent tablets are popular because in addition to their

---

medicinal value, they provide to the public a unique dosage form, which is interesting to prepare. Also, it produces a flavoured carbonated drink, which helps to mask tastes of certain drugs. Depending upon the intended use of solution that is prepared from the tablet, the effervescent tablets can be either for internal use or for external use.

Raw materials :

Two properties of the raw materials for effervescent tablets are extremely important in addition to the normal requirements of any tablet raw material -

i. The moisture content: The effervescent reaction is catalysed by presence of even trace amounts of moisture; therefore in order to avoid the reaction during processing, the raw materials should be used in their anhydrous forms. If used in hydrous form, they must be dried properly prior to use.

ii. Solubility: As the tablet is intended to be dissolved prior to administration, all the excipients and the drug must be water soluble to produce a clear solution.

Acid sources : They are either food acids, acid anhydrides or acid salts.

Food acids

Citric acid : It is readily available, inexpensive, highly water soluble, has high acid strength but is hygroscopic.

Tartaric acid : More soluble than citric acid but also more hygroscopic. Its acid strength is less.

Malic acid : Hygroscopic, readily soluble, acid strength is less. It has a smooth taste which does not burst in flavour.

Fumaric acid, Adipic acid, Succinic acid: These acids are rarely used as they are not cost effective.

Acid anhydrides : When mixed with water, they release the corresponding acid. Water cannot be used in manufacturing of products containing acid anhydrides, since they will be converted to acid prior to product use. Commonly used substance is succinic anhydride.

Acid salts : Sodium dihydrogen phosphate, disodium dihydrogen phosphate, or sodium bisulphite may aslo be used as acid sources.

Carbonate sources.

Sodium bicarbonate : Completely soluble in water, inexpensive, abundant and available in five particle sizes ranging from fine powder to granules. It is the mildest of sodium alkalies, producing solutions of pH 8.3 at 0.85 per cent concentration. It yields around 52 per cent carbon di oxide.

Sodium carbonate : Produces solutions of pH 11.5 with 1 per cent concentration. It has a tendency to absorb moisture preferentially, preventing initiation of effervescent reaction. Therefore it is used as stabiliser.

Potassium bicarbonate and carbonate : They are less soluble and more expensive than their sodium counterparts. They are specially used when sodium is not desired.

Others : Sodium sesquicarbonate, sodium glycine carbonate.

Other effervescent sources:

1. Materials like anhydrous sodium perborate evolve oxygen when mixed with water. It is used in tablets used as denture cleansers.
2. Chlorine compounds liberate hypochlorite on contact with water.

Lubricants:

Effervescent granulations are difficult to lubricate, due to the rapid tablet disintegration usually required.

Powdered sodium benzoate and micronised PEG- 4000 and 6000 are effective water soluble lubricants. Sodium stearate and sodium oleate are soluble in low concentration; therefore, may be used in small amounts in combination. Polyvenyl pyrrolidone, powdered sodium acetate and boric acid powder are also used as soluble lubricants. L-Leucine is an amino acid, which is very effective as water-soluble lubricant, though very expensive.

Sodium lauryl sulphate and magnesium, lauryl sulphate and MgLS may also be used as water soluble lubricants, but they drastically increase the disintegration time.

Binders and Granulating agents:

The use of any binder, though water-soluble, retards disintegration of an effervescent tablet. In granulations which require a binder, proper balance must be maintained between granule cohesiveness and tablet disintegration time.

Conventional binders like acacia, tragacanth, starch paste are not effective as they retard tablet dissolution. Dry binders like lactose, dextrose and mannitol can be used, but are not effective in low concentrations normally permissible in effervescent tablets. Polyvinyl pyrrolidone is an effective binder and is either used dry or as a solution with aqueous, alcoholic or hydro alcoholic fluid.

Diluents

Effervescent materials themselves are used in large quantity as fillers, unless they unnecessarily extra effervescence and pH variation.

Sources of carbon dioxide-

Na-bicarbonate

It is an odourless, white crystalline powder with a salty, slightly alkaline taste. A variety of particle size grades are available. CO_2 yield is approximately 52 per cent w/w at room humidity less than 35 per cent. Moisture content is less than 1 per cent. Upon heating, at 250-300°C, $NaHCO_3$ decomposes and is converted into anhydrous $NaHCO_3$, which consolidates by plastic deformation, and not by fragmentation and hence tablets show low strength; thereby needing a binder. In order to overcome poor flow properties and compressibility, spray drying technique may be used.

PROCESSING OF EFFERVESCENT TABLETS

Environmental Conditions:

Low room humidity and moderate to cool temperatures in processing areas is required to prevent picking up of moisture from atmosphere. A maximum of 25 per cent relative humidity and controlled room temperature of 25°C is satisfactory.

Wet granulation

1. With heat : This involves the release of water from hydrated formulation ingredients at a low temperature to form a workable mass. The ingredient most often used for this purpose is hydrous citric acid, which, when fully hydrated, contains 8.5 per cent water. This process is difficult to control to achieve reproducible results and hence is rarely used.

2. With non-reactive liquids : Granulating fluids like ethyl alcohol or isopropyl alcohol, in which most of the ingredients are insoluble, are used. Binders may be added to the non-reactive liquid if soluble in it, or can be added to dry ingredients and activated as the mass is wetted.

3. With reactive liquids : This involves addition of small amounts of water, about 0.1-0.5 per cent to the blend of raw materials. Water is usually incorporated in the form of a fine spray. The free flowing granulations are then compressed.

Dry granulation techniques, which either employ roller compaction or slugging may also be used.

Tablet Evaluation:

i) Physical properties: Disintegration time is the most important characteristic since the visual effect of dissolving tablet and its subsequent carbonation are the main reasons for use of effervescent systems. A properly formulated effervescent tablet will disintegrate and dissolve rapidly - usually within 1-2 minutes. Temperature and volume of water depend on the product being used. Effervescent tablets often float on water when the density of the tablet mass and adhering bubbles becomes less than the liquid. Hardness, friability & weight variation are some other evaluation parameters.

ii) Chemical Properties: A unique chemical property is the pH generated when the tablet dissolves. Due to the nature of the effervescent components, buffer systems are formed which generate a very specific pH. Consistent measurement of solution pH is a sign of good distribution of raw materials within the tablet. Solution pH is measured with suitable instruments in standardised water volumes and temperatures.

Effervescence Stability

Methods of achieving stability:

1. Tablets should be manufactured in controlled low relative humidity atmosphere.
2. Proper types of anhydrous raw materials should be selected.

3. Finely divided anhydrous sodium carbonate is an effective stabilising agent when incorporated at about 10 per cent w/w of sodium bicarbonate concentration.
4. Sodium bicarbonate used in the formulation is heated so that 2-10 per cent w/w of it is converted to sodium carbonate.
5. Substances which decrease hygroscopicity of the effervescent system can also be incorporated. Encapsulation of the acid or base phases, mixing of sodium bicarbonate with a dilute solution of guar gum, or addition of 0.5 per cent albumin can be done.

Stability testing and shelf-life :

Arrhenius plots are used for stability prediction. Each tablet is hermetically sealed in an aluminium foil laminate. Pouches are placed at 25, 37, 45 and 60°C, and the thickness of the tablet and foil pouch is measured. If decomposition occurs, small volumes of carbon dioxide are evolved causing the pouch to swell. The degree of swelling is measured as increase in wall thickness of the pouch. An increase of less than 1/16th of an inch is considered negligible.

An alternative method is to assay the tablets for total carbon dioxide content. The method uses a liquid volume displacement apparatus known as Chittick Apparatus. A tablet sample is crushed, weighed and placed in a flask, into which is introduced an acid water solution. Amount of carbon dioxide evolved is measured volumetrically by displacement of a solution contained in a graduated cylinder.

In process quality control : It is not possible every time to place samples of each batch at elevated temperature. Since decomposition is triggered by trace amounts of water, several methods have been devised to measure residual water content either directly or indirectly.

Conventional LOD methods are not satisfactory as the heat generated will drive off carbon dioxide. Karl Fischer methods are also not satisfactory as the water to be analysed is too low to be assayed accurately. A better method is vacuum drying over concentrated sulphuric acid, but it is time-consuming and not satisfactory. One acceptable method is use of Parr calorimeter. Tablets are sealed in a chamber fitted with a pressure gauge with scale ranging from 1-60 lb/sq. inch. Enough tablets should be placed in the chamber so as to leave minimum space. Heat is applied externally from a constant temperature source, trace amounts of water will be liberated, causing the effervescent reaction to begin and release carbon dioxide. Pressure of the evolved gas is measured on a pressure gauge, this being directly related to the amount of water.

PACKAGING :

Effervescent tablets must be protected from atmospheric moisture. They are packaged in multiple use containers, such as tubes or bottles of glass, plastic or metal or in individual foil pouches, joined to form a strip of tablets. For individual pouches, usually, aluminium foil laminates composed of several layers of different materials bonded together are used. Outer layer is typically of some paper, allowing surface for printing. Next layer is polyethylene, followed by aluminium foil and again polyethylene.

Two sheets of the laminate converge and pass between a pair of matching heated cylinders, each containing exactly corresponding cavities appropriate in depth and dimensions to the tablet. Tablets are fed between the converging sheets synchronously with the cylinder cavities, so that they are not crushed. Two sheets of laminate around each cavity are heated by contact with the cylinder surface and are subjected to pressure between the cylinders, forming the heat seal. As the formed pouch leaves the cylinders, temperature of the laminate falls causing the two heat seal layers to bond. The sheet is then cut and perforated.

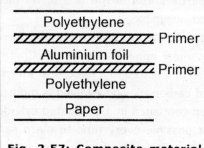

Fig. 2.57: Composite material used for packaging effervescent tablets

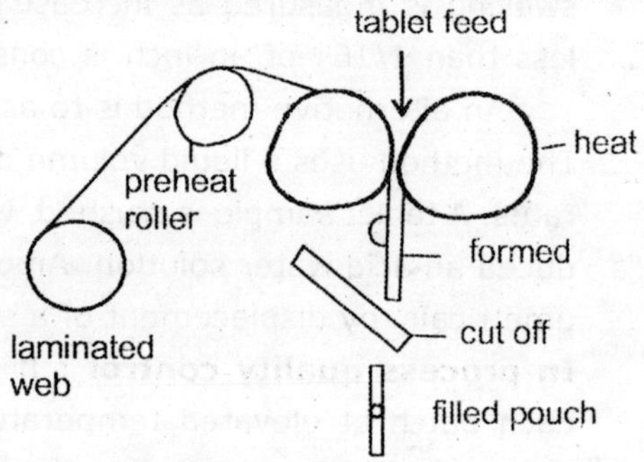

Fig. 2.58: Strip packing machine for effervescent tablets.

Table 2.23: Special evaluation tests for effervescent Tablets

- pH determination
- Water content determination using Parr calorimeter
- Accelerated stability testing to test change in thickness of foil laminates
- Accelerated stability testing to assay total carbon dioxide content by using Chittick apparatus
- Package integrity testing using vacuum underwater method detection of tracer material sealed within the pouch or purging with a detectable gas.

Package Integrity testing:

i) Vacuum underwater method : Vacuum is applied to the pouches to be tested. They are placed in a water filled chamber under a weighted plate to keep them from floating. Chamber is sealed and vacuum is drawn for 3 minutes. Vacuum is then slowly released. Seal and foil defects can be located by small stream of bubbles arising from a particular point on the pouch.

---

ii) Detection of trace material sealed within the pouch : A tracer material such as dry carbon dioxide or helium is sealed into the pouch with the tablet. Pouches are placed in a small sealed chamber to which a vacuum is applied. Effluent from the chamber is passed through an IR spectrophotometric sensing device, calibrated for that particular tracer. If a leak exists, a tracer is detected and alarm is sounded.

iii) Purging with a detectable gas : This method is similar to the second method, except that the pouches are placed in a vessel which is subsequently pressurised with the tracer gas. If the pouches have seal or foil defects, the gas will enter the pouch and mix with the contents. Pressure is released and pouches are tested as described above.

LAYERED TABLETS

Layered tablets consist of two or three layers of granulations compressed together. They can separate two incompatible substances with a layer of inert material between them. They can be used for sustained release with the immediate release portion of drug in one layer and slow release portion in the second.

Advantages of layered tablets over compression coated tablets -
-    They are easier to produce.
-    They require less material, weigh less and are thinner.
-    Monograms may be impressed on layered tablets.
-    Colouring of separate layers provides unique identity
-    There is no transfer of tablet to second set of punches and dies unlike compression coated tablets. Odd shapes present no tooling problems.

Disadvantages-
-    Requires two or more granulations for each product
-    Layered tablets are thicker and difficult to swallow
-    Layered tablet presses have low outputs.

LAYER TABLET PRESSES

There are two types of layer presses which differ mainly in the way the layers are removed for weight and hardness checking. In first type, the first layer or the first two layers are removed for weight and hardness checking. In this, the first layer or the first two layers are diverted from the machine and in the other, the first layer is made so hard that the second layer will not bond to it, or will bond only weakly. Upon ejection of the complete tablet, the two layers can be separated easily and tested individually.

The figure 2.59 represents operation of a three layer press. The line A represents the die table. A granulation is placed in the first hopper and flows into the feed frame B. The volume of granulation is adjusted by the weight adjustment cam C. The upper and lower punches are brought together by the pre-compres-

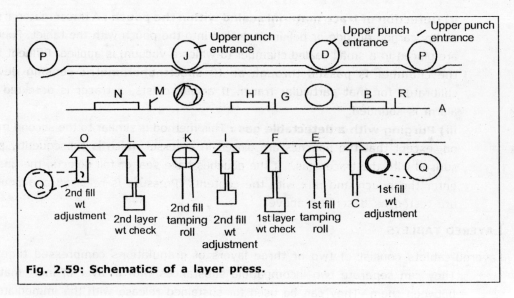

Fig. 2.59: Schematics of a layer press.

sion rollers D and E to form a weak compact. Part of the lower cam track F is then raised hydraulically to eject the first layer, which is swept off the die table by a swipe-off blade G affixed to the back edge of the second feeder H. Samples are weighed and hardness is determined. The operator makes necessary corrections. When conditions are satisfactory, the ejection cam is lowered, and the entire procedure is repeated for the second layer, using feed frame H, weight adjusting cam I tamping rollers J and K ejection cam L and swipe-off blades. The weight of the second layer is determined by difference in the two layers. The sequence is again repeated for third layer of tablets by means of feed frame N, weight adjustment Cam O and final compression rolls P and Q with the completed tablet being removed by the wipe off blade R (Which is to the right of the first feed frame B).

The second type of machine is similar to the first one except for the manner in which weight checking is handled. Instead of a cam arrangement for ejecting the layers, pressure on the first layer is increased and the layer is made so hard that it cannot bond to the next layer. Thus both layers are easily separated for weighing.

Formulation

Similar to the compression-coated tablets, granulation for layered tablets should be readily compressible. Dust-like fines should be kept to a minimum to keep the scrape off clean at each sweep-off. Lubricants, however, must be finely divided and therefore their quantity should be kept to a minimum. Metallic stearates present difficulty in bonding. Stearic acid and hydrogenated fats are better lubricants.

IN-LAY TABLETS (DOT/BULLS EYE TABLET)

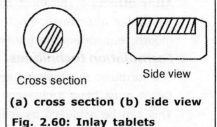

(a) cross section (b) side view
Fig. 2.60: Inlay tablets

Instead of the core tablet being completely surrounded by the coating, its top surface is completely exposed. For preparation of such tablets, top layer of coating is eliminated. Only the bottom layer is deposited and the core is placed on it. The compression rolls then embed the core in the granulation and finally press the entire tablet. The feed frame and hopper, which supply top layer granulation, should not be installed in case of Colton model. In case of Manestry Drycota, which uses two compartment feed frame for coating, it is necessary to block off the second part.

Advantages over compression-coated tablets

- Requires less amount of coating material
- Core is visible, so coreless tablets are easily detected
- Tablets are thinner

CHEWABLE TABLETS

These are the tablets to be chewed in buccal cavity prior to swallowing. Chewable tablets are an important dosage form for following two reasons-

1. They are convenient and have acceptance amongst young as well as geriatric patients, who cannot swallow tablets easily.
2. They have rapid onset of action due to disintegration of tablet prior to entering GIT.

Formulation factors :

The most important formulation attribute is the flavour and mouthfeel without compromising on the normal attributes like stability and efficacy. The organoleptic properties are of primary concern in formulation. The drug substance must be converted to a form having acceptable taste and odour. Thus extremely bad tasting drugs are difficult to formulate. Following factors must be considered while improving organoleptic properties. :

Taste and flavour : Many organic medicinal compounds have bitter taste. Most saccharides, some disaccharides and some aldehydes are sweet. Aspirin is sour, while salts are salty. The term 'flavour' refers to a combined sensation of taste and smell, e.g. sugar has sweet taste but no flavour, while honey has sweet taste and a characteristic odour, which combined together, is called honey flavour.

Aroma : Pleasant smells are called aromas. Orange flavoured tablet has a sweet and sour taste and an aroma of fresh orange.

Mouthfeel : It is the sensation or touch that a tablet produces in the mouth upon chewing. Gritty, e.g. calcium carbonate, or gummy textures are undesirable. Soothing and cooling sensation and smooth texture is required.

After-effects : The most common after-effect is the after-taste, e.g. saccharin has bitter after-taste. Another common effect is the numbing sensation in the mouth, e.g. promethazine HCL.

Formulation techniques:

The formulation problems involve bad taste, bad mouth-feel or after-taste. The tablet must have a pleasant taste, soothing mouthfeel and good compressibility. This can be achieved by following techniques-

i) Microencapsulation

ii) Adsorption on inert substrates that mask the taste, but release the drug in stomach, e.g. dextromethorphan hydrobromide on magnesium trisilicate.

iii) Ion-exchange resins (cationic and anionic) may be used to complex the drug of opposite charge.

iv) Spray drying and spray congealing, using appropriate coating agents, e.g. mono and diglycerides of edible fatty acids used to coat thiamine mononitrate.

v) Formation of less soluble salts or derivatives of drug, to render it less soluble in saliva and thereby less stimulating for taste buds.

vi) Coating by conventional granulation, where the drug is granulated with a relatively sweet excipient.

vii) Use of amino acids and protein hydrolysates to reduce bitterness of penicillins.

Directly Compressible vehicles :

In addition to the desired quantities of directly compressible vehicles, like flow properties, compressibility and compatibility, directly compressible vehicles for chewable tablets should have sweet taste and good mouth feel. For this pur- pose, monosaccharide and disaccharide classes of sugars and polyols may be used. Monosaccharides and disaccharides like sucrose, dextrose, fructose and lactose; while polyols like mannitol and sorbitol may be used. Gluconolactone and maltose are used rarely. Most of these vehicles are commercially available as mixtures of two or three entities under a brand name,

e.g. Sugartab (90-93 % sucrose + 7-10% invert sugar)

Di Pac (97% sucrose + 3% modified dextrins)

Nu Tab (95% sucrose + 4% invert sugar+cornstarch + magnesium stearate)

Mannitol is the most popularly used vehicle for chewable tablets. It is sweet in taste, possesses good mouthfeel and has a negative heat of dissolution, which gives a pleasant cooling sensation in the mouth. Its high cost is offset by these properties.

Most of the direct compression vehicles are commercially available as free flowing granules of controlled particle size. Their choice depends on compatibility with drug quantity of drug per tablet, degree of bad taste and properties of the vehicle.

Flavouring of Chewable tablets :

While formulating a chewable tablet, attempt should be made not only to mask a bad taste, but also to produce a tablet with a good taste. Generally, flavouring includes the initial impact, mouthfeel, after-effects and associated olfactory sensations. Unflavoured tablets containing at least two different formulation techniques and two different chewable vehicles should be prepared as 'baseline' formulation to further formulate with different flavours. Following criterion must be considered while choosing a flavour for chewable tablets-

i) Therapeutic classification : Antacids are generally chalky in taste, while vitamins are pungent and oily. They should have a pleasant initial taste with a sweet flavour. After sometime, when the tablet comes in contact with the back of the tongue, where the chalky or oily taste is perceived, a second flavour must be released.

Table 2.24: Common vehicles for chewable tablets.

Vehicle	Brand name	Composition
Brown sugar	–	Sucrose, invert sugar
Sugar	Sugartab	Sucrose, invert sugar
Sugar	Di-Pac	Sucrose, dextrins
Dextrose	Emdex	Dextrose, maltose higher saccharides
Fructose and dextrose	Sweetrex	
Mannitol	Mannitol	Mannitol
Sorbitol	Sorbitol	D-sorbitol - granular
Gluconolactone	Gluconolactone	D-Glucuronic acid δ-lactones and/or γ-lactones
Xylitol	Xylitol	Xylitol

ii) Active ingredient : Knowledge of the taste characteristic of the active ingredient in baseline formulation helps in at least eliminating certain flavours. Primary amine type drugs should not be formulated with reducing sugars as they undergo Schiff base formation. Most of the flavours are aldehydes, ketones, esters, alcohols or ethers chemically. Chemical incompatibilities of drugs with such flavours should be considered. Table 2.25 recommends guidelines for selection of flavours based on the taste of the active drug.

iii) Formulation: Some element of sweetness usually exists due to the chewable vehicle, which should be enhanced by appropriate choice of flavour. The cooling sensation and good mouthfeel of mannitol or sorbitol based diluents is enhanced by mint, menthol, wintergreen or peppermint type of flavours. If saccharine is used as a sweeter, its bitter aftertaste must be masked. Citric or tartaric acid may be used to enhance the sweet and sour taste of vitamin C tablets.

Table 2.25: Flavour selection guideline.

Taste of baseline formulation	Recommended flavour
Sweet	Mixed fruit and berries, vanilla, maple, honey
Sour	Citrus, fruit beer, anise, liquorice, raspberry cherry, strawberry
Bitter	Anise, mint, nut, cherry, chocolate, spice
Salty	Melon, raspberry, mixed citrus, mixed fruit, maple, butterscotch
Alkaline	Mint combination, chocolate, cream, vanilla, custard
Metallic	Grape, lemon, lime

iv) Dose per tablet and frequency of administration : The amount of flavour per tablet depends on the amount of drug per tablet and its relative bitterness. If frequency of administration is more, it may affect flavour selection since certain flavours are fatiguing on repeated use.

v) Intended patient population : Intensely sweet flavours are popular with children and elderly. Citrus and spicy flavours are preferred by adults.

vi) Marketing preference : If the product is being positioned against a competitive product, either the competitors flavour is improved (by choosing a flavour in the same class) or a totally different flavour is chosen. If it is an over-the-counter product, intensely sweet or extremely intense flavours should be avoided as there is a danger of losing repeat customers.

Flavours for pharmaceutical use are available in following physical forms :-

natural oils

spray dried powders

adsorbed powders

Flavours are incorporated generally by blending with final granulation, prior to lubrication. Sometimes, it is required to pre-screen the flavours to avoid large agglomerates. Several tablets are formulated using different flavours. Flavour selection panels are set up and final selection of first and second choice flavours is done through systematic evaluation. The stability studies are performed and a flavour is finally selected.

Sweeteners for chewable tablets

The vehicles selected for chewable tablets are sweet and have an ability to mask the bad taste of drugs. But sometimes it is necessary to incorporate an auxiliary sweetener. Sometimes the degree of bitterness or dose of drug is so high that it would require unreasonably high quantities of vehicle. Saccharin (450 times sweeter with respect to sucrose), aspartame (250 times sweeter) or cyclamate sodium (50 times sweeter) may be used as auxiliary sweeteners.

Colours for chewable tablets

Suitable D&C or FD&C colours may be used for colouring of chewable tablets. Usually the colours are selected according to the choice of flavours as indicated in the following table.

Table 2.26: Colour - flavour combinations for chewable tablets.

Colour	Flavours
Pink to red	Cherry, tutti-frutti, raspberry, strawberry, apple
Brown	Chocolate, maple, honey, butterscotch, walnut, caramel
Yellow to orange	Lemon, lime, orange, custard, banana
Green	Lime, mint, menthol, peppermint, spearmint
Off white to white	Vanilla, custard, banana
Violet to purple	Grape, plum, liquorice
Blue	Mint, blueberry, plum
Speckled	Colour of specks or background corresponding to flavour chosen.

Examples of Chewable tablet formulations:

Antacid tablets : Antacid tablets are conveniently formulated as chewable tablets for following reasons-

1. Antacids are most beneficial in suspension form as they neutralise the gastric acid. Smaller the particle size of suspended antacid, larger is the surface area available for neutralisation of acid. But suspensions are difficult to handle and transport. If the antacids are formulated as chewable tablets, the tablet is broken up into granules during chewing and the granules mix with saliva before swallowing, thus rendering the antacid into a 'suspension form'. Thus chewable antacid tablets have the convenience of handling, as that of tablets, and good neutralising capacity as that of suspensions.

2. Antacids have large doses. Normal compressed tablets are large in size and are difficult to swallow. Hence they are conveniently formulated as chewable tablets.

Example 1: Chewable antacid tablets (Wet granulation)

		Qty.per/tablet (mg)
Active	Magnesium trisilicate	450
ingredient	Aluminium hydroxide dried gel	200
Vehicle	Mannitol powder	300
Binder	Starch paste (7% w/w)	q.s.
Flavour and		q.s.
Sweetener	(e.g. peppermint sodium saccharin)	
Lubricant	Cornstarch	10
Glidant	magnesium stearate	10

Pharmaceutics- Formulation and Processing of Conventional Dosage Forms / 121

Mix magnesium stearate and aluminium hydroxide with mannitol. Dissolve saccharin sodium in water and combine with starch paste. Granulate the mixture with starch paste, dry at 60°C and screen through 16 # screen. Add flavour and cornstarch-magnesium stearate premix by passing through 20 # screen. Mix for 10 minutes. Allow the granules to stand for at least 24 hours before compression.

Vitamin tablets

Chewable vitamin tablets are intended for children between ages of 2 and 12 years. Additionally, chewable single vitamin tablets are also very popular.

Example : Chewable vitamin E tablets.

		Qty/tablet
Active ingredient	Dry vitamin E acetate	412 mg
Glidant	Colloidal silicon dioxide	25 mg.
Vehicle	Di-Pac/Sugartab/Emdex	255 mg.
Flavour		5 mg.
Colour		1 mg.
Lubricant	Magnesium stearate	2 mg.

Mix all ingredients, except vehicle and lubricant, and pass through screen #20 perforated plate at slow speed, knives forward. Add vehicle and blend for 15-20 minutes. Add the lubricant. Blend for 3-5 mins, compress.

Evaluation of Chewable tablets

In addition to the evaluation parameters tested for normal compressed tablets, some special tests are performed for chewable tablets.

i) Organoleptic evaluation:

Organoleptic evaluation is performed at various stages in formulation development of a chewable tablet. This is indicated in [table 2.27] below.

Table 2.27: Stages of organoleptic evaluation for chewable tablets.

Sr. No.	Evaluation	Description
i	Evaluation of drug	Characterisation and comparison of drug in absolute sense or against a known reference
ii	Evaluation of coated or treated (e.g. adsorbed) drug	comparison with pure drug and different drug coatings or treatment approaches
iii	Evaluation of unflavoured baseline formulation	Comparison amongst different vehicles or proportion of vehicles
iv	Evaluation of flavoured baseline formulation	Comparison amongst different flavoured formulations
v	Final selection and acceptance	Comparison between two 'top candidate' formulations

ii) Stability evaluation: Three major areas of stability evaluation are physical stability, chemical stability and organoleptic stability. The stability evaluation protocol is similar to that for normal compressed tablets. But following facts. Should be considered-

The flavours that are used in the chewable tablets are mixtures of as many as 50 chemicals. The flavours are incorporated in the tablets, which in turn consist of active ingredients and additives. Exposure of tablet to high temperatures is highly damaging to the product. The volatile oils may be lost preferentially. High humidity may cause desorption of adsorbed flavours. Flavours may react with the active ingredients or additives. Sometimes the flavours are picked up by plastic containers. While designing the stability protocol, all these points must be considered to evaluate physical chemical and organoleptic stability of the tablets.

FAST DISSOLVING TABLETS (Mouth Dissolving Tablets/Orodispersible tablets)

Fast dissolving tablets have advantage of solids and liquids. They can be defined as dosage forms for oral administration, which when placed in mouth, disintegrate rapidly or dissolve and can be swallowed in the form of a liquid.

Advantages
1. Ease of administration to patients who are mentally ill, disabled and unco-operative
2. Require no water intake
3. Quick disintegration and dissolution
4. Taste masking of unacceptable taste of drugs
5. Can be designed to leave minimal or no residue in mouth after administration and provide pleasant mouth feel.
6. Allow high drug loading

Characteristics of fast dissolving tablets :

Taste of the medicament : These tablets release the active ingredient in the mouth which directly comes in contact with the taste buds. Therefore, taste masking of the drug is required for better patient compliance.

Hygroscopicity : Several fast dissolving tablets are hygroscopic and cannot maintain physical integrity under normal conditions of temperature and humidity. Therefore, dehumidified conditions during processing as well as specialized product packaging is required.

Friability : In order to make them dissolve fast in mouth, these dosage forms are made of either very porous and soft moulded matrices, or compressed into tablets with very low compression force, which makes the tablets friable and brittle. Therefore, require specialised peel-off blister packs.

Techniques used in manufacturing :

i) Tablet moulding : In this method the delivery system is prepared by using water soluble additives to allow the tablets to dissolve completely in mouth. All ingredients are finely sieved, dry blended, wetted with a hydroalcoholic solvent and then compressed into tablets having low compression forces. Solvent present is removed by air drying. The so formed moulded tablets contain a porous structure which enhances dissolution. The mechanical strength of such tablets is low and hence a binding agent like sucrose, polyvinyl pyrrolidone, HPMC may be added to the solvent system.

ii) Spray drying : Spray drying can be used to prepare highly porous, fine powders. A composition containing a diluent, (e.g. mannitol / lactose) a superdisintegrant (Sodium starch glycollate/croscarmellose sodium) and the drug, which are spray dried and compressed together, show fast disintegration.

iii) Lyophilisation : Lyophilisation results in preparations which are highly porous and dissolve rapidly.

iv) Sublimation : A sublimed salt may be added to the powder mixture, the tablets are compressed and then the salt is removed by sublimation by exposing the tablets to reduced atmospheric pressure. Sublime salts that can be used are ammonium carbonate, ammonium bicarbonate and ammonium acetate.

v) Use of superdisintegrants : Super disintegrants absorb large amount of water, several times their actual weight, by capillary action and effectively disintegrate the tablets. Superdisintegrants like microcrystalline cellulose, crosslinked sodium carboxymethyl cellulose, crosslinked polyvinyl pyrrolidone and partially substituted hydroxypropyl cellulose may be used.

Table 2.28: Patented technologies for fast disintegrating tablets.

Name of technology	Principle used	Description
Zydis	Freeze drying	Water-soluble carrier & drug are filled in preformed pockets of blisterpack & lyophilised. The blisters are then immediately sealed.
Orasolv	use of effervescent disintegrant	Taste masked drug & effervescent disintegrant are mixed & directly compressed & packaged in a specialised package.
Durasolv	disintegrants	Drug & fillers & lubricants are compressed by conventional tabletting technology.
Flash dose	Flash heating	Consist of self binding shearform matrix prepared by flash heating.
Wowtab	Super disintegrants	Drug & a low mouldability saccharide (rapid dissolution) & high mouldability saccharide (good binding) is compressed.
Flash	Rapid disintegration by forming of active ingredient in the forming of micro-crystals	Drug microgranules prepared by conventional techniques, mixed with excipients & compressed.

EVALUATION OF TABLETS :

Tablets are evaluated by performing several tests. Table 2.29 lists some compendial & some non compendial (in house) quality control tests for teblets.

Table 2.29: Compendial and non-compendial quality control tests for tablets

Non-compendial tests	Compendial tests
- Size and shape	- Weight variation
- Colour	- Disintegration
- Odour	- Dissolution
- Physical defects	- Content uniformity
- Hardness	- Uniformity of active ingredient
- Friability	

General Appearance :

General appearance, visual identity and overall elegance should not differ from lot-to-lot and batch-to-batch of tablets.

i) Size and Shape : Thickness of the tablet is the only dimension. The crown thickness of individual tablets may be variable with a micrometer. Other technique used is placing 5 or 10 tablets in a holding tray, where their total crown thickness is measured. Tablet thickness should be controlled within ±5 per cent variation of a standard value. Any variation in the tablet thickness may cause difficulties in the use of unit dose and other packaging equipments.

ii) Unique identification markings: The identification markings include the company name or symbol, product code, product name, or potency, which are either embossed, engraved or printed.

iii) Organoleptic properties: The colour of the tablets should be uniform within the tablet, from tablet-to-tablet and from lot-to-lot. This is essential not only for aesthetic appeal, but also because colour variation may be related by consumers with non-uniformity of contents. It is difficult to judge the colour with the naked eye. In addition, visual colour comparisons require that a sample be compared against some colour standard. Colours can be quantified by use of reflectance spectrophotometry or microreflectance spectrophotometer.

Presence of some unusual odour in the tablet may be indicative of some instability. Taste is important in case of some tablets, like chewable tablets or lozenges. Companies employ taste panels to judge the performance of different flavours and flavour levels in the development of a product.

A tablet's level of flaws, such as chips, cracks, contamination from foreign solid substances, surface texture and appearance, are also noted.

Hardness and Friability:

Tablets require a certain amount of strength or hardness and resistance to friability, to withstand mechanical shocks of handling, manufacturing, packaging and shipping. Adequate tablet hardness and resistance to powdering and friability are necessary requisites for consumer acceptance.

Tablet hardness is defined as force required to break a tablet in a diametric compression test. To perform the test, a tablet is placed between two anvils, force is applied to the anvils and the crushing strength that just causes the tablet to break is recorded. Hardness is thus sometimes termed as the crushing strength. Several devices, namely Monsanto Strong-Cobb, Pfizer, Erweka or the Schleuniger hardness testers are used for this purpose.

Monsanto hardness tester was the earliest tester used to evaluate tablets. It consists of a barrel containing a compressible spring held between two plungers (fig. 2.62). The lower plunger is kept in contact with the tablet and a zero reading is taken. The upper plunger is then forced against a spring by turning a threaded bolt until the tablet fractures. As the spring compresses, a pointer rides along a gauge in the barrel to indicate the force. The force of fracture is recorded and the zero force is deducted from it.

The Pfizer hardness tester resembles a pair of pliers (fig 2.63). As the pliers' handles are squeezed, the tablet is compressed between a holding anvil and a piston connected to a direct force reading gauge. The dial indicator remains at the reading when the tablet breaks and returns to zero on pressing the reset button.

The Strong-Cobb tester eliminates the manual nature of the Monsanto hardness tester. The tablet is held between two jaws and the pressure is applied by a small hydraulic pump and the fracture is indicated by a needle on a calibrated dial.

However, since hardness is strain-rate dependent and dictated by the operator; in these methods, the results can be variable depending upon how quickly the load is applied. In erweka tester, the tablet is placed on the lower anvil, and the anvil is then adjusted so that the tablet just touches the upper test anvil. A suspended motor driven weight moves along a rail, which slowly and uniformly transmits pressure onto the tablet. A pointer moving along a scale provides the breaking

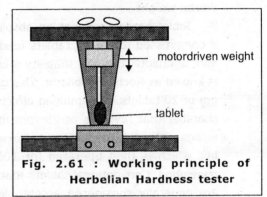

Fig. 2.61 : **Working principle of Herbelian Hardness tester**

strength value in kgs. The Schleuniger tester operates in a horizontal manner (Herbelian). Sometimes the testers are also calibrated in Strong-Cobb units.

1SCU = 714KP

Test for hardness

Though even though referred to as 'tablet hardness', the term is a misnomer. 'Hardness' implies that a tablet possesses a surface that is to be penetrated. But the test carried out to measure the hardness involves breaking or crushing of the tablet by application of a load. Hence, a better name to describe the test

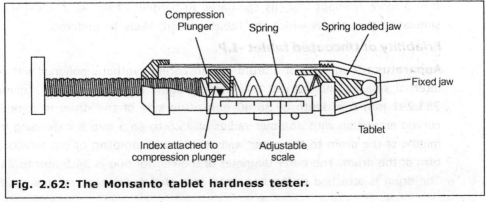

Fig. 2.62: **The Monsanto tablet hardness tester.**

would be test for breaking strength or crushing strength.

Crushing strength is part-ly governed by the rate at which the force is applied. Manually operated testers, like Monsanto or Pfizer testers, may give errors. Hence in so-phisticated hardness testers, namely Schleuniger and Erwe-ka hardness testers, load is applied uniformly by a motor driven weight.

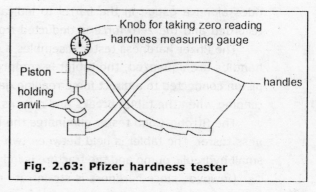

Fig. 2.63: Pfizer hardness tester

Tablet hardness is not an absolute indicator of strength, since some tablets if compressed to harder tablets tend to cap on attrition. Therefore another mea-sure of tablets strength, friability is often measured. The laboratory friability tester is known as Roche Friabilator. This device subjects a number of tablets, usually 6 gm or 20 tablets, to combined effects of abrassion and shock by utilising a plastic chamber that revolves at 25 rpm, dropping the tablets through a distance of 6 inches with each revolution. A pre-weighed tablet sample is placed in the cham-ber which is then operated for 100 revolutions. Tablets are then dusted and reweighed. Conventional tablets that lose less than 0.5-1 per cent of their weight are generally considered acceptable.

Low, acceptable moisture content, is required, which acts as a binder in tablet. Very dry granulations often produce more friable tablets; therefore, man-ufacturing of chemically stable tablets that contain some hydrolysable drugs that are mechanically sound, is difficult.

Test for Friability : A tablet is unlikely to be exposed to a compressive load, large enough to fracture it. But it is often subjected to tumbling motion, e.g. during coating, packaging or transport. This may abrade fine particles from its surface. To examine the resistance to abrasion, friability test has been devised. It is a more relevant test, as compared to hardness test, as it is carried out by simulating that stress which the tablet is more likely to undergo.

Friability of Uncoated tablet -I.P.

Apparatus : It consists of a drum of transparent synthetic polymer with polished internal sufaces and subject to minimum static build up. It has a diameter of 283.291 mm & a depth of 36-40 m.m. One side of the drum is removable. A curved projection with an inner radius of 75.5 to 85.5 mm & extending from the middle of the drum to the outer wall enables the tumbling of the tablets at each turn of the drum. The outer diameter of the central ring is 24.5 mm to 25.5 mm. The drum is attached to the horizontal axis of a device that rotates at 25 (±) 1 rpm. It should be ensured that with every turn of the drum the tablets roll or slide and fall into the drum wall or onto each other.

Method : For tablets with an average weight of 0.65g or less take a sample of whole tablets corresponding to about 6.5 g and for tablets with an average weight of more than 0.65g take a sample of 10 whole tablets.

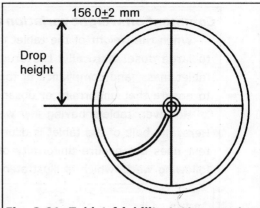

Fig. 2.64: Tablet friability test apparatus

Dedust & weigh the required number of tablets. Place the tablets in the drum & rotate it 100 times. Remove the tablets, remove any loose dust from them and weigh them accurately. The test is run only once. If the results are difficult to interpret or if the weight loss is greater than the targeted value, the test is repeated twice & the mean of the three tests is determined. A maximum loss of weight, not more than 1.0 per cent is acceptable for most tablets. If obviously cracked, chipped or broken tablets are present in the sample, the sample fails the test.

Weight Variation test :

With a tablet designed to contain a specific amount of drug, in a specific amount of tablet formula, the weight of the tablet being made is routinely measured to if enough, that the tablet contains the proper amount of drug.

Usually composite samples (20 tablets) are taken and weighed combinedly. The weight divided by 20, gives average weight for each tablet. But the individual tablets may deviate from the average weight. To help overcome this problem, I.P. provides limits for weight variation for individual tablets expressed as a percentage of average weight.

The I.P. weight variation test is run by weighing 20 tablets selected at random and determining the average weight. Not more than two of the individual weights deviate from the average weight by more than the deviation shown in the tablets and none deviates by more than twice that percentage.

Table 2.30: Official Weight variation tests

Average weight of tablet as per I.P.	% deviation	Avg. wt. of tablet as per U.S.P.
< 80 mg.	+ 10	< 130 mg
> 80 mg but < 250 mg	+ 7.5	> 130 mg but < 324 mg
> 250 mg	+ 5	> 324 mg

Comment on weight variation test :

When the weight of the tablet is more, it contains a drug having moderate to large dose. Naturally, the drug substance forms the greater part of the tablet mass, and compliance of the tablet with the weight variation test helps to ensure that uniformity of dosage is achieved.

However, tablets having low weights, usually contain highly potent drugs. Here, the bulk of the tablet is diluent and compliance with the weight variation test does not ensure uniformity of weight. This point can be exemplified by following work, which is illustrated in the figure given below.

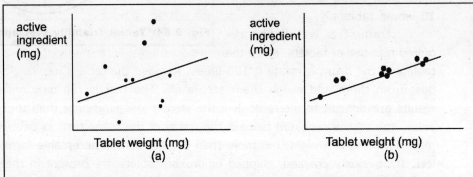

Fig. 2.65 : Relationship between tablet weight and drug content.
   (a) Drug content 23% of tablet weight
   (b) Drug content 90% of tablet weight

When the tablet contains 90 per cent of active ingredient, then a perfectly linear relationship exists between tablet weight and drug content. When the tablet contains only 23 per cent of the active ingredient, the relationship is insignificant.

This fact explains the need of having more stringent limits of percentage deviation in weight variation test for tablets having larger weights than for low weight tablets.

Disintegration :

For most tablets the first important step toward dissolution is tablet disintegration. The time that is required for a tablet to disintegrate is measured in a device known as Disintegration Time apparatus. One should not automatically expect a correlation between Disintegration Time and dissolution. However, since the dissolution of a drug from a fragmented tablet partially or competely controls the appearance of the drug in the blood, Disintegration Time is used as a guide by formulator in preparation of an optimum tablet formula.

Table 2.31: Compendial tests for tablets at a glance.

Weight variation test	Tests the deviation in tablets weight from average weight.
Disintegration test	Tests the time required for the tablets to break into fine particles of a particular size.
Dissolution test	Tests the amount of the drug that goes into solution from the tablets after specific time period.
Content of active ingredient	Determines the average amount of active ingredient in each tablet of sample and finds out the deviation from the label claim.
Content uniformity ingredient	Determines the actual amount of active ingredient in each tablet in the sample and finds out the deviation from the average amount. Performed only for low-dose tablets.

Disintegration test-I.P. : The test is provided to determine whether uncoated and coated tablets disintegrate within a prescribed time, when placed in a liquid medium under prescribed experimental conditions. Disintegration is defined as that state in which any residue of tablet, except fragments of insoluble coating, remaining on the screen of the test apparatus, consists of a soft mass having no palpably firm unmoistened core.

Disintegration test

Following points should be noted about this test

1. Pharmacopoeial disintegration tests do not mimic conditions in human G.I.T. with respect to fluid composition or agitation.
2. The temperature of medium is low for effervescent and dispersible tablets (room temperature), as they do not disintegrate in G.I.T.
3. A variation of $+ 2^0C$ is permissible, as far as the temperature of the medium is concerned.

Apparatus

a) A rigid basket-rack assembly supporting six cylindrical glass tubes
b) The tubes are held vertically by two superimposed transparent plastic plates perforated by six holes, which accommodate the tubes. To the underside of the lower plate, woven gauze with nominal mesh aperture of 2 mm (8 # mesh) is attached.
c) The plates are held vertically by two rods, one at the periphery and one at the centre. The central rod facilitates the attachment to a mechanical device which raises and lowers the assembly at a constant frequency of 28-32 cycles/min. through a distance of 50-60 mm.
d) Sometimes discs are placed on tablets to submerge them in liquid.
e) The assembly is suspended in liquid medium in 1000 ml beaker. Volume of

liquid is such that the wire mesh, at its highest point, is at least 25 mm below surface of liquid and, at its lowest point, at least 25 mm above the bottom of the beaker.

f) A thermostat for maintaining temperature between 35-39ºC.

General procedure:

Place one tablet each in tubes and operate the apparatus. At the end

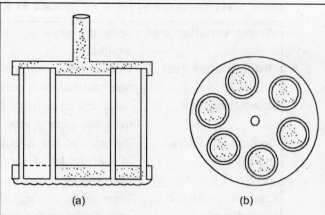

Fig. 2.66: Basket rack assembly of Disintegration test apparatus
a) Front view B) Top view

of the specified time, lift the basket from the liquid and observe the tablets. The tablets pass the test if all 6 have disintegrated. If one or two fail to disintegrate, repeat the test on 12 additional tablets. Not less than16 of the 18 tested tablets should pass the test.

Limits

Table 2.30: Limits for disintegration test for tablets according to I.P.

Type of tablet	Medium	Temperature	Limit
Uncoated	Water	37 ± 2ºC	15 mins or as indicated in monograph
Coated	Water	37 ± 2ºC	60 mins or as indicated in monograph
	if 1-2 fail	37 ± 2ºC	60 Mins or as indicated monograph
	0.1 M HCl		
Film Coated	Water	37 ± 2ºC	30 mins or as indicated monograph
Enteric Coated (If tablet has a soluble external coat immerse in Water for 5 minutes)	0.1M HCl	37 ± 2ºC	Should not disintegrate at the end of 2 hours
	Phosphate buffer pH 6.8	37 ± 2ºC	1 hr
Hard Capsules	Water	37 ± 2ºC	30 mins
Soft capsules	Water	37 ± 2ºC	60 mins
Dispersible/soluble	Water	24 to 26ºC	< 3 mins

For effervesceut tablets :

Place one tablet in 250 ml beaker with water at 20-30°C. Gas bubbles evolve. When they cease, tablets should have disintegrated (either dissolved or disintegrated.) Repeat the test for 5 tablets. Each should disintegrate within 5 minutes. All should pass the test.

Uniformity of dispersion for dispersible tablets :- Place 2 tablets in 100 ml water in a beaker. Stir gently until completely dispersed. A smooth dispersion is obtained, which passes through a sieve with nominal mesh aperture of 710 μ (# 22).

Disintegration Test U.S.P. : The apparatus is similar to that described for I.P. Table 2.33 indicates the acceptance criteria for disintegration test as per USP.

Table 2.33: U.S.P. Limits for disiutegration test for tablets according to USP.

Type of tablet	Medium	temperature	limit
Uncoated	Water	37 ± 2°C	As per individual monograph
Coated	Water	37 ± 2°C	As per individual monograph
Enteric coated (If soluble coat, immerse in water for 5 min.	Simulated gastric fluid (NaCl+ Pepsin HCl + Water)	37 ± 2°C	Should not disintegrate in 1 hr
	Simulated intestinal fluid (monobasic potassium-phosphate + pancreatin + 0.2 MHCl + water)	37 ± 2°C	Individual monograph
Buccal tablets	Water	37 ± 2°C	4 hrs
Sublingual	Water	37 ± 2°C	As per individual monograph
Hard gelatin capsule	Water	37 ± 2°C	As per individual monograph
Soft gelatin capsule	Water	37 ± 2°C	As per individual monograph

Dissolution Test - I. P. :

The test is designed to determine compliance with the dissolution requirements of tablets. I.P. prescribes two different apparatii for carrying out dissolution tests. Use apparatus I unless otherwise specified.

Apparatus I - An assembly consisting of following:

a.   A cylindrical 1000 ml vessel A, made up of boro

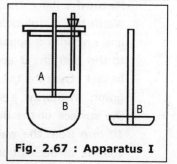

Fig. 2.67 : Apparatus I

silicate glass or any other transparent material. The vessel may be flat bottomed or have a hemispherical bottom. It is fitted with a lid which has a number of openings.

b. A variable speed motor, which causes the paddle to rotate in the vessel. The mother consists of a drive shaft and blade forming a paddle, B.

c. The paddle blade passing through the diameter of the shaft so that the bottom of the blade is flush with the bottom of the shaft. The lower edge of the blade is 23 to 27 mm from the inside bottom of the vessel. The apparatus operates in such a way that the paddle rotates smoothly.

c. A water bath set to maintain the dissolution medium at 36.5 to 37.5^0C.

d. Vessel is equipped with a suitable device for withdrawal of samples from a point approximately halfway between basket wall and wall of vessel.

Apparatus II - The apparatus is similar to apparatus I. But the stirring element i.e. the paddle is replaced by a basket D. The metallic shaft rotates smoothly.

The top part of the basket is fitted with three spring clips. The lower dettachable part is made of welded steam cloth with 0.381 mm openings, formed into a cylinder.

Apparatus suitability : An apparatus that permits observation of the preparation under the examination and the stirrer during the test is preferable. Use apparatus I unless otherwise stated.

Dissolution medium : Use the medium specified in the individual monograph. If the medium is a buffered solution adjust its pH within 0.05 units of the specified pH.

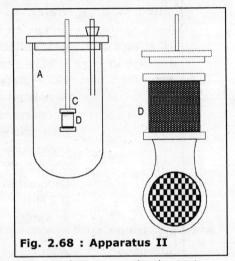

Fig. 2.68 : Apparatus II

Time : When a single time is specified in the individual monograph, the test may be concluded in a shorter period of time if the requirement for minimum amount dissolved is met. If two or more times are specified, specimens are withdrawn only at the stated times.

Method : Place the stated dissolution mediumin the vessel of the apparatus. Warm the dissolution medium to 36.5 to 37.5^0C. Unless otherwise stated, place one unit in the apparatus. If apparatus I is used allow the tablet/capsule to sink to the bottom. If apparatus II is being used, place a tablet/capsule in the dry basket. Operate the apparatus at the speed specified in the individual monograph. Withdraw a sample at the time specified from a zone midway between the surface of the dissolution medium and top of rotating basket, not less than 10 mm from the wall of vessel. Except in the case of a single sampling, add a volume of dissolution medium equal to the volume of the samples withdrawn.

Perform the analysis by method given in the individual monograph. Repeat the whole operation five times.

Acceptance criteria

Conventional release dosage form

Unless otherwise specified, the requirements are met if the quantities of active substances dissolved from the dosage units conform to table.

Level	number tested	Acceptance creteria
S_1	6	Each unit is not less than D* + 5%**
S_2	6	Average of 12 units (S_1 + S_2) is equal to or greater than is greater than or equal to D, and no unit is less than D-15%**
S_3	12	Average of 24 units (S_1+S_2+S_3) & if no unit is less than D-25%
*		D = amount of dissolved active ingredient specified in the individual monograph, expressed as a percentage of labelled content.
**		Percentage of the labelled content

If the results do not conform to the requirements at stage S_1 given in the table, continue testing with additional dosage units through stages S_2 and S_3 unless the results conform at stage S_3.

Capsules : If capsule shells interfere with the analysis, remove contents of not less than 6 capsules as completely as possible, and dissolve the empty capsule shells in the specified volume of the dissolution medium. Perform analysis as stated in individual monograph. Make any necessary correction. Correction factors should not be greater than 25% of the stated amount.

Dissolution Test for tablets-USP

Apparatus : Apparatus I is the basket assembly and Apparatus II is paddle. i.e. I.P. Apparatus I is USP apparatus II and vice versa

USP reference standards :

1) USP Prednisolone Tablets RS - disintegrating type

2) USP salicylic acid Tablets RS - nondisintegrating type

Apparatus suitability test : Individually test 1 tablet of the USP dissolution calibrator, disintegrating type and 1 tablet of USP dissolution calibrator,non disintegrating type. The apparatus is suitable if the results obtained are within the acceptable range stated in the certificate for that calibrator in the apparatus tested.

Medium : Same as I.P.

Time : Same as I.P.

Procedure : Same as I.P.

Acceptanc criteria : Same as I.P. The amout of dissolved active ingredient specified in the individual monograph, is called 'D' according to I.P. and 'Q' according to USP

Uniformity of contents of single dose preparations :

This test is based on the assay of the individual contents of active substances of number of single dose units to determine whether the individual contents are within limits set with reference to the average content of the sample.

Method : Determine the content of active ingredients in each of 10 dosage units taken at random using the method given in the monograph or by any other suitable analytical method.

Acceptance limit : For tablets, powders and suspensions : The preparation complies with the test if each individual content is 85 to 115% of average content. The preparation fails to comply with the test if more than one individual content is outside these limits or if one individual content is outside the limits of 75 - 125% of average content.

If one individual content is outside the limits of 85-115% of average but within the limits of 75-125% repeat the determination on using another 20 dosage units. The preparation complies with the test if not more than one of the individual contents of the total sample of 30 dosage units is outside 85-115% of average content and none is outside the limits of 75-125% of average.

Apparatus III - Consists of a cylindrical flat bottomed glass vessels, a set of glass reciprocating cylinders, stainless steel fitting & screens. The cylinders reciprocate vertically inside the vessels. The vessels are partially immersed in water bath at 37 $\pm$ 0.5°c.

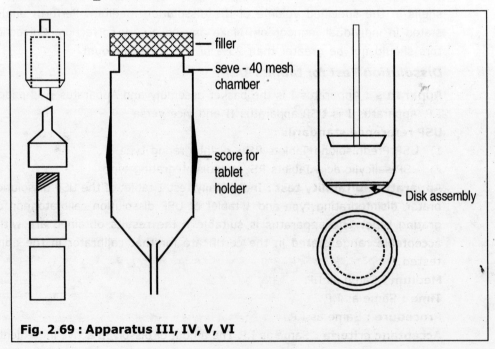

filler

seve - 40 mesh chamber

score for tablet holder

Disk assembly

Fig. 2.69 : Apparatus III, IV, V, VI

Apparatus IV - Flow through cell

Apparatus V - Paddle over disc for transdermal drug delivery systems. It consists of a disc to hold the transdermal patch in a paddle type vessel like apparatus 2.

Apparatus VI - It is uses the assembly from apparatus 1, except to replace the basket with a SS cylinder stirring element. The dosage unit is placed on the cylinder at the begining of each test.

Test for Content Uniformity I.P.:

For tablets containing more than one active ingredient, carry out the test for each active ingredient.

Determine content of active ingredients in each of 10 tablets taken at random using method given in monograph. The tablets comply with the test if not more than one of the individual value thus obtained is outside the limits 85-115 per cent of the average value and none is outside the limit of 75-125 per cent of average. If 2 or 3 of the individual values are outside 85-115 per cent of average, and none is outside 75-125 per cent, repeat the determination for 20 more tablets. The tablets comply with the test if, in the total sample of 30 tablets, not more than one of the individual values are outside the limits 85-115 per cent and none is outside the limits 75-125 per cent average value.

Content Uniformity USP :

This test applies to both the dosage units containing a single active ingredient or more than one active ingredient. It applies individually to each active ingredient in the product. It is required to be performed for tablets containing 50 mg or more of an active ingredient that comprises 50% or more by weight of one tablet.

Dissolution test

Apparatus consists of following :

1.   A cylindrical, covered 1000 ml vessel of glass or any other inert transparent material. The vessel may be flat bottomed or have a spherical shape. It is fitted with a lid, which has a number of openings.

2.   A variable speed motor, which causes a basket to rotate in the vessel. Speed of the motor should be capable of being varied between 25-150 rpm. The motor drives a basket by means of a shaft. It is so positioned that its axis is not more than 2 mm at any point from vertical axis of vessels.

3.   A cylindrical SS basket assembly made of woven wire cloth with a nominal aperture size of 425 μm. The top of the basket is attached to the disc on the driving shaft by three clips.

4.   Vessel is equipped with suitable device for withdrawal of samples from a point approximately halfway between the surface of dissolution medium and bottom of the vessel and halfway between basket walls and wall of vessel. Sampling should not disturb flow of medium.

5. Vessel is clamped in a waterbath to maintain its temperature at 37 + 0.5ºC

Method - as per I.P. : Unless otherwise stated in the monograph, introduce 1000 ml water in the vessel previously warmed to 36.5-37.5ºC. Place the specified number of tablets/capsules in the apparatus and assemble the apparatus, adjusting the distribution between bottom of the basket and bottom of vessel to between 23 mm and 27 mm.

Start the motor, adjust speed to 100 rpm/or speed in monograph. Withdraw stated volume of solution at 45 minutes or at the time specified. Filter immediately through an inert medium with nominal pore size of 1μ or less. Determine amount of active ingredient by method given in monograph. Repeat the complete operation four times.

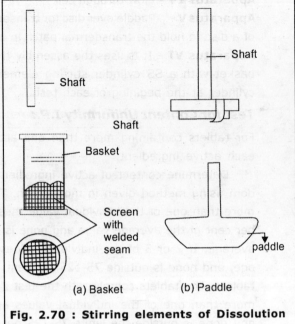

Fig. 2.70 : Stirring elements of Dissolution test apparatus.

Interpretation: Requirements of test are met if, in all the five tablets/capsules tested (in those cases where one tablet/capsule is directed to be placed in basket), the amount of active ingredient in solution is not less than 70 per cent of the stated amount. Where two or more than two tablets/capsules are directed to be placed, the amount of active ingredient in solution per tablet/capsule, in each test, is not less than 70 per cent of stated amount unless otherwise specified in the monograph. No re-test is permitted.

U.S.P.

Apparatus II : Instead of using a basket, a paddle formed from a blade and a shaft is used.

Medium : Solvent specified in monograph

Procedure : Same as I.P.

Comment on Dissolution test

1. The constitution of the dissolution fluid is specified in the individual monograph. If it is not specified, water is the medium of choice. The dissolution fluid is chosen by considering nature of drug substance and sensitivity of assay procedure.

---

2. The specified temp. is 37 + 0.5°C. The tolerance of only + 0.5°C is allowable in the temperature of the medium. The effect of temperature on solubility of a substance is well known. Hence to avoid false positive or false negative results, the tolerance in the temperature is kept narrower, unlike the disintegration test, where it is + 2C.
3. The general dissolution requirement as per IP is 70% dissolved in 45 mins, whereas, as per USP, the general requirement is 75% dissolved in 45 mins.

For determination of dosage unit uniformity by assay of individual units, select not less than 30 tablets and proceed.

Uncoated/coated/hard/soft capsules: Assay 10 units individually as directed.

1. Prepare a composite specimen of a sufficient number of dosage units to provide the amount of specimen called for in the assay in the individual monograph, plus the amount required for the special procedure for content uniformity by finely powdering the tablets.
2. Assay separately, accurately measured portions of the composite specimen of tablets, both (a) as directed in the assay and (b) using the special procedure for content uniformity mentioned in the monograph.
3. Calculate the weight of active ingredient equivalent to 1 average dosage unit by (a) using the results obtained by the assay (b) using results obtained by the special procedure.
4. Calculate correction factor, F by formula- $F = A/P$

Where,

A = weight of active ingredient, equivalent to 1 average dosage unit obtained by assay procedure

P = weight of active ingredient, equivalent to 1 average dosage unit obtained by special procedure

If, $\dfrac{100 \, |A - P|}{A}$ is > 10, use of correction factor is not valid.

5. A valid correction my be applied if F is not less than 1.030 not greater than 1.100, or not less than 0.900 nor greater than 0.970 to if F is between 0.970 & 1.030, no correction is required.

6. If F lies between 1.030 & 1.100 or between 0.900 & 0.970 calcuate the weight of active ingredient in each dosage unit by multiplying each of the weights found using special procedure by F.

If amount of active ingredient in each of 10 dosage units, as determined by weight variation or content uniformity method, lies within the range of 85-115 per cent of the label claim. If 1 unit is outside the range of 85-115 per cent of label claim, and no unit is outside the 75-125 per cent of label claim, test 20 additional units. If not more than 1 unit of the 30 is outside the range of 85-115 label claim, and no unit is outside range of 75-125 per cent, the requirement is met.

Content of active ingredient - USP

To assure uniform potency for tablets of low dose drugs, a content uniformity test is applied. In this test, 30 tablets are randomly selected for the sample, and at least 10 of them are assayed individually. Nine of the 10 tablets must contain not less than 85 per cent or more than 115 per cent of the labelled drug content. The 10th tablet may not contain less than 75 per cent or more than 125 per cent of the labelled content. If these conditions are not met, the remaining tablets, from the 30 selected, must be assayed individually, and none may fall outside of the 85-115 per cent range in evaluating a particular lot of tablets, several samples of tablets should be taken from various parts of the production run.

PACKAGING OF TABLETS

Tablets are either packaged in a multiple dose container of glass or plastic, or unit dose packaging, i.e., strip or blister packaging.

Strip packaging

A strip package is formed by feeding two webs of heat sealable flexible film through a heated crimping roller. The product is dropped into the packet formed prior to forming the final set of seals. A continuous strip of packet is formed, generally several packets wide, depending on the packaged machine's limitations. The strip of packets is cut to the desired number of packets in length. The product sealed between the two sheets of film usually has a seal around each tablet, with perforations usually separating adjacent packets. A number of different packaging materials are used. For high barrier applications, a paper/polyethylenefoil / polyethylene lamination is commonly used. When product visibility is important, heat sealable cellophane or polyester can be used.

Blister packaging

It is used extensively for pharmaceutical packaging for several good reasons. It is capable of providing good environmental protection with aesthetically pleasing appearance. It also provides user functionality in terms of convenience, child resistance and tamper resistance.

Blister packaging is formed by heat-softening a sheet of thermoplastic resin, and vacuum drawing the softened sheet of plastic into a contoured mould. After cooling, the sheet is released from the mould and proceeds to the filling station of the packaging machine. The semi-rigid blister previously formed is filled with product and lidded with a heat-sealable backing material. The backing material can be of either a push-through or peelable type. For a push-through type of blister, the backing material is usually heat seal coated aluminium foil. The coating must be compatible with the blister material to ensure satisfactory sealing, for product protection and for tamper resistance. Peelable backing materials are used for child resistant packaging. This type of backing must have a degree of puncture resistance to prevent a child from pushing the product through the backing, but should allow it to be pulled away from the blister, by a grown up, even when it is strongly adhered to it. Material such as polyester or paper is used as component of lid material. Foil is used when moisture protection is required.

Material used for blister : Polyvinyl chloride / Polyethylene combination, polystyrene/polypropylene.

LAYOUT OF TABLETTING SECTION:

In a pharmaceutical manufacturing unit, several tablets are made at a given time. Each tablet-manufacturing operation involves numerous steps. This increases the possibility of cross-contamination and product mix-ups. To eliminate this risk, a separate booth is recommended for each step. Each booth/room is to be thoroughly cleaned between operations. Thus the space, maintenance and labour costs increase.

The need for carrying out each step in granulation process in separate compartment, fragments the operation and increases space, capital and labour cost. Being a multi-step process, granulation cost is more than the tabletting cost. Therefore, each operation in the granulation area should be designed to reduce the cost and improve the process. Fig. 2.71 shows a layout of a typical granulation room.

A washing facility is provided for cleaning portable equipments, such as FBD. Each room should be provided with floor drains and patched floor. Provision should be made for supply of hot and cold water and steam for special cleaning purpose. If the room is not air-conditioned, all the windows should be

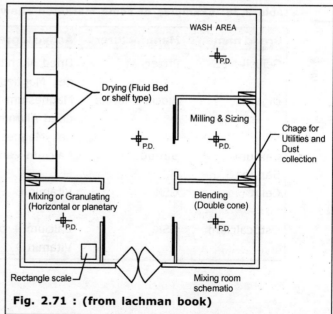

Fig. 2.71 : (from lachman book)

screened for protection against insects. Racks and trays in the drying ovens should be rust free and designed for easy cleaning.

Separate rooms or booths should be provided for tablet compression machines to avoid cross-contamination. When dehumidified conditions are required for special products like effervescent tablets or tablets containing moisture sensitive drug, a chemical unit containing lithium or silica gel is provided for relative humidity levels below 20 per cent. The walls should be specially treated for low water vapour transmission rates. The room should be supplied with air locks.

Since each tablet press is to be placed in its own separate location, the rooms can be all of same size, or may vary in size to accommodate the smallest and largest press.

The booth walls should extend from floor to ceiling and may be made of tiles upto 4-5 feet level, with a glass or transparent partition above it, extending upto the ceiling. Hard surfaces should be used sparingly, as they contribute to the noise level. Space should be provided for placing in-process quality control equipments, such as hardness testers, balances, friabilators, etc.

The number of compression rooms is usually less than the number of booths, since all the presses are not being used at a time. Once a batch is complete the machine is removed from the booth and replaced with one that has been cleaned and prepared for the next product. Each press should be mounted on metal frames so that it can be moved by lift trucks into the cleaning area. A room should be made available nearby for cleaning of presses and replacement of punches and dies.

Table 2.38: Examples of some marketed chewable tablets

Brand name	Manufacturer	Active ingredient	Category
Gelusil-MPS	Pfizer	Dried Aluminium hydroxide gel, Magnesium	Antacid
Digene	Biocia Pharma	Magnesium hydroxide, dried Aluminium hydroxide gel, Magnesium oxide	Antacid
Calcium Sandoz	Sandoz	Calcium carbonate	Calcium supplement
Celin	GSK	Vitamin C	Vitamin C supplement
Ostocalcium	GSK	Calcium + phosphorus + Vitamin D$_3$	Calcium supplement

Table 2.39: Examples of some mouth-dissolving tablets

Brand name	Manufacturer	Active ingredient	Category
Celact-MD	Sun Pharma.	Celecoxib	Cox-2 inhibitor
Nimulid-MD	Panacea Biotech	Nimesulide	NSAID
Avomine-MD	Nicholas Piramal	Promethazine	Antiemetic
Zofer-MD	Sun Pharma	Ondansetron	Antacid

Table 2.40: Examples of some commercially available effervescent tablets

Brand name	Manufacturer	Active ingredient	Category
Disprin	Reckitt Benckister	Aspirin	Analgesic/ antipyretic
Colsprin	Reckitt Benckister	Aspirin	
Histac-EVT	Ranbaxy	Ranitidine	H-2 receptor blocker

Table 2.41: Examples of some commercially available dispersible tablets

Brand name	Manufacturer	Active ingredient	Category
Domstal DT	Torrent	Domperidone	GI Prokenetic
Ketorol DT	Dr. Reddy's	Ketorolac	Analgesic
Voveran D	Novartis	Diclofenac sodium	Analgesic
Mox-DT	Rexcel	Amoxycillin	Antibacterial
Althrocin DT	Alembic	Erythromycin	Antibacterial

Table 2.42 : Examples of some commercially available layered tablets

Brand name	Manufacture	Active ingredient	Category
Alerid-D	Cipla	Cetinizine	Antiallergic
		Phenylpropanolamine HCl	Anticold
Gluformin-Gl	Nicholas	Glimepiride Metformin	Antidiabetic
Gluconorm-G	Lupin	Metformin	Antidiabetic
Gemer forte-2	Sun Pharma	Metformin	Antidiabetic

Example : Effervescent antacid tablets by wet granulation method with reactive liquid

Ingredients	Quantity
1. Citric acid anhydrous (granular)	1180 gm
2. Sodium bicarbonate (granular)	1700 gm
3. Sodium bicarbonate (powder)	175 gm
4. Citrus flavour (spray-dried)	50 gm
5. Water	30 gm

Thoroughly blend citric acid anhydrous (granular), sodium bicarbonate (granular), citrus flavour (spray-dried) and water in a planetary mixer. Quickly add all the four ingredients and mix until a workable mass is formed. Granulate through a 10# mesh screen using oscillating granulator, spread evenly on a paper-lined drying tray and dry in oven at 70 per cent for 2 hours. Cool and re-granulate through 16# mesh screen. Place granulations in a tumble blender and add ingredient sodium bicarbonate (powder). Mix well. Compress into flat faced, bevelled-edge tablets, each weighing 3.10 g.

Example : Effervescent Analgesic tablets by direct compression.

Ingredients	Quantity
1. Aspirin (80# granular)	325 gm
2. Monobasic calcium phosphate (powder)	165 gm
3. Sodium bicarbonate (granular)	1700 gm
4. Citric acid anhydrous	1060 gm

Convert sodium bicarbonate (powder) to 7-9 per cent sodium carbonate by placing in oven at 100°C for 45 minutes with two mixings at 15 minutes intervals. Cool and mix with monobasic calcium phosphate (powder) and citric acid anhydrous in a tumbler blender. Add aspirin (80# granular) and mix for 10 minutes. Compress Aspirin (80# granular) in diameter flat-faced, bevelled-edge tablets, each weighing 3.25 gm. Stabilise tablets in the oven at 60°C for 1 hour. Cool and package.

Example : Effervescent Denture cleanser tablets
(Wet granulation with non-reactive liquid)

Ingredients	Quantity
1. Potassium monopersulfate	800 gm
2. Citric acid anhydrous (granular)	575 gm
3. Sodium bicarbonate	800 gm
4. Sodium Chloride	320 gm
5. Sodium perborate monohydrate	320 gm
6. Sodium Sulfate	225 gm
7. Polyvenyl pyrrolidone	100 gm
8. Isopropyl alcohol	170 gm
9. Sodium lauryl sulfate	10 gm
10. Colour	2 gm
11. Peppermint Oil	16 gm
12. Magnesium stearate	20 gm

Blend Sodium bicarbonate, Sodium Chloride, Sodium perborate monohydrate, Sodium Sulfate and Polyvenyl pyrrolidone in a planetary mixer. Add Isopropyl alcohol and mix until the mass is wet. Spread the mixture on trays about 1 inch' deep. Dry in forced draft oven at 68°C for 16 hours. Pass through 18# screen. Mix Potassium monopersulfate and Citric acid anhydrous (granular) in a tumble blender. Add 1500 gm of dried screened granulation and tumble until well mixed. Distribute Sodium lauryl sulfate, Colour and Peppermint Oil on 265 gm dried screened granulation and add to tumble blender and mix well. Compress 1 inch diameter, flat faced bevelled-edge tablets, weighing 3.19 gm each.

Example : Phenobarbital tablets (Wet Aqueous granulation)

Ingredients	Quantity per tablet
Phenobarbital	65 mg
Lactose	40 mg
Starch (as starch paste)	04 mg
Starch (dry)	10 mg
Talc	10 mg
Mineral Oil, 50 cps	04 mg

Mix phenobarbital and lactose and moisten with 10 per cent starch paste to proper wetness. Granulate by passing through a 14 mesh screen and dry at 140°F. Pass through 20 mesh screen, add dry starch and talc, mix well and add mineral oil. Mix again and compress.

Example : Thiamine Hydrochloride Tablets (Aqueous wet granulation)

Ingredients	Quantity per tablet
Thiamine HCl	55 mg
Lactose	200 mg
Tartaric acid	5 mg
Starch (as paste)	6 mg
Sterotex	8 mg
Alginic acid	10 mg

Formula includes 10 per cent excess thiamine HCl. Mix thiamine HCl, lactose and tartaric acid and moisten with starch paste. Pass through 14 mesh screen to granulate Dry at 120°F. Pass through 20 mesh screen. Add alginic acid and sterotex. Mix and compress.

Example :   Acetaminophen tablets (Non-aqueous wet granulation)

Ingredients	Quantity per tab
Acetaminophen (powder)	325 mg
Ethyl cellulose (10 cps) (5% in alcohol)	q.s.
Starch	20 mg
Guar gum	15 mg
Magnesium stearate	12 mg

Moisten Acetaminophen with ethyl cellulose solution. Granulate by passing through 14# screen. Air-dry. Add Magnesium stearate. Pass through 918# screen. Add starch and guar gum. Mix in a twin shell blender for 3 minutes, compress.

Example : Phenobarbital sodium tablets (dry granulation)

Ingredients	Quantity per tablet
Phenobarbital sodium	65 mg
Lactose (granular, 12- mesh)	26 mg
Starch	20 mg
Talc	20 mg
Magnesium stearate	0.3 mg

Mix all the ingredients. Compress into slugs. Grind and screen to 14-16# mesh granules. Compress using a 9/32 inch concave punch.

Example : Vitamin B complex tablets (dry granulation)

Ingredients	Quantity per tablet
Thiamine mononitrate*	0.733 mg
Riboflavin *	0.733 mg
Pyridoxine HCl	0.333 mg
Calcium pantothenate	0.4 mg
Nicotinamide	5 mg
Lactose (powder)	75.2 mg
Starch	21.9 mg
Talc	20 mg
Stearic acid (powder)	0.701 mg

* Includes 10 per cent excess of label claim. Mix all ingredients thoroughly. Compress into slugs. Grind and screen to 14-6# mesh granules. Recompress into tablets, using a ¼ inch concave punch. Use sufficient tartaric acid to adjust the pH to 4.5

Example : Aspirin Phenacetin caffeine tablets (direct compression)

(Direct compression) Ingredients	Quantity per tablet
Aspirin (40- mesh crystal)	224 mg
Phenacetin	160 mg
Caffeine, anhydrous	32 mg
Di-Pac	93.4 mg
Sterotex	7.8 mg
Silica gel	2.8 mg

Blend all ingredients in a twin shell blender for 15 minutes, compress.

Example : Ascorbic acid tablets (Direct compression)

Ingredients	Quantity per tablets
Ascorbic acid, USP (Fine crystals)	255 mg
Avicel	159 mg
Stearic acid	9 mg
Colloidal silica	2 mg

Blend in a suitable blender. Compress.

Examples of Compression, Coated tablets

Example : Typical core granulation

Ingredients	Quantity
Active ingredient	q.s.
Starch U.S.P.	5%
Magnesium stearate U.S.P.	0.5%
Lactose U.S.P. anhydrous	q.s.
	100%

Example : Typical core granulation

Ingredients	Quantity
Active ingredient	q.s
Microcrystalline cellulose (100??)	30%
Magnesium stearate U.S.P.	0.5%
Lactose U.S.P. (spray dried)	q.s.
	100%

Example : Typical coating granulation

Ingredients	Quantity
Lactose U.S.P. (spray dried)	q.s
Confectioners sugar U.S.P.	2%
Acacia U.S.P. (spray dried)	2%
PEG 6000	4%
Talc U.S.P.	3%
Magnesium stearate U.S.P.	0.5%
Soluble dye	q.s.
purified water U.S.P.	q.s. 100%

Blend all ingredients except the dye and PEG in a double arm mixer. Dissolve dye in minimum amount of water and the PEG in 1.2 times its weight of water at 50°C. Combine the two solutions and add slowly to mixed powders. Mix for 30 minutes. Spread on trays and dry at 45°C. The granulation is ready for compression.

Example : Typical coating granulation (moisture resistant)

Ingredients	Quantity
Calcium sulfate dihydrate	q.s.
Mannitol NF	10%
Tragacanth	2%
Acacia U.S.P.	3%
Talc U.S.P	5%
Magnesium stearate U.S.P	2%
Colorant	q.s.
Purified water U.S.P	q.s

Blend calcium sulphate, mannitol, tragacanth, talc, Magnesium stearate and Colorant. Make mucilage of acacia with water and add to the mixed powders. Granulate. Spread on trays and dry in oven at 45°C size by passing through a 20# screen.

Example of layered tablets

Layer 1	Quantity per tablet
Phenylpropanolamine HCl NF	12.5 mg
Lactose U.S.P.	76.5 mg
Sucrose U.S.P.	2.0 mg
Talc U.S.P.	3.0 mg
Tragacanth U.S.P.	2.0 mg
PEG 6000 U.S.P.	4.0 mg
Purified Water U.S.P.	q.s
Anhydrous alcohol	q.s.

Blend phenyl propanolamine, lactose, sucrose, talc and tragacanth, combine purified water and alcohol and dissolve PEG in the mixed powders. Continue mixing till the mass is evenly moistened and granular.

Dry in an oven. Pass through a 20 # screen.

Layer 2	
Lactose U.S.P.	48 mg
Confectioners sugar U.S.P.	24 mg
Starch U.S.P.	7 mg
FD and C Colour	0.002 mg
Purified water U.S.P.	q.s.
Stearic acid U.S.P.	0.998 mg

Pass lactose and sugar through a 20# screen and blend with starch. Dissolve colour in water and add to the powders. Continue mixing till colour is uniformly distributed. Dry in oven at 40-45°C.

Add stearic acid. Blend for 10 minutes.

Layer 3	
Aspirin-starch (20# granules, 10% starch)	90 mg
Talc U.S.P.	10 mg

Blend in suitable mixer for 10-15 minutes. Compress the three layers together using 3/8 inch diameter flat faced, bevelled-edge punches. Weight of each layer is-

Compression	Quantity
First layer	100 mg
Second layer	80 mg
Third layer	100 mg

Tablet Coating

INTRODUCTION

Coated tablets are defined in Indian Pharmacopoeia 96 as 'Tablets coated with mixtures of various substances such as resins, gums, inactive and insoluble fillers, sugars, waxes, etc.' The coating may also contain medicaments. Tablet coating, as a pharmaceutical unit process, has its origins in ancient Egypt. Refined sugar became more widely available in the middle of 19th century. Modern sugar coating process evolved around this time. Sugar coating processes for tablets were developed by modifying processes used to produce coated confectioneries. The sugar coating process remained essentially unchanged till 1950's. In 1953, first filmcoated tablet was marketed. Concurrently, an Air Suspension coater that efficiently applied film coatings was patented by Dr. Wurster in 1950s.

TYPES OF TABLET COATING -

There are three types of tablet coatings-
   1. Sugar Coating   2. Film Coating
   3. Compression Coating (Press Coating)
Sugar coating was employed most extensively. But it is now being replaced by film coating.

REASONS BEHIND TABLET COATING :

TABLETS MAY BE COATED FOR FOLLOWING REASONS:
   1. To protect the drug from environment, particularly from light and moisture.

2. To mask taste, colour or odour of the drug.

3. Coating has an added advantage as it increases mechanical strength of the tablet core and improves handling of tablets on high speed machine.

4. To incorporate another drug or formula adjuvant in the coating to avoid chemical incompatibilities or to control release of drug from the tablet.

5. To protect the drug from the stomach's gastric environment with an acid resistant enteric coating.

   Depending upon the aforementioned uses of tablet coating, specific functions of coating may be divided into three main groups (Table 3.1).

Table 3.1: Aspects of tablet coating

General Aspects	Function
Therapy	
Avoid bad taste	Insulation
Avoid oesophageal irritation	Insulation, slow release
Avoid irritation to stomach	Gastroresistance
Avoid inactivation in stomach	Gastroresistance
Avoid flash release	modified release (slow)
Improve drug efficacy	Modified release (Time controlled, pulse release)
Improve drug action in distinct sections	Modified release (site controlled, pH-specific)
Prolong dosing intervals	Modified release (slow, special release)
Improve patient compliance	Modified release
Technology	
Avoid dust formation	Insulation
Reduce influence of moisture	Insulation
Reduce influence of atmosphere (oxygen, CO_2)	Insulation
Improve drug stability	Insulation
Prolong shelf life	Insulation
Marketing	
Avoid bad taste, odour	Insulation
Improve product identification	Color coating
Improve appearance	Insulation, color coating, polishing
Improve patient compliance	Modified release

1. Insulation which does not influence the release pattern and does not change the tablet appearance markedly.
2. Modified release with specific requirements.
3. Colour coating which provides insulation or is combined with modified release coating.

TABLET PROPERTIES ESSENTIAL FOR COATING

Tablets must have following proper physical characteristics for effective coating :

1. Tablets experience intense attrition as they roll in the coating pan or the air suspension coater. The tablets must be robust enough to tolerate this attrition.
2. Tablets should not be brittle, get softened in presence of heat or get affected by coating composition.
3. Shape of tablets: When tablets are sprayed with a coating composition, they are covered with a tacky polymeric film. As the tablets are dried, the applied coating changes from a sticky liquid to a tacky semisolid and then to a non-tacky dry surface. Tablets must be in constant motion to avoid agglomeration in early stages of drying. Tablets should preferably have rounded surfaces rather than flat faces with minimum edge thickness, to avoid sticking together.
4. The coating composition must wet the tablet surfaces so that it adheres to the face. Hydrophobic tablet surfaces are difficult to coat with aqueous coatings.

COATING EQUIPMENTS

COATING PANS:

The pan serves as a container for a batch of tablets and keeps them in continuous motion throughout the process. Designs of coating pans have undergone some major changes during the last 30 years.

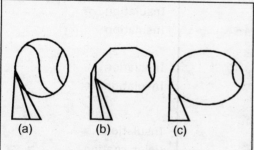

Fig. 3.1: Conventional coating pan
hapes a) Spherical,
b) Hexagonal,

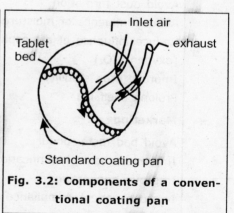

Standard coating pan

Fig. 3.2: Components of a conventional coating pan

A. Conventional Coating Pans:

The term is used to describe spherical, hexagonal or pear shaped pans as shown in Figure 3.1. The pan is mounted angularly on a stand. It is 8-60 inches in diameter.

The Pan is rotated on its horizontal axis by a motor. Hot air is directed inside it and onto the tablet bed; and spent air is let out via an exhaust, by means of ducts positioned through the front of the pan. Coating solutions are applied to tablets by ladling (pouring) or by spraying. Spraying significantly reduces drying time between two consecutive applications of coats.

1. Drying takes place mostly on the surface of the material and therefore, drying efficiency is low.

2. Mixing efficiency is poor. Many dead spots may exist in the product bed.

3. Improper balance between inlet and exhaust air can, with organic based solvent coatings, cause the solvent vapour to leak into the general coating area, posing health hazard and increasing risk of explosion.

B. Modified conventional coating pans:

Pellegrini pan: It is an angular coating pan that rotates on a horizontal axis. The pan has baffles and a diffuser that diffuses the air for drying uniformly. Access to the interior of the pan is both from front and back sides. Newer models are completely enclosed, which increases their drying efficiency. Mixing efficiency is improved due to baffles and drying efficiency is improved due to the diffuser. But drying is somewhat conventional.

Glatt immersion sword system: Drying Air is introduced through a perforated metal sword. This air flows upward from the sword through the tablet bed. There is intimate mixing of the drying air with the wet tablets, thus increasing efficiency of drying. Coating solution is sprayed by an atomised spray system.

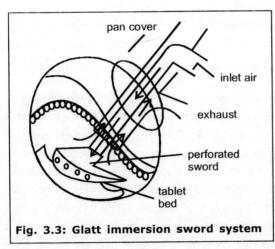

Fig. 3.3: Glatt immersion sword system

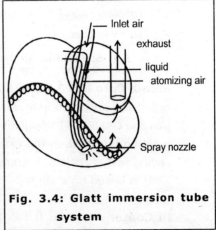

Fig. 3.4: Glatt immersion tube system

Glatt immersion tube system (Fig. 3.4): Drying air is introduced through a tube that is immersed in the tablet bed. Air flows up through the tablet bed. A spray nozzle is built in at the tip of this tube, which simultaneously sprays coating solution.

Both, the immersion sword and immersion tube systems can be adapted for conventional pans.

C. Perforated/side vented coating pans

In this system, the pan is perforated or partially perforated, angularly mounted and has baffles. Air is introduced into the interior of the pan, drawn through the product being coated and ultimately vented. Various approaches of handling airflow in side vented systems are shown in Figure 3.5.

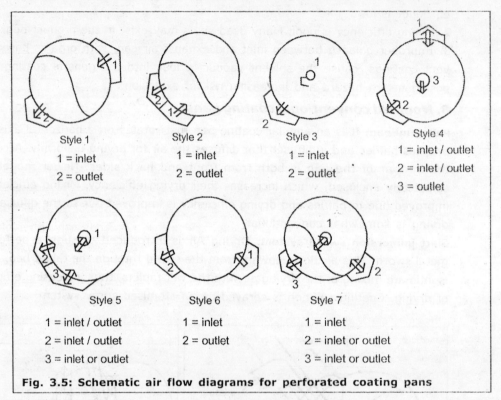

Style 1	Style 2	Style 3	Style 4
1 = inlet	1 = inlet	1 = inlet	1 = inlet / outlet
2 = outlet	2 = outlet	2 = outlet	2 = inlet / outlet
			3 = outlet

Style 5	Style 6	Style 7
1 = inlet / outlet	1 = inlet	1 = inlet
2 = inlet / outlet	2 = outlet	2 = inlet or outlet
3 = inlet or outlet		3 = inlet or outlet

Fig. 3.5: Schematic air flow diagrams for perforated coating pans

Accela Cota (Fig. 3.6): Air flow through the pan is facilitated by a fully perforated cylindrical portion of pan. Air is introduced by a plenum attached to the top of the pan and circulated through the pan and tablet bed. The air is then exhausted through a plenum located on the exterior of the pan in a position immediately below cascading bed of tablets. It conforms with airflow style no. 1. A modification of Accela Cota is based on style no. 2 for facilitating coating of granules. It is called Multi-Cota.

Hi Coater (Fig. 3.7): It has four perforated segments, located at a 90° angle to each other in the pan. Each of this perforated section acts as the opening to an

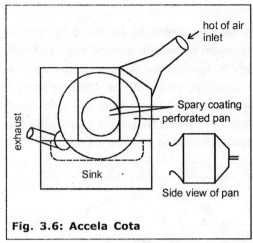

Fig. 3.6: Accela Cota

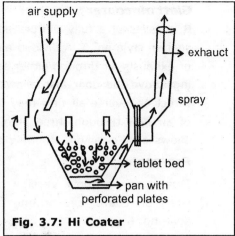

Fig. 3.7: Hi Coater

exhaust air duct fixed to the outside of the rotating pan and each duct makes contact with an exhaust plenum as the pan rotates. The exhaust plenum is designed to permit venting when the pan is between the 6 and 9 o'clock positions, as it rotates. Drying air is introduced through an opening located immediately above the door. Air flow conforms with style no. 3.

Driacoater (Fig. 3.8): Driacoater pan is nonagonal in shape. Attached to each of the nine flat sections is a perforated rib. This rib is linked via a duct to the exterior of the pan to one of the two air handling systems. Each of these air handling systems can produce positive or negative air flow, i.e., they can either blow air into, or exhaust air away, from the pan. A third air handling system present is connected to an opening at the back of the pan. This is capable only of exhausting air. This conforms with style no. 4 of the air handling system. It can achieve one of the three types of air flow mentioned below:

Direct air flow : Air enters the top through perforated ribs and out through ribs located below tablet bed.

Reverse air flow A : Air gets in through ribs located below tablet bed and gets out through ribs at the top of the pan.

Reverse air flow B : Air gets in through ribs located below tablet bed and gets out through plenum connected to opening at the back of the pan.

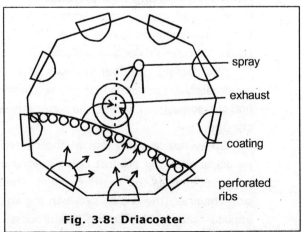

Fig. 3.8: Driacoater

Glatt air coater :

It consists of a fully perforated pan conforming to air handling capabilities as seen in style no. 5. A divided air plenum below the moving bed of tablets admits or exhausts air through either section. Another air plenum connected to an opening above the door also allows the air to blow into or exhaust from the pan. Direct or reverse air flow may be accomplished by any of the nine combinations of air flow through three plenums. The pan consists of gull-wing door, which allows easy cleaning. Its main drawback is that it is very expensive.

Pro-coater

This is an economy version of Glatt air coater conforming to style no. 6.

Huttlin Butterfly Pan

It consists of a series of large, angled, slotted openings in the pan wall at the junction of the cylindrical portion with each of the front or back panels. These openings exhaust the air from the pan. They are angled in such a way that during normal rotation, the tablets are prevented from entering the exhaust system. When coating is complete, reversal of pan causes the product to be emptied through the same slotted openings.

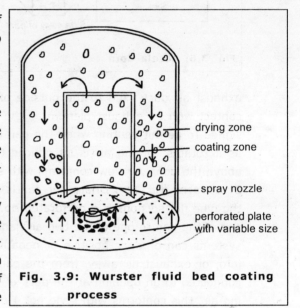

drying zone

coating zone

spray nozzle

perforated plate with variable size

Fig. 3.9: Wurster fluid bed coating process

Fluid-Bed Coating Equipments

Fluidised bed dryers, after addition of spray nozzles, can be used for granulation. Air suspension process specially modified for coating purpose was patented as 'Wurster Process' in 1950s.

The coating chamber consists of an inner partition whose diameter is approximately 50 per cent that of the coating chamber. Air distribution plate at the bottom consists of larger diameter holes at the centre than the ones at the periphery.

Spray nozzle is present at the center of the air distribution plate. Fluidising air accelerates the product being coated up through the inner partition. This can be considered as the coating region. The tablets decelerate in the outer expansion chamber (the region between the walls of the chamber and the insert). The applied coating dries during this process. The tablets move down quickly to the bottom of the coating chamber where they again enter the coating zone and receive next layer of coating.

Geometric limitations of Wurster design prevent the diameter of insert exceeding 9 inches. Therefore, in order to increase the capacity of the equipment, larger units are based on multiples of 9 inch, e.g. the 32 inch unit has a diameter of 32 inch, but contains three 9 inch inserts.

COATING EQUIPMENT ACCESSORIES

SPRAY APPLICATION SYSTEMS

There are mainly two types of spray application systems: High pressure airless spray systems and low pressure air atomised systems.

In airless spray, liquid is pumped at high pressure (250-3000 psig) through small orifice (0.009-0.02 inch id). If suspended solids are present in the coating formulation, they may block the small orifice.

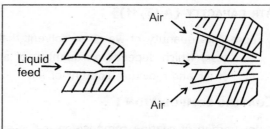

Fig. 3.10: Spray application systems
a) High pressure, airless,
b) low pressure, air automised

In low pressure air atomised system, liquid is pumped through a larger orifice (0.02-0.06 inch) at relatively low pressure (5-50 psig). Low pressure air (10-100 psig) contacts the liquid stream at the tip of the atomiser.

METERING/DELIVERY EQUIPMENT

These are the equipments used for delivering coating liquids from bulk tank to the application systems. They can be of following types-

- Pressurised Containers
- Gear pumps
- Peristaltic pumps
- Piston pumps

ANCILLARY EQUIPMENT

They include following equipments-

1. Equipments to prevent escape of organic solvents and particulate matter to atmosphere.
2. Recovery systems for organic solvents.
3. Tanks, filters and mixers for solution preparation.
4. Colloid mill/Ball mill for homogenising, coating liquid containing dispersed solids.
5. Jacketed kettles to keep solutions at elevated temperature.

PROCESS PARAMETERS:

The equilibrium between application of coating solution and evaporation of solvent should be maintained. The balance of coating process may be given as –

Inlet A (T_1, H_1) + $C_1(S)$ + pSA_1 —E-= A (T_2, H_2) + C_2 + pSA_2 Exhaust

Where,

A (T_1, H) = air capacity,

C(S) = coating composition

pSA = tablet surface area

E = efficiency of machine

AIR CAPACITY {A (T, H)} :

It represents quantity of water or solvent that can be removed during the coating process, which depends on quantity of air flowing through tablet bed, temperature of air and moisture content of air.

COATING COMPOSITION :

Major portion of coating composition is the solvent. Inlet air provides heat to evaporate the solvent and exhaust air becomes cooler as it contains the evaporated solvent. Tablet cores are permeable to solvents, thus causing coating difficulties.

If however, high temperatures are used to remove the solvent, it may be detrimental to the tablet core. The coating application may be continuous or intermittent. The drying characteristics of the film should be considered. Generally, viscous, aqueous-based coating utilise the movement of tablets outside the application zone, to produce partial distribution of coating, thereby requiring longer drying periods. Hence, intermittent coating application may be used. Thin, rapidly drying formulations dry quickly and require continuous application.

TABLET SURFACE AREA (pSA) :

With increase in tablet weight, tablet surface area per unit weight decreases rapidly. Therefore, application of film with the same thickness requires correspondingly less coating composition. Presence of atomised coating droplet must be smaller as the features to be coated become smaller.

COATING EFFICIENCY (E) :

It is obtained by dividing net increase in coated tablet weight by total non-volatile coating weight applied to tablets. Ideally, 90-95 per cent of applied coating should be deposited on tablets. Coating efficiency of sugar coating is low as compared to that of film coating (60 per cent). This is because application rate is too slow for coating conditions (large tablet surface area high air flow, high temperature). This results in drying of part of the coating composition before it reaches the tablet surfaces, so that it is exhausted as dust.

SUGAR COATING :

Sugar coating is one of the oldest pharmaceutical processes. Even though the process of sugar coating has modernised in recent years, it is still considered to be an art rather than a technology.

The process of sugar coating has experienced declining popularity, because of following reasons:

1. Efficiency of sugar coating largely depends on operator's skills.
2. There is a large increase in size and weight of the finished product.
3. The sugar-coated tablets are brittle.
4. The final gloss is achieved by polishing, which makes imprinting difficult.
5. The process is complicated and therefore, its automation is difficult.

But despite all these shortcomings, sugar coating is still being used for tablet coating because of the following reasons:

1. Equipments required are simple and inexpensive.
2. Raw materials have very few regulatory problems.
3. The main raw material (sugar) is inexpensive and easily available.
4. The coated tablets have excellent gloss and very good aesthetic appeal.

RAW MATERIALS

The major ingredient used is sugar. Apart from sugar, a variety of additives are needed for different steps of sugar-coating process.

Fillers :	Calcium carbonate, titanium dioxide, talc.
Film formers :	Acacia, gelatin, cellulosics.
Colorants :	Dyes, aluminium lakes, iron oxides, titanium dioxide.
Antiadherants :	Talc.
Flavours.	
Surfactants :	As suspending agents and wetting agents.

PROCESS

A sugar coating process goes through the following steps-

1. Sealing
2. Sub-coating
3. Grossing or syrup Coating
4. Colour coating
5. Polishing
6. Imprinting

The process requires repeated application of coating liquid. Each application, followed by a period, during which tablets are allowed to tumble to allow a complete distribution of coating material, followed by a drying period.

1. Sealing:

Most of the sugar-coating formulations are aqueous, while the tablet cores are porous, highly adsorbent and formulated to disintegrate on contact with water. If these cores are not protected, this ultimately affects the product stability. Sealing is done to offer this primary protection and to avoid migration of some of the core ingredients onto the surface.

Sealing is done by application of polymer, based in coating materials, viz., shellac, zein, polyvinyl phthalate (PVP), hydroxypropyl methylcellulose (HPMC), polyvenyl acetate phthalate (PVAP), cellulose acetate phthalate (CAP). They are prepared as 15-30 percent solution in some organic solvent.

Shellac undergoes polymerisation on storage and increases dissolution and disintegration time. This can be minimised by addition of PVP to shellac formulation or changing the sealant.

Sealing polymers must be used in minimum quantity to avoid increase in disintegration time. When seal coat is applied by ladling, de-tacking agents, such as talc, are used to avoid clumping or twinning.

If the final product is to have enteric properties, CAP or PVAP is used as sealant.

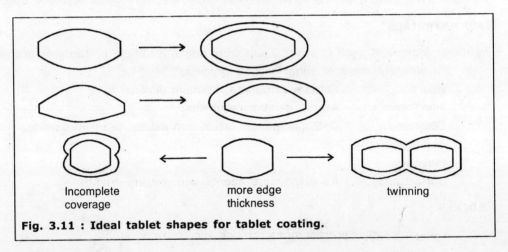

Incomplete coverage   more edge thickness   twinning

Fig. 3.11 : Ideal tablet shapes for tablet coating.

2. Sub-coating:

Sub-coating is done for rounding off the tablet edges and building up the core weight. It also provides a foundation for the remaining sugar coating process. In order to build up the weight, sub-coating formulations always contain high amounts of fillers, like Calcium sulphate, calcium carbonate, talc, kaolin and ancillary film formers, such as gelatin, acacia, tragacanth.

During sub-coating, effective coverage of the coating material must be achieved over the tablet edges. For this, selecting an appropriate shape for tablets, which minimises the number of corners, is important. Convex tablet shape is preferred over flat faced tablets. The convex shape minimizes the points of contacts of the adjacent tablets. It is also necessary to minimise the tablet edge thickness to avoid twinning and incomplete covering of the edges.

Two main approaches to the process of sub-coating are: Lamination process and suspension sub-coating.

Lamination process : This involves alternate applications of binder solution and dusting powder until the required level of coating is achieved. A careful balance should be maintained between relative amounts of binder solution and dusting powder. Under utilisation of dusting powder increases risk of sticking and twinning, over-dusting can give rise to tablets with brittle coating. Moreover, the process requires skilled operators as it is messy and difficult to operate.

Example of sub-coating formulation: in lamination process

Binder solution -

Gelatin -	3.3 %
Gum acacia -	8.7 %
Sucrose -	55.3 %
Distilled water-	32.7 %

Dusting powder -

Calcium Carbonate -	40 %
Titanium dioxide -	5 %
Talc -	25 %
Sucrose (powder) -	28 %
Gum acacia -	2 %

Suspension sub-coating process: In this, binder and powders are combined together. This decreases complexity of the process and it can be carried out by less skilled operators. It is also easy to automate the process.

Example of suspension sub-coating formulation

Sucrose -	40 %
Calcium carbonate -	20 %
Talc -	12 %
Titanium dioxide -	1 %
Gum acacia -	2 %
Distilled water -	25 %

3. Grossing (smoothening):

The surface of sugar coating must be smooth and free from irregularities prior to the application of colour coat. Sometimes, if some surface defects are seen even after sub-coating, further smoothening is necessary. Depending on the degree of smoothening, the formulation may consist of 70 percent sucrose syrup, often containing Titanium dioxide (TiO_2) as opacifier and possibly tinted with small concentration of colorant to provide a good base for subsequent application of colour coat. If substantial amount of coating is required, other additives such as talc, calcium carbonate ($CaCO_3$) or corn starch may be used in low concentrations.

4. Colour coating :

It is the most important step as it gives the final visual impact.

Two different approaches to colour coating exist. They use either water-soluble dyes or insoluble pigments.

Dye coating : Prior to 1950s, soluble dyes were used extensively. The process required high skill and was time consuming (2-3 days). And if not handled properly gave rise to mottled tablets since soluble dye can migrate during drying. Colour consistency from batch to batch was not predictable and sensitivity to light, with subsequent fading, was also a problem.

Pigment coating : This uses insoluble certified lakes. In this, colour migration on drying is eliminated, light stability is improved, mottling is rarely observed and coating time is shortened. A number of shades can be achieved by combining lakes with Titanium dioxide (TiO_2). The dispersion of colour must be uniform. To avoid non-uniformity of dispersion, nowadays, predispersed, opacified, ready to use colour concentrates are available.

However, pigment coated tablets are not as bright and clean looking as that of dye coated tablets.

5. Polishing (Glossing) :

Freshly colour-coated tablets are dull and mottled, and hence need to be polished to achieve the required gloss. Glossing can be carried out in various equipments, including canvas or wax lined pans and equipment used for sugar coating itself. Polishing systems include-

i) Organic solvent based solutions of waxes, beeswax, carnauba wax or candelilla wax.

ii) Alcoholic slurries of waxes.

iii) Finely powdered mixtures of dry waxes

iv) Pharmaceutical glazes (alcoholic solutions of shellac waxes).

6. Printing :

Printing is an optional step used for identification. It involves application of pharmaceutical branding ink to tablet surface by a process known as offset rotogravure.

Tablets may be printed before or after polishing. If printed before polishing, ink adheres well to tablet surface, but it may be subsequently removed by friction or contact with organic solvent during polishing. If printed after polishing, print rub-off problems do not exist, but ink does not always adhere well to polished tablets.

QUALITY PROBLEMS WITH SUGAR-COATED TABLETS :

1. Problems with tablet core :
Hardness, friability and lamination tendency of the tablet cores is very important. If not taken care of, tablet fragmentation may take place. The broken tablets may get glued to the surface of the undamaged tablets, thus spoiling significant amount of the batch.

2. Chipping of coat:
Sugar coatings are brittle and may undergo chipping. Addition of small concentrations of polymers, like PVP, cellulosics, acacia or gelatin to coating formulation helps avoid chipping.

3. Cracking of coats:
Tablet cores that expand, either during or after coating are likely to cause the coating to crack. The expansion of the tablet core may be a result of moisture absorption by core or stress relaxation of the core after compaction. Moisture sorption can be resolved by use of a seal coat and expansion after compaction can be resolved by extending the time between compaction and sugar-coating.

4. Non-drying coating:
Non-drying, sucrose-based sugar coatings are indication of presence of more than 5 percent of invert sugar. Inversion of sucrose is catalysed by keeping the sugar syrups at elevated temperatures, under acidic conditions, for extended periods of time. Such conditions occur when sugar coating solutions containing Aluminium lakes are kept hot for too long, or such sugar coating formulations are constantly reheated to re-dissolve sugar that is beginning to crystallise out.

5. Twinning (or build up of multiples):
Sugar coatings become very sticky when they begin to dry and allow the adjacent tablets to stick together. This becomes a problem when tablets being coated have flat surfaces, which can easily come in contact with each other. Appropriate choice of tablet shape can solve this problem.

6. Uneven colour (mottling):
This problem is observed particularly with darker shades. Many factors contribute to this problem.
i)   Poor distribution of coating liquid due to poor mixing of tablets or inadequate amount of coating liquid to coat completely the surface of every tablet in batch.
ii) Colour migration of soluble dyes during drying.
iii) Uneven surface of sub-coat when using dye-coating: This causes variation in thickness of the transparent colour layer that is perceived as different colour intensity.

---

iv) Washing back of pigment colour coatings:Pigments do not migrate on drying. But if excessive quantities of coating liquids are applied, there is a tendency of the previously applied and dried coating to re-dissolve and get distributed non-uniformly, giving rise to non-uniform appearance. This problem is particularly observed with Aluminium lake coatings, i.e., dark colours, where level of opacifier is low.

v) Excessive drying between colour applications causes erosion of colour layer and contributes to unevenness of the colour coat.

7. Blooming and Sweating :

Residual moisture in the finished sugar coated tablets can create problems. This moisture can diffuse out over a period of time and affect the quality of the product. Moderate levels of moisture cause the polished surface to take on a fogged appearance, which is called as 'blooming'. Higher levels of moisture may appear as beads of perspiration on tablet surface and is called 'sweating'. This may lead to sticking together of tablets stored in closed containers. Proper care must be taken by allowing drying at the end of each application of coating liquid.

8. Marbling:

The colour must be uniformly distributed, and at the same time a smooth coating surface must be obtained. If the surface is not sufficiently smooth, wax is collected in small surface depressions of a rough coating and is particularly evident by darker colourations.

FILM COATING

Film coating can be described as the process of application of thin (20-200 µm) polymer-based coating to tablets. Following conditions are essential for an efficient film coating process:

1. Balance between the rate of addition of coating liquid and the rate of drying.
2. Uniform distribution of coating liquid on the tablet surface.
3. Optimum aesthetic and functional qualities of the final coated product.

Film coating is now most commonly done by spray application systems.

The advantages of film coating over sugar coating processes are as follows-
1. Minimal weight gain in core tablets (only 2-3%)
2. Process is quicker compared to sugar-coating.
3. Process efficiency and output is excellent.
4. Core tablets become more resistant to chipping and cracking.
5. Formulation of film coating liquids is more flexible.

In the early years of film coating, organic solvents were being used more frequently due to their greater volatility and lesser drying times. But use of organic solvents led to many potential problems mentioned below:

1. Hazards due to their inflammable nature.
2. Toxicity hazards to personnel and environment.
3. Cost of solvents and added cost of using explosion-proof equipments.

But now film coating processes can be carried out successfully by using water as a solvent.

DEVELOPMENT OF FILM COATING FORMULATIONS :

The purpose of tablet coating must be clearly understood before one starts formulation of film coated tablets, i.e., whether film coating is being done for masking the colour, taste and odour or whether it is for sustained release. The shape, size and colour of tablets being coated should also be taken into account.

Different film coating formulations under consideration must be screened. The films are prepared by casting (spreading the coating formula on a teflon, glass or aluminium surface) or spraying. These films may then be tested using the following parameters-

1. Visual inspection - for separation of colorant or opaquant
2. Water vapour permeability - if the purpose of coating is to provide a sealed coat.
3. Tensile strength - elasticity and breaking strength is evaluated to study effect of varying concentrations of plasticizer.

COATED FILM EVALUATIONS :

Once the films are evaluated for screening, the coated tablets are evaluated for studying coating core interactions. Following tests are performed-

1. Adhesion tests with tensile strength testers are used to study the force required to peel the coating away from tablets.

2. Diametral crushing strengths are measured with hardness testers. Comparison with that of core tablets gives an idea about the increase in strength provided by coating.

3. Rate of disintegration is studied. Unless the tablet is for controlled release, the coating should not affect the rate of disintegration and dissolution.

4. Stability studies are carried out to study effect of moisture and temperature on film stability. Tablets are exposed to increasing humidity and moisture and weighed to study increase in weight.

5. Surface roughness, hardness and colour uniformity is examined visually. Many times, tablets are rubbed on white paper and checked for any colour that may get transferred to the paper.

MATERIALS USED IN FILM COATING

The coating material may be a physical deposition of the material on the tablet core or they form a continuous film. Ideal features of a film coating material are-

1. It should have an adequate solubility for the desired purpose, e.g. free water solubility for normal coated tablets, slow solubility for sustained release and pH-dependant solubility for enteric coating.
2. It should be soluble in desired solvent of the coating formulation.
3. It should produce an elegant film.
4. It should be stable in presence of heat, light, temperature, humidity, air and the tablet core.
5. It should be compatible with common coating formula ingredient.
6. It should be tasteless, colourless and odourless.
7. It should be non-toxic and should have no pharmacologic activity.
8. It should provide adequate moisture, light or odour barrier if required.
9. It should be resistant to cracking.
10. It should not fill the embossed monograms.
11. It should provide ease of printing.

The film coating liquids consist of polymers, solvents, plasticizers, colorants, opaquant extenders and some miscellaneous ingredients.

1. *Film formers-*

Table 3.2 lists some polymers used as film formers in conventional film coating

Table 3.2: Polymer used in conventional film coatings

Class	Example
1. Cellulosics	Hydroxypropyl methylcellulose, Hydroxypropyl cellulose Hydroxyethyl cellulose, Methylhydroxyethyl cellulose Methyl cellulose, Ethylcellulose, Sodium carboxymethyl cellulose
2. Vinyls	Polyvinyl pyrrolidone
3. Glycols	Polythylene glycols
4. Acrylates	Dimethylaminoethyl methacrylate - methylacrylate acid ester copolymer, Ethylacrylate - methylmetacrylate copolymer

i) Hydroxy Propyl methyl Cellulose : Prepared by reacting alkali treated cellulose first with methyl chloride and then with propylene oxide to introduce propylene glycol ether groups. It has good solubility characteristics in gastrointestinal fluids and in aqueous and non-aqueous solvent systems. Its advantages are-

- It does not interfere with tablet disintegration and drug availability.
- It is flexible, resistant to chipping, tasteless and odourless.
- It is stable in presence of heat, light, air and small quantities of moisture.
- Colour and other additives can be easily incorporated to it.

It is widely accepted for non-enteric film coating and if used alone, has a tendancy to fill and bridge the engravings. Therefore, used with other polymers or plasticizers.

ii) Methylhydroxyethyl cellulose : Prepared by reacting alkali treated cellulose first with methyl chloride and then with ethylene oxide. Being Structurally similar to HPMC, it is expected to have similar properties. Because of its solubility in only a few organic solvents, it is not used frequently.

iii) Ethylcellulose : It is manufactured by reaction of ethyl chloride or sulfate with cellulose dissolved in NaOH. Depending on the degree of ethoxylation, different viscosity grades are available commercially. They are completely insoluble in water and gastrointestinal fluid, therefore cannot be used alone. When combined with various aqueous soluble polymers, they are used for sustained release. It is soluble in a wide variety of organic solvents, is non-toxic, tasteless, colourless and odourless. Unplasticised films are brittle.

iv) Hydroxypropyl cellulose: It is manufactured by treatment of cellulose with NaOH, followed by reaction with propylene oxide at elevated temperature and pressure. It is soluble in water below 40°C, in gastrointestinal fluid and many polar organic solvents. Being extremely tacky as it dries, it may be used for subcoat, but not for colour coat. It is usually used in combination with other polymers to improve film characteristics.

v) Sodium Carboxymethyl Cellulose: It is manufactured by reacting soda cellulose with sodium salt of monochloroacetic acid, it is available in low, medium, high and extra high viscosity grades. It is easily dispersible in water to form colloid as solutions, but insoluble in most organic solvents. Films are brittle, but adhere well to tablets. Partially dried films are tacky and should be modified.

vi) Povidone: It is a synthetic polymer consisting of linear 1-vinyl-2-pyrrolidinone groups. Available in various molecular weight ranges and four different viscosities, i.e. K-15, K-30, K-60 and K-90 having approximate molecular weight of 10,000; 40,000, 1,60,000 and 3,60,000 respectively. It has excellent solubility in wide variety of organic solvents, water and in gastrointestinal fluids. Films are clear, glossy and hard. Polymer is extremely tacky, but can be modified by plasticizers or other polymers. It can be cross-linked with other polymers to produce films with enteric properties.

vii) Polyethylene glycols (PEGs): PEGs are manufactured by reaction of ethylene glycol with ethylene oxide in presence of NaOH at elevated temperature and pressure. Materials with low molecular weight (200-600) are liquid at room temperature and are used as plasticizers for coating solution films. Materials with high molecular weights (900 to 8000) are waxy solids. They are used with other polymers to modify film properties. Combination with Cellulose acetate phthalate provide films soluble in gastric fluids. Coats produced with high molecular weight PEGs are hard, smooth, tasteless and non-toxic, but somewhat sensitive to elevated temperatures.

viii) Acrylate Polymers : They are marketed under the trademark Eudragits. Eudragit E is the only material that is freely soluble in gastric fluid upto pH 5. It is available either as 12.5 percent organic solution in isopropyl alcohol/acetone or as a solid or 30 percent aqueous dispersion. Eudragit RL and RS are available only as organic solutions and solid materials. They are used for delayed action (pH-independent) coatings.

2. *Solvents*

After the rise in importance of aqueous film coating, the question of solvent selection got eliminated. But certain types of film coating processes require use of some organic solvents.

A solvent dissolves or disperses the polymers and other additives, conveying them to the substrate surface. Ideal features of a solvent are-

1. It should either dissolve or disperse the polymer.
2. It should disperse the other coating components as well.
3. A small concentration of polymer should not result in highly viscous solution.
4. It should be colourless, odourless, tasteless, inexpensive, non-toxic, inert and non-inflammable.
5. It should have a rapid drying rate.
6. It should be environmentally safe. Some commonly used solvents are listed in Table 3.3

Table 3.3: Commonly used solvents in film coating.

Class	Example
1. Water	-
2. Alcohols	Methanol, Ethanol, Isopropanol
3. Esters	Ethyl acetate, Ethyl lactate
4. Ketones	Acetone
5. Chlorinated hydrocarbons	Methylene chloride, 1:1:1 Trichloroethane

3. *Plasticizers*

The film quality can be modified by internal or external plasticising. Internal plasticising is the chemical alteration in the polymer to change its physical properties. This can be accomplished by controlling degree of substitution, type of substitution and polymer chain length. Alternatively the film properties can also be modified by adding external plasticizer, which is either non-volatile liquid or a second polymer. It is incorporated along with the primary polymer to alter its film flexibility tensile strength and adhesion properties.

After removal of solvent, polymeric materials pack to form a 3-D honeycomb like matrix structure. The plasticizer solvates the polymer and alters polymer-polymer interactions. When incorporated in correct proportions, plasticizers impart flexibility by relieving molecular rigidity. The type of plasticizer and its concentration, in relation to the polymer, should be optimized.

A combination of plasticizers may also be used. Its concentration depends on chemistry of polymer, method of application and other additives. The drying rate and temperature can also affect the plasticizer. Presence of colorants, flavours and other additives also affect the plasticizer. Recommended concentrations of plasticizer range from 1-50 percent by weight of the film former. Some commonly used plasticizers are castor oil, glycerin, propylene glycol, polyethylene glycol of 200-400 series and surfactants like tweens (polysorbates) and spans (sorbitans) and organic acid esters. Polyethylene glycol and propylene glycol are aqueous based plasticizers. Castor oil and spans are used for organic coatings.

The plasticizer and the film former must be at least partially soluble in the solvent.

Table 3.4: Plasticizers used in conventional film coating

Class	Example
1. Polyhydric alcohols	Polyethylene glycols, Glycerin, Propylene glycol
2. Acetate esters	Glyceryl acetate (Triacetin), Triethyl citrate
	Acetyl triethyl citrate
3. Phthalate esters	Diethylphthalate
4. Oils	Castor oil, Mineral oil

4. *Colorants*

Colorant may be soluble in solvent or may be dispersed.

They are used for product identification and aesthetic appeal. For proper distribution, the colorants must be finely powdered (<10m). The dye content, crystal form of dye and particle size distribution should be controlled to control batch-to-batch variation in colour.

The widely used colorants are-

Food, Drug & Cosmetic (FD&C) and D&C dyes- either dyes, or lakes of these dyes, precipitated on alumina or talc. More reproducible colours are achieved with lakes and therefore they are preferred. Lakes may contain 10-30 percent and sometimes 50 percent of the dye. Sometimes the solvent system may leach out the dye from the lake, depending on temperature and time. In such cases, pure dyes should be used.

Concentration of the colorant depends on the shade desired, type of colourant, i.e., dye or lake and concentration of opaquant extender. The concentration may range in between 0.01-2 percent. Lakes contain lesser amount of colour and therefore require higher concentration in solution.

Inorganic colourants, e.g. iron oxides and natural colorants (anthocyanins, caramel, carotenoids, chlorophyll, flavones, indigo, turmeric and carminic acid) may also be used.

Newly developed colorants are non-absorbable colourants. They are prepared by attaching dyes to long, high molecular weight polymers, which are too big to be absorbed in gastrointestinal tract and yet are resistant to degradation.

Some commercial colorants are available as colour concentrates, which do not require additional milling equipments, e.g. Opalux, Opaspray, Opadry

5. *Opaquant Extenders*

These are fine inorganic powders used to achieve pastel shades and increase film coverage. They provide a white coating or mask the colour of the core. Opaquants are much cheaper than colorants and less colorants are required if opaquants are used.

Most commonly used opaquants are Titanium dioxide; other materials are silicates (talc, aluminium silicate), magnesium carbonate, calcium sulfate, magnesium oxide and aluminium hydroxide.

6. *Miscellaneous* -

i)   Flavours and sweeteners.

ii) Surfactants to solubilise insoluble ingredients.

iii) Oxidants to stabilise dye to oxidation and colour change

iv) Antimicrobials to prevent microbial attack on coating formulation during preparation and storage.

v)   Suspending agents.

MODIFIED RELEASE / FUNCTIONAL FILM COATINGS

Film coating technique may be used to modify the release of the active ingredient from the tablet. Two types of dosage forms may be considered as modified release dosage forms:

    A. Enteric release

    B. Sustained/Controlled release.

A. ENTERIC FILM COATINGS -

Enteric coating may be done for stabilising the drug in acidic pH of gastrointestinal tract (GIT) or protection against local irritation by or for the drug release in specific part of GIT.

Stomach pH is around 1-3 and intestinal pH is significantly higher. The GIT time for passage of dosage form through the stomach varies, depending on its size and presence of food. Most drugs are absorbed in upper part of the intestine due to its large surface area. Enteric coating may be of different types:

One layer system : Coating formulation applied in one layer which can be white, opaque or coloured. Only one application is required.

Two layer system: To prepare enteric tablets of high aesthetic appeal, enteric formulation is applied first followed by coloured film. Both layers may contain an enteric polymer, or only basic layer contains enteric polymer.

For pH sensitive drugs such as enzymes, the usual pH 2-3 of aqueous dispersion of Eudragit may be increased to 5.2 by neutralising 6 mole per cent of carboxylic groups, to prevent inactivation of drug by penetration of acid into core during coating.

Reasons for enteric coating are-

1. To protect acid-labile drugs from gastric environment, e.g. enzymes
2. To prevent gastric distress or nausea due to irritation from drugs, e.g. sodium salicylate.
3. For local action of drugs in intestine, e.g. intestinal antiseptics.
   To deliver drugs which are better absorbed in small intestine.
4. To provide the delayed release component for repeat action tablets.

The ideal properties of an enteric coating material are :
i) Resistance to gastric fluids and ready permeability to intestinal fluids.
ii) Compatibility with coating solution components and additives.
iii) Stability alone and in coating solutions.
iv) Formulation of continuous film.
v) Non-toxicity.
vi) Low cost.
vii) Ease of application.
viii) Ease of printing.

The enteric coating materials range from water resistant films to pH sensitive materials. Some are digested or emulsified by intestinal fluids, while some slowly swell and fall apart when solvated. Many times a combination of these two mechanisms is used.

U.S.P. disintegration test for enteric coated tablets requires the tablets to remain intact for one hour in simulated gastric juice and then to disintegrate within two hours in a simulated intestinal fluid. But passing U.S.P. test does not ensure optimum bioavailability of the drug from a tablet. pH of stomach varies 1.5 to 4.0, from person to person and for the same individual from time to time. Gastric residence time may vary from less than half an hour to four hours, depending on time of administration, presence of food and type and quantity of food. Several commercial enteric coated products, although having passed U.S.P. disintegration test, release varying amounts of drug in enteric fluid. Acid labile drugs require protection between pH 1 and 5 and should be released when pH of pylorus, i.e., 5, is achieved. Therefore an ideal enteric polymer should dissolve near pH 5.

The retardant type of polymers, having non pH-dependent solubility, act by mechanical hydrophobicity. If the dosage form travels too fast from stomach to intestine, and if the coating film is too thick, solubilisation of polymer in intestine is never achieved.

Table 3.5: Commonly used polymers for enteric film coating

1.	Cellulose acetate phthalate (CAP)
2.	Cellulose acetate trimellitate (CAT)
3.	Polyvinyl acetate phthalate (PVAP)
4.	Hydroxypropyl methylcellulose phthalate ((HPMCP)
5.	Hydroxypropyl methylcellulose succinate (HPMCAS)
6.	Poly (Methacrylic acid - Methylmethacrylate) 1:1
7.	Poly (Methacrylic acid - Methylmethacrylate) 1:2

1. Cellulose acetate phthalate (CAP):

It has a disadvantage of dissolving only above pH 6. It is hygroscopic and relatively permeable to moisture and gastric fluid. CAP films may lose phthalic and acetic acid groups on hydrolysis, which changes the film's properties. They are brittle and usually formulated with hydrophobic materials to achieve a better film. An aqueous coating material is available as Aquateric. It is a reconstituted colloidal dispersion of latex particles. It is composed of solid or semisolid polymer spheres of CAP ranging in size from 0.05-3 μ.

2. Acrylate polymers:

Two forms of acrylates used are Eudragit L and Eudragit S. Both produce films resistant to gastric fluid and soluble in intestinal fluid at pH 6 and 7 respectively.

3. Hydroxypropyl methyl cellulose (HPMCP) phthalate :

They are available as three enteric coating polymers obtained by reaction of HPMC by esterification with phthalic anhydride and are marketed as HP-50, HP-55 and HP-55-S. They dissolve at a lower pH (5-5.5) than CAP or acrylate and therefore may provide better bioavailability of some specific drugs. They are quite stable compared to CAP because of absence of labile groups.

4. Polyvinyl acetate phthalate (PVAP):

It is obtained by esterification of partially hydrolysed PVA with phthalic anhydride. It is similar to HP-55 in stability and pH dependent solubility.

B. SUSTAINED RELEASE/CONTROLLED RELEASE FILM COATINGS:

Drug release from sustained release dosage forms is moderated by polymers, which act as membranes that allow infusion of gastrointestinal fluids and the outward diffusion of dissolved drug. Table 3.6 lists some materials used in sustained release film coatings:

Table 3.6: Film forming polymers for sustained release

Class	Example
Fats and Waxes (beeswax, carnavba, wax, Cetyl alcohol, cetostearyl alcohol)	Permeable and Erodible
Shellac	Permeable and soluble
Zein	Permeable and soluble
Ethyl cellulose	Permeable
Cellulose esters	Semipermeable
Silicone elastomers	Permeable (with PEG)
Acrylic esters	Permeable

QUALITY CONTROL OF COATED TABLETS

STANDARDS FOR COATED TABLETS :

The evaluation procedures for tablets have been already discussed in depth in Chapter 2. Although, there are some differences in standards for coated and uncoated tablets as per U.S.P. and I.P. as follows- The evaluation parameters that differ for coated and uncoated tablets are discussed here. The evaluation parameters that are not mentioned here remain the same for uncoated and coated tablets.

1. I.P. procedure for Sugar/Film Coated Tablets :

If the coated tablets have a soluble external coating, they are to be immersed in water at room temperature for five minutes. And then the disintegration test is carried out in water at 37 $\pm$ 2°C for 30 minutes for sugar-coated tablets and 60 minutes for film-coated tablets. Unless otherwise indicated in individual monograph, if the tablets fail to disintegrate in water, the test is to be repeated using 0.1 N Hydrochloric acid as immersion medium.

2. U.S.P. procedure for Sugar/Film Coated Tablets:

If the coated tablets have a soluble external coating, they are to be immersed in water at room temperature for five minutes. Then the disintegration test is carried out in simulated gastric fluid at 37 $\pm$ 2°C for 30 minutes. If the tablets fail to disintegrate, the medium is replaced with simulated intestinal fluid at 37 $\pm$ 2°C. The test is continued for total period of time, including previous exposure to water and simulated gastric fluid, equal to the time specified in individual time plus 30 minutes.

3. I.P. Procedure for Enteric Coated Tablets:

If the tablet has soluble exterior coating, it is to be immersed in water for 5 minutes at room temperature. Then, the test is continued using 0.1 N HCl at 37 $\pm$ 2°C as immersion fluid. The tablets must not disintegrate within 2 hours. After two hours, immersion fluid is replaced with phosphate buffer pH 6.8 at 37 $\pm$ 2°C. The tablets must disintegrate within one hour, unless otherwise specified in the individual monograph.

4. U.S.P. Procedure for Enteric Coated Tablets:

If the tablet has soluble external coating, it is to be immersed in water for 5 minutes at room temperature. Then the test is continued using simulated gastric fluid at 37 $\pm$ 2°C as immersion fluid. The tablets must not disintegrate within one hour. The immersion fluid is now replaced with simulated intestinal Fluid. The tablets should now disintegrate within time specified in the individual monograph.

Table 3.7: Comparison of disintegration time test for uncoated tablets and coated tablets as per I.P. and U.S.P.

	Uncoated tablet	Coated tablet I.P.	Coated tablet U.S.P.
Immersion medium	Water	i) Water at room temperature ii) 0.1N HCl at 37 + 2°C	i) Water at room temperature ii) Simulated gastric fluid at 37 $\pm$ 2°C iii) Simulated intestinal fluid at 37 $\pm$ 2°C
Limit	15 minutes (I.P.) As per individual monograph (U.S.P.)	- 30 minutes for sugar coated - 60 minutes for film coated	As per individual monograph

Table 3.8: Comparison of disintegration time test for enteric coated tablets as per I.P. and U.S.P.

	I.P.	U.S.P.
Immersion medium	1. Water at room temperature 2. 0.1N HCl at 37 $\pm$ 2°C 3. Phosphate buffer pH 6.8 at 37 $\pm$ 2°C	1. Water at room temperature 2. Simulated gastric fluid at 37 $\pm$ 2°C 3. Simulated intestinal fluid at 37 $\pm$ 2°C
Limit	1. Tablets must not disintegrate in 0.1N HCl with 2 hours 2. Tablets should disintegrate in phosphate buffer within 1 hour	1. Tablets must not disintegrate in simulated gastric fluid within 1 hour 2. Tablets should disintegrate in simulated intestinal fluid in time as indicated in individual monograph.

STABILITY TESTING

For determination of shelf-life and expiry date of coated products under normal and exaggerated storage conditions, Accelerated Stability Test (AST) may be carried out at elevated temperature, humidity and light exposure. Potency data is evaluated by using Arrhenius plots.

In the developmental stage, stability program may be used to test variation in formulation process. On ageing, a particular variation may give rise to physical instability of film, i.e., colour changes or chemical degradation of active ingredient.

DEFECTS IN FILM-COATED TABLETS

Several types of defects may be observed in film coated tablets due to following reasons-

1. Replacement of organic solvents with water. Water has more latent heat of evaporation and therefore, drying must be closely monitored.
2. Improper porosity and surface texture of core tablet.
3. Viscosity and surface tension of coating liquid.
4. Low strength of core or coating film.

Commonly found film coating defects are as follows-

A. STICKING AND PICKING :

Sticking and picking is a result of sticking of tablets with each other or with the coating pan due to over-wetting of tablets or excessive tackiness of the coating solution. After drying, the tablets may separate with a piece of film remaining adhered to the coating pan or to the other tablet, at the point of contact. In extreme cases, flat faced tablets may remain permanently attached to each other, causing a defect called 'twinning'.

Over-wetting may take place when the spray rate is excessive. Spray nozzles used may also cause localised over-wetting. The problem can be resolved by reducing the spray application rate, increasing the number of spray nozzles or increasing the drying air temperature or volume.

Certain types of formulations are inherently tackier, giving rise to this problem.

B. ROUGHNESS :

When the coating formulation is being applied as a spray, some of the spray droplets may become dry even before they reach the tablet bed. These dried particles are deposited on the tablet bed rather than droplets, giving the tablet a rough appearance.

Formation of excessively fine droplets is the reason for this defect. It may be resolved by using nozzles with larger aperture size, or moving the nozzles away from the tablet bed.

Surface roughness may also be caused due to higher concentration of pigments and polymers in coating formula.

C. Orange Peel Effect :

Inadequate spreading of the coating solution before drying causes a bumpy, uneven tablet surface. Inadequate spreading may be a result of too rapid drying or too high solution viscosity.

D. Edge Wear (Chipping) :

Tablets have to undergo attrition stress when they tumble in coating pans. Tablet edges are the most susceptible parts to this attrition. Thus fractures may develop at these points, exposing the tablet core.

This problem arises due to tablet cores having high friability, worn out tablet punches or brittle film coatings.

E. Blistering:

Coated tablets sometimes require further drying in ovens. Too rapid solvent evaporation from the core may cause blisters. Milder drying conditions should be used to combat this problem.

F. Hazing/dull film (Bloom):

The film coating may look dull when exposed to excessively high temperatures. The problem is particularly evident when coating polymer is a cellulosic, being applied in an aqueous medium. Exposure of tablets to high humidity also causes this defect due to partial solution of films.

G. Cracking:

When the internal stress that develops within the coating during drying exceeds the tensile strength of the coating, the film may develop cracks. These problems are absolutely unacceptable when the applied coating is functional. The problem is mainly due to brittleness of coating or significant differences in coefficients of expansion of the core and coating.

Tensile strength of film may be increased by using higher molecular weight polymers or polymer blends and adjusting the plasticizer type and concentration.

H. Logo bridging (Intagliation):

During drying, the internal stress in the film becomes so high that it causes partial or complete detachment of the coating in the region of the logo. Legibility of logo is significantly reduced. The problem may be solved by improving film adhesion or reducing stress within the film.

I. IN FILLING OF LOGOS:

It is visually similar to logo bridging. But the reason for this problem is the application of high amount of solution or at excessive rate, resulting in a thick film that fills the monogram.

J. COLOUR VARIATION:

The problem may arise due to processing or formulation defects. Improper mixing of the colouring pigment, uneven spraying and insufficient coating may cause this problem. Soluble dyes, plasticizers and other soluble components may migrate during drying, giving a mottled appearance to the tablet. Use of a lake instead of a dye, or reformulation with different plasticizers is a solution to overcome this problem.

SPECIALISED COATING

A. COMPRESSION COATING :

Compression coated tablets have been discussed in detail in Chapter 2.

B. ELECTROSTATIC COATING :

A strong electrostatic charge is applied to the surface. The charge is opposite to the charge on the ionic species present in the coating material. Complete and uniform coating on corners and monograms may be achieved. Pharmaceutical tablets are relatively non-conductive species. Therefore this process can be rarely used.

C. DIP COATING:

Coating is applied by dipping the tablet cores in coating solution. Tablets are then dried in conventional coating pans. Alternative dipping and drying operations are carried out. This process lacks speed, versatility and reliability.

D. VACUUM FILM COATING :

This is a new technique used for coating. A specially designed pan is used. The pan has baffles and is jacketed for holding hot water. It can be sealed to create vacuum. After sealing the pan, air is removed and displaced by nitrogen till the vacuum is drawn. Coating material is sprayed with the help of airless spray systems. Instead of using high speed, hot air drying is carried out in heated pan. Thus energy requirements are low and efficiency is high. Organic solvents may be used conveniently with minimum environmental and safety considerations and can be recycled.

Capsules

INTRODUCTION

The word 'capsule' in English language is derived from the Latin word *capsula*, which means a small box or a container. In pharmacy, capsule is the word used to describe a solid dosage form which consists of a container, usually made of gelatin, filled with a medicinal substance. The word can be used to refer either to the gelatin container itself or to the whole object container plus the drug.

TYPES OF CAPSULES :

Capsules are basically categorised into two different classes, hard and soft. The hard gelatin capsules consist of two separate parts that are semi-cylindrical in shape. One part is called the cap, which is shorter and has a slightly larger diameter than the other, called the body. The cap fits closely over the body to form a closed unit.

Soft gelatin capsule is a one-piece container having a variable shape and either has a seam along its axis or is seamless. Glycerol is used as plasticiser in the shells of soft gelatin capsules, to make the shell soft and elastic.

Mothes and Dublanc, two Frenchmen, are credited with the invention of gelatin capsules. James Murdock of London, invented the two piece telescopic capsule in 1848 that was patented in 1865.

ADVANTAGES :

Capsules as pharmaceutical dosage forms have following advantages:-
1. They provide a smooth, slippery and tasteless dosage form for drugs.
2. They efficiently mask the bad taste, colour or odour of drugs.

3. They are elegant and available in wide range of colours.
4. They are economical to produce in large quantities.
5. They are easy to use and portable.
6. They are easy to swallow due to their elongated shape.
7. The contained drug becomes readily available as the shell is highly soluble.
8. Minimum excipients and little pressure are required to compact the material, as opposed to tabletting.

DISADVANTAGES

Capsules have following disadvantages-
1. They cannot be used for highly soluble materials like potassium chloride or ammonium chloride, since the sudden release of these compounds into the stomach may cause irritation.
2. They cannot be used for highly efflorescent materials as they cause the shell to soften.
3. They cannot be used for deliquescent materials as they dry the capsule shell to excessive brittleness.
4. Capsules are not tamperproof and if any tampering is done with the contents, it is not evident.

MATERIALS :

The empty capsule shells are made principally of gelatin and may contain small amounts of plasticisers, colorants and preservatives.

GELATIN :

Gelatin is the major component of the capsules. Several other materials have been tried for making capsules. But gelatin is the only material that has proved to be successful. Following are the reasons for this:
1. Gelatin is readily soluble in biological fluids at body temperatures.
2. It is a good film-forming material.
3. It is non-toxic. It is used in food stuffs and is acceptable for use in all countries in the world.
4. Solution of glycerin in water undergoes a phase change from sol to gel, at a temperature that is slightly above the ambient temperatures. Many other polymers used for forming films require either evaporation of large amounts of volatile organic solvents or large quantities of heat. Therefore, film formation is relatively easy with gelatin.

Gelatin is a substance of natural origin. But it does not occur as such in nature. It is derived from the fibrous protein collagen, which is the principal constituent of

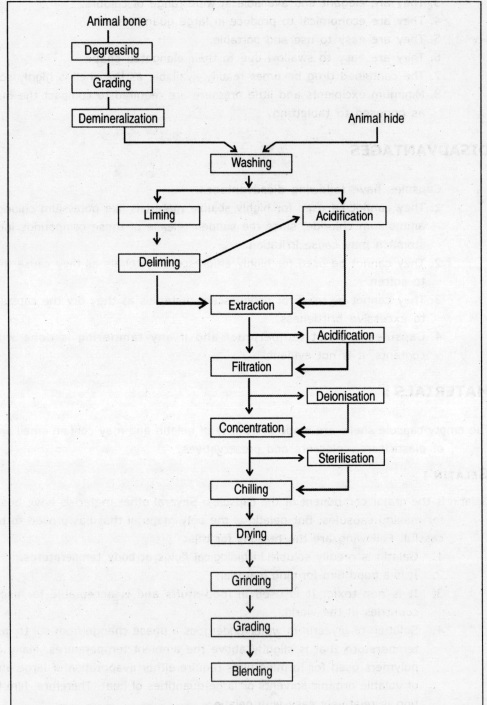

Figure 4.1 A flow sheet of the commercial process for conversion of collagen into gelatin.

animal skin, bone and connective tissue. Gelatin is obtained by irreversible hydrolytic extraction of collagen. Physicochemical properties of gelatin mainly depend on the parent collagen, method of extraction, pH value and electrolyte content. The main raw materials for sources of collagen are cattle skin (hide), cattle bones and pigskin. Depending upon the method of hydrolysis, it is either Type A gelatin or Type B gelatin.

Type A gelatin is manufactured by acid hydrolysis and Type B gelatin is prepared by base hydrolysis. The choice of method depends on the nature of raw materials. Skins are usually acid hydrolysed, while bones are base hydrolysed.

Type B gelatins are usually derived from animal bones. Either dried bones or fresh bones ('green' bones) may be used as raw materials. Bones are milled. Fresh bones require a pretreatment to remove adhering moisture and fat which is called degreasing. After degreasing, bones are graded into hard bones, soft bones and sinew fraction. The graded bones are then demineralised to free collagen from the inorganic portion (calcium phosphate and carbonates). This is achieved by treatment with dilute hydrochloric acid. This dissolves tricalcium phosphate to the monocalcium salt :

$$Ca_3(PO_4)_2 + 4HCl \longrightarrow Ca(H_2PO_4)_2 + 2\,CaCl_2$$

After demineralisation, the collagen is limed to condition it, so that gelatin with the desired physical properties is obtained in good yield. Collagen stock is soaked in slaked lime slurry (2-5 per cent) for 4-8 weeks. Liming hydrolyses collagen. After the liming process, the lime is removed by washing with water for about 24 hours. The pH at this stage is 9-10. The material is now neutralised to pH 5-6.5 by washing with acid.

Soaking collagen in acid (9 per cent HCl), prior to liming, significantly reduces the liming period.

Type A gelatins are usually derived by acid treating the animal skins. The collagen is brought to low pH by treating with acid for 24 hours. The process, therefore, is much shorter than liming process. But it is usually restricted to animal skins to achieve reasonable yields and quality.

The gelatin so formed is now extracted by either acid extraction or neutral extraction. The extract contains suspended collagen particles and fat globules. It is clarified and pressure-filtered through sterile compressed pads of cellulose pulp. The filtered gelatin is concentrated by evaporation under vacuum. The concentrated extract is dried by chilling to form a gel which is then air-dried. The dried gelatin films are now milled to form crumbs, sieved and then packed.

Type A gelatin shows an isoelectric point in the range of pH 9; whereas, type B gelatin has its isoelectric point in the range of pH 4.7. The usual practice is to use a mixture of both types, taking into consideration their availability and cost. Blends of bone and pork skin gelatins, of relatively high gel strength, are normal-

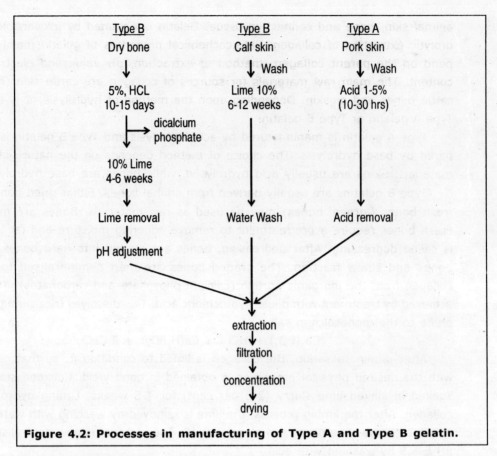

Type B	Type B	Type A
Dry bone	Calf skin	Pork skin
	↓ Wash	↓ Wash
5%, HCL 10-15 days	Lime 10% 6-12 weeks	Acid 1-5% (10-30 hrs)

→ dicalcium phosphate

10% Lime
4-6 weeks

Lime removal → Water Wash → Acid removal

pH adjustment

→ extraction
→ filtration
→ concentration
→ drying

Figure 4.2: Processes in manufacturing of Type A and Type B gelatin.

ly used for hard capsule production. Bone gelatin produces tough, firm films that are hazy and brittle. Pork skin gelatin films are more plastic and clear.

Table 4.1 : Specifications of gelatin for soft and hard capsules as per IP and USP

Test	USP	IP
Clarity, colour (in solution)	Slightly opalescent	Opalescent
Odour (2.5% solution)	not disagreeable	very slight
pH (1% solution)	--	Betn 3.8 to 7.6
Gel strength, (g)	--	150 to 250 g
Ash % max	2.0	3.25
Sulphur dioxide, ppm max	40	200
Arsenic, ppm max	0.8	2
Heavy metals, ppm max	50	50
Microbiological standards		
Total count, orgs/gm, max	1000	1000
E. Coli	*absent in 10 gm*	*absent in 1 gm*
Salmonellae	absent in 10 gm	absent in 10 gm

Two recent developments in gelatin production are-

1. Use of 'green' or fresh bones, as already mentioned.
2. Processing of 'acid bone gelatin' by techniques used for type A gelatin.

Tests and Specifications for gelatin :

The properties of gelatin that are most important for capsule manufacture are gel strength (bloom strength) and viscosity.

Bloom strength is determined by measuring the load in grams required to depress the surface of a 6.67 per cent w/w gel, matured at 10°C for 16-18 hours, by a distance of 4 mm, using a flat-bottomed plunger, 12.7 mm in diameter. Gelatin used for hard capsules is high bloom strength (230-275 gm) and that for soft capsules is low bloom strength (150-195 gm).

Viscosities of gelatin solutions are routinely measured of 6.67 per cent w/w solution at 60°C using Ostwald or Pipette viscometer. Viscosity should be around 4.3-4.7 millipoise (mPs) for hard capsules and 2.7-3.6 mPs for soft capsules. Table 4.1 shows specifications of gelatin for soft and hard capsules, as per I.P. and U.S.P.

PLASTICISERS

A plasticiser reduces the rigidity of the capsule wall and makes it pliable. Hard gelatin capsules are hard and firm, while soft capsules are more soft and flexible. Soft gelatin capsule is manufactured and filled in one operation, which results in the pressure of the contents maintaining the capsule shape. Hard capsules may or may not contain less than 5 per cent w/w of plasticisers; whereas, soft capsules contain around 20-40 per cent w/w of plasticiser.

Glycerin is the most widely used plasticiser. Its concentration is varied to produce capsule for different applications (Table 4.2).

Table 4.2 : Plasticiser content of soft capsules

Glycerol : gelatin ratio (parts of dry glycerol per part of dry gelatin	Applications
0.35	Oral capsule for filling oils where final capsule is hard.
0.46	Oral capsule for filling oils where final capsule is elastic.
0.55 - 0.65	Oil containing capsules with added surfactants of hydrophilic liquids.
0.76	Oral capsules with chewable shell.

Sorbitol, propylene glycol, sucrose and acacia may also be used as plasticisers. Certain other materials have been claimed to enhance the effect of the main plasticiser in concentrations of 2.6 per cent. These include glycine, mannitol, acetamide, formamide and lactamide.

Colouring agents :

Capsules are coloured for aesthetic effects, for identification and for psychological effects on patients. Colorants used for capsules are synthetic water soluble dyes, pigments and certain dyes of natural origin. Synthetic soluble dyes used are azo, indigoid, quinophthalone, triphenylmethane and xanthene dyes. They can be blended to achieve different shades.

Pigments used are of two types. The one which is used most widely, titanium dioxide, is also an opacifier. The other class of pigments are inorganic oxides. Black, red and yellow oxides of iron are the most widely used.

Curcumin and Carotenoids are the naturally occurring colorants that may be used for capsules.

The list of permitted colours varies from country to country. Ten most widely accepted colorants are listed in Table 4.3.

Table 4.3 : Ten most acceptable colorants worldwide

Dye	Colour	Dye	Colour
Titanium dioxide	White	Tartrazine	Yellow
Erythrosine	red	Yellow iron Oxide	Yellow
Indigo carmine	blue	Black Iron Oxide	Black
Red iron Oxide	red	Ponceau 4 R	Red
Sunset yellow FCF	orange	Canthaxanthine	Orange

Preservatives :

Gelatin, in presence of moisture, is a good medium for bacterial growth. Sulphur dioxide is most widely used as a preservative, added in the form of a solution of sodium sulphate, or sodium metabisulphite. Quantity used is less than 1000 ppm, calculated as sulphur dioxide.

Table 4.4 Materials for manufacturing of empty gelatin capsule shells.

Class	Examples
1. Gelatin	Cattle skin gelatin, bone gelatin, pig skin gelatin
2. Plasticisers	Glycerin, sorbitol, propylene glycol, sucrose, acacia
3. Colouring agents	
a) Synthetic dyes	Erythrosine, tartrazine, ponceu 4R, sunset Yellow
b) Pigments	Titanium dioxide
c) Natural dyes	Curcumin, carotenoids
4. Preservatives	Sodium sulphite, Sodium metabisulphite, Methyl Paraben, Propyl paraben, Benzoic, Propionic, sorbic acid and their sodium salts.
5. Process aids	
surfactants :	Sodium lauryl sulphate
aid enteric release	Silicone fluid
6. Performance aid :	flavouring agents Vanillin, peppermint oil, menthol

Methyl paraben and propyl paraben in a 4:1 ratio is used upto 0.2 per cent w/v concentration. Organic acids such as benzoic, propionic and sorbic acids and their sodium salts may be used upto 1 per cent w/v concentration.

Process and Performance Aids :

Substances used to aid in the manufacturing process (process aids) are of two types - surfactants which help the gelatin solution to take the shape of the moulds better and substances that enable the capsules to be further processed, e.g. silicone fluid for formaldehyde treatment of capsules for sustained release.

Performance aids improve patient acceptability, e.g. flavouring agents such as vanillin or volatile oils, added to the gelatin capsule shells, to mask the objectionable odour of fill material such as antibiotics. Table 4.4 summarises different materials in manufacturing of empty gelatin capsules.

HARD GELATIN CAPSULES

CAPSULE SIZES, SHAPES AND TYPES

The size and shapes of capsules are fixed according to the standard chart.

Sizes

Eight sizes of hard gelatin capsule are commercially available. Figure 4.3 shows the sizes and fill volumes. Most widely used sizes are 0-4. Capsule sizes of 00 and 000 are difficult to swallow and are rarely used for human consumption. They are preferred for veterinary use. Size 5 poses difficulties in an automatic filling process.

Determination of Capsule Fill Weight :

To choose the size of capsule for the given fill volume, following relation is used-

$$\text{Capsule fill weight} = \frac{\text{Tapped bulk density}}{\text{of formulation}} \times \frac{\text{Capsule}}{\text{Volume}}$$

Example: Weight of a formulation to be filled in each capsule (theoretical fill weight) is 500 mg and its tapped bulk density is 0.8 gm/ml.

$$\text{Volume occupied by fill weight} = \frac{0.5}{0.8} = 0.625 \, ml$$

From Figure 4.3, it is found that a size 0 capsule has a fill volume of 0.67 ml. Therefore, it is the appropriate choice for this formulation. If the formulation having a fill volume of 0.625 ml is to be filled in a capsule having fill volume of 0.67 ml, then,

0.67 - 0.625 = 0.045 ml volume remains unoccupied.

A diluent is added to the formulation to make up this volume. If the tapped bulk density of this diluent is 0.7 gm/ml,

Quantity of diluent required per capsule = 0.7 x 0.045 = 31.5 mg.

Therefore, additional 31.5 mg

No.	Actual size	Volume in ml
5	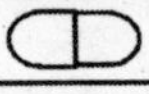	0.13
4	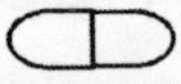	0.20
3	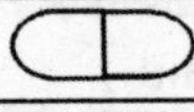	0.27
2	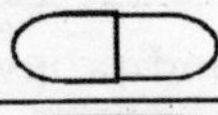	0.37
1	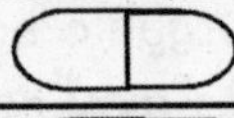	0.48
0	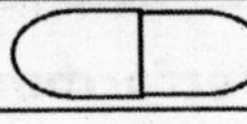	0.67
00	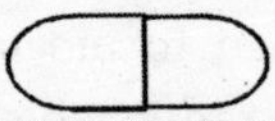	0.95
000	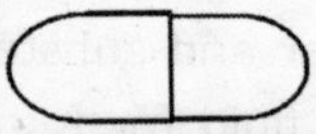	1.36

Figure 4.3: Hard gelatin capsule (sizes and full volumes.)

of a diluent is to be added to the formulation to use 0 size capsule as the most appropriate capsule to fill the given formulation.

TYPES OF HARD GELATIN CAPSULES

Whosoever is the manufacturer of the empty gelatin capsules, the sizes and specifications of capsules are very similar, so that they can be used on any standard automatic filling machine. The capsules are dot sealed or banded, so that the cap and body does not separate after filling. Self-locking capsules were developed as an alternative to this. **Lok-Cap** and **Posilok** capsules were produced by Eli Lilly, **snap** fit and Coni-Snap capsules by Parke Davis and **Star-Lok** and **Lox-It** capsules by R.P. Scherer. Figure 4.4 shows the snap fit principle. A development of this design is the Coni-Snap shown in Figure 4.5.

In Coni-Snap capsule, the cap is so designed that after filling and closing, only the tip of the body is visible.

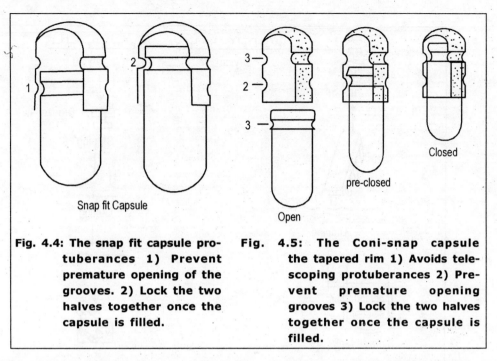

Fig. 4.4: The snap fit capsule pro-
    tuberances 1) Prevent
    premature opening of the
    grooves. 2) Lock the two
    halves together once the
    capsule is filled.

Fig. 4.5: The Coni-snap capsule
    the tapered rim 1) Avoids tele-
    scoping protuberances 2) Pre-
    vent premature opening
    grooves 3) Lock the two halves
    together once the capsule is
    filled.

R.P. Scherer produced Star-Lok (standard) and Lox-It capsules, shown in Figure 4.6.
    A Posilok capsule is illustrated in Figure 4.7 the pre-lock feature is designed to
prevent the cap and body from separating during transit.

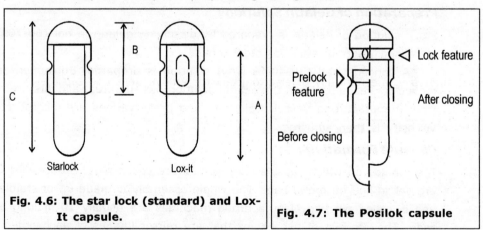

Fig. 4.6: The star lock (standard) and Lox-
    It capsule.

Fig. 4.7: The Posilok capsule

METHOD OF PRODUCTION OF EMPTY HARD GELATIN CAPSULES

The manufacturing process for empty gelatin capsules can be summarised as
follows: Gelatin solution containing colorants and additives is prepared. Capsules are made by dipping them in the solution and then dried. Dried capsules
are removed from moulds and assembled. Assembled capsules are sorted, printed and packaged as shown in Figure 4.8.

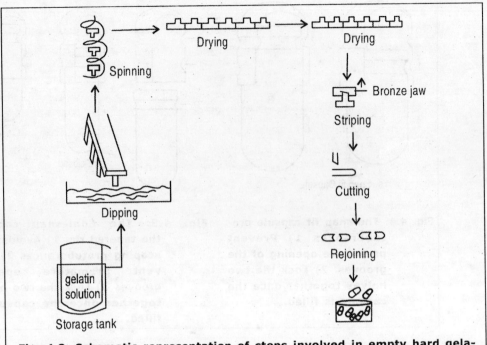

Fig. 4.8: Schematic representation of steps involved in empty hard gelatin capsule production

Preparation of Gelatin Solution :

Stock solution of gelatin is prepared by dissolving gelatin in hot (60-70°C) demineralised water in stainless steel tanks.

A concentrated (30-40 % w/w) solution is prepared. Entrapped air is removed by vacuum. When the gelatin solution has matured, aliquots are removed from manufacturing vessel. Colorants and preservatives are incorporated. The viscosity is then adjusted.

Capsule Formation :

The moulds on which capsules are formed are called pins. Groups of these pins are set in line on metal bars. The whole assembly is made up of stainless steel and is called pin bar. Manufacturing machines are usually 10 m long and 2 m wide. They consist of two halves that are mirror images of each other. On one half, caps are made and on other half, bodies are made. Machine is divided into upper and lower level.

Gelatin solution is transferred to a jacketed, heated, stirred container on the manufacturing machine called a 'dip pan' or 'dip pot'.

The pin bars (at room temperature) are gently lowered into the gelatin solution, then slowly withdrawn. Gelatin is picked up on the mould pins. Quantity of gelatin is governed by viscosity of gelatin solution. A film is formed on the pins.

Pins are rotated during their transfer to upper level of machine to form a film of uniform thickness (spinning). As they rise, they pass through a current of cold air, which helps to set the gelatin solution and fix the film on the mould.

Drying :

Pin bars are passed through a series of drying kilns for gradual and precisely controlled removal of water. At the rear end of the machine, the bars are transferred to lower level and passed through drying kilns to the front side of the machine. Air is heated only upto a few degrees, as higher temperatures cannot be employed, because the moulds have to return to the correct operating temperature for re-dipping.

Capsule removal and assembly :

Gelatin films formed on the pins are longer than required. The lower edges of the films are feathery and of variable thickness. They need to be trimmed into a good clean edge at the required length. Capsule shells are removed from pins by sets of metal jaws, which are placed around each pin on a bar. The jaws transfer the film from the shell into a metal holder. The holder rotates against a knife which is adjusted to cut the capsule part to a specified length. The two halves of the capsule are then joined by transferring them to a joining block. The capsules are then carried by a conveyor belt into a receiver.

Thickness of capsule shells may be controlled by controlling viscosity of gelatin solution, speed and time of dipping, rate of spinning, mold pin dimensions, rate of drying and the machine control related to cut lengths.

Capsule Sorting :

Capsules now pass through a series of sorting and checking processes. They are inspected manually, mechanically or electronically to remove defective capsules.

Capsule Printing :

Variety of information may be printed on capsules, such as product name, approved chemical name, strength, company name and logo or symbol. The process used is 'offset gravure' using an edible pharmaceutical ink on an automatic machine. The printing can be laid along the long axis of the capsule. This is called axial printing. Alternatively, the inscription can be placed perpendicularly to the long axis of the capsule. This is called radial printing. Figure 4.9 indicates four arrangements of axial printing on capsules.

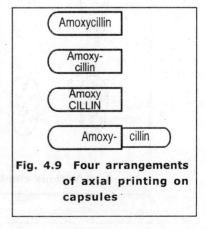

Fig. 4.9 Four arrangements of axial printing on capsules

Packing and Storage :

The capsules are packed and stored in polythene-lined fiber drums or cardboard boxes in heat sealed polythene bags.

STANDARDS FOR EMPTY HARD CAPSULES

Dimensions:

Although capsules are made in standard sizes, but they are standard enough to fit all the standard capsule filling machines. The lengths of individual cap and body, their length after closing the two halves and the diameters of cap and body are critical.

Solubility:

Pharmacopoeial solubility tests are performed on filled capsules. The American Federal Standard requires empty capsules to remain undissolved after immersion in water, at 25ºC for 15 minutes, but to completely dissolve or disintegrate after immersion in 0.5 per cent w/w HCl, at 36-38ºC for 15 minutes.

Moisture content and brittleness:

Moisture content should be normally 13 to 16 per cent to prevent brittleness determined by drying at 105ºC.

The brittleness can be checked by applying pressure at the centre of the capsule against a smooth, hard surface, the capsule must not shatter.

Odour:

The capsule shells must be free from any foreign odour. This is determined by checking a sample after storage in a sealed bottle for 24 hours at 30-40ºC.

Filling of Hard Gelatin Capsules

Powders are normally filled in hard gelatin capsules. However, other preparations, or combination of preparations, may also be filled in capsules. Figure 4.10 illustrates various possibilities.

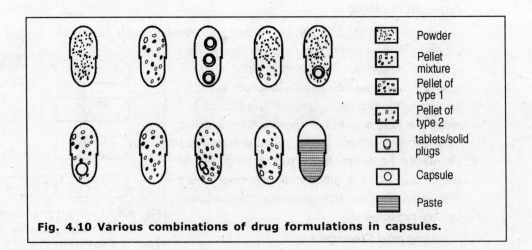

Fig. 4.10 Various combinations of drug formulations in capsules.

Filling hard capsules with powders :

The filling machine performs basically four operations. It rectifies the capsules, separates the body from the cap, fills the body and replaces the cap. Figure 4.11 indicates basic operations in hard gelatin capsule filling. The method of putting powder into the capsule varies greatly from manufacturer to manufacturer. Following mechanisms may be used:

Plate method : The figure 4.12 illustrates a block containing three capsule bodies and a quantity of powder filling them, with some excess material covering the top of the block. When the powder

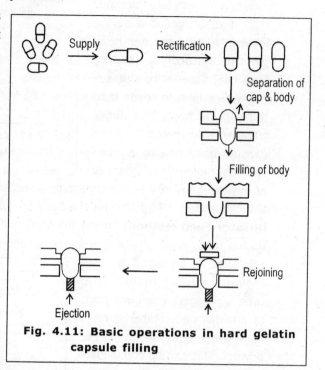

Fig. 4.11: Basic operations in hard gelatin capsule filling

is formulated for a certain size of capsule and is of reasonably uniform density, the material is spread over the capsule bodies to fill them completely. The excess powder remaining after the capsules are filled is removed before replacing the

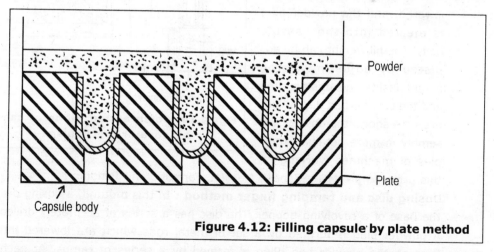

Figure 4.12: Filling capsule by plate method

caps. Some machines apply a form of vibrations to the block, inspite of possibility of segregation. Machines working on this principle are Tevopharm and Banapace.

Auger Feed Method: It is a modification of plate method. (Fig. 4.13) Auger is a device located in the powder hopper. An agitator is used to feed the material to the auger, which in turn feeds it to the capsule body. The auger transfers the material to the capsule body due to its mechanical movement. Quantity

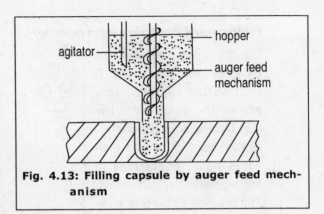

Fig. 4.13: Filling capsule by auger feed mechanism

of powder delivered is dependent on speed of revolution, design of auger, quantity of powder in hopper and the time for which body remains under hopper.

Dosator Feed Method: This is the most widely used mechanism. It consists of a dosing tube, which contains a spring loaded piston inside. The internal volume of this tube is changed by this movable piston inside. The tube is plunged, open end first, in powder bed. Material rises up in the tube to form a plug of powder. This can be consolidated farther by applying pressure to the piston. The assembly is then raised and positioned over capsule body. Piston is lowered, and the powder plug is ejected into the capsule body. The fill weight can be adjusted by adjusting piston height inside the dosing tube and the powder bed depth. Figure 4.14 shows the dosator assembly in more details. Examples of machines working on

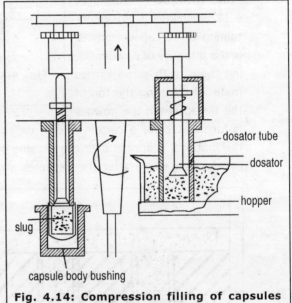

Fig. 4.14: Compression filling of capsules by dosator mechanism

this principle are MG2, Zanasi, Macofar, Farmatic and Pendini.

Dosing disc and tamping finger method : In this method, a dosing disc forms the base of a revolving hopper. The disc has a series of accurately drilled holes. A powder plug is formed by a set of metal rods which are lowered into holes through the powder bed. Plug is formed by a series of tamps. At each tamp, fingers push the material into holes before they index into the next position. At the sixth position, plug is pushed out into the capsule body. Fill weight can be

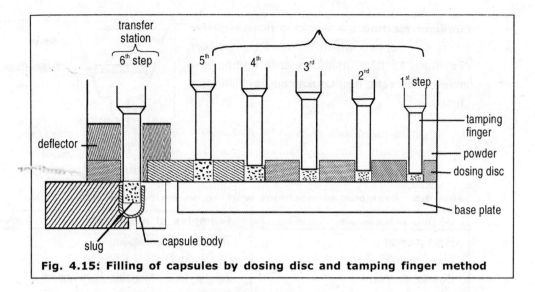

Fig. 4.15: Filling of capsules by dosing disc and tamping finger method

varied by adjusting thickness of dosing disc, movement of the tamping finger and pressure applied on the tamping fingers. The technique is used in fully automatic machines.

Vacuum filling (Accofill) : Perry industries developed a method based on their idea of using vacuum to fill powders in vials by a technique called Accofil. The powder is drawn into the dosator by suction, applied through a filter pad. Material is held in place by vacuum until the dosing tube is positioned over the capsule body, where the powder is ejected by releasing the vacuum, e.g. Perry capsule filling machine.

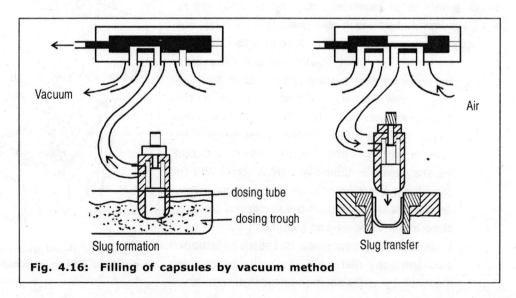

Fig. 4.16: Filling of capsules by vacuum method

Fluidiser Method : A vibrating plate is placed inside the hopper, which fluidises the powder, causing it to flow inside capsule bodies at a uniform flow rate, e.g. Osaka capsule filling machines.

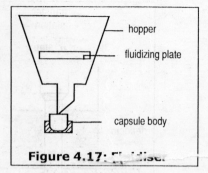

Figure 4.17: Fluidiser

Table 4.5 : Examples of machines working on various dosing principles

Dosing mechanism	Examples of machines
Plate method	Tevopharm, Bonapace
Auger method	Lilly/Parke-Davis, Elanco
Dosator method	Zanasi, MG2, Macofar, Farmatic, Pendini, Bonapace
Dosing disc and tamping finger	Hofliger Karg, Harrohofliger
Vacuum (Accofil)	Perry
Fluidiser	Osaka

CAPSULE FILLING MACHINES

HAND OPERATED CAPSULE FILLING MACHINE

Small quantities of capsules (from 50-10,000) are required to be filled in community pharmacies, hospital pharmacies and for clinical trials. There are a number of small hand operated machines available for this purpose, viz., Feton and Labocaps. They consist of sets of plastic plates that have predrilled holes to take 30-100 capsules. Empty shells are fed into the holes either manually or with a simple loading device. The bodies are locked in their place by a screw and the caps fixed by their holders are removed. Powder is filled by placing on the surface of the body plate and spreading and leveling it by means of a spatula. The cap plate is then repositioned over the body plate and the capsules rejoined together by exerting manual pressure.

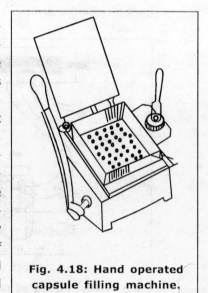

Fig. 4.18: Hand operated capsule filling machine.

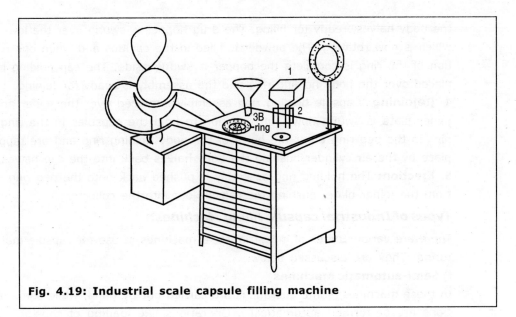

Fig. 4.19: Industrial scale capsule filling machine

INDUSTRIAL MACHINES

The machines for the large scale filling of hard gelatin capsules are available in number of sizes and shapes: semi-automatic to fully automatic, with continuous and inter-mittent motion and varying in output from 5,000-1,50,000 per hour. The basic method of capsule handling is same in every case and they mainly differ in the method of powder dosing, as already described.

A basic design of a capsule filling machine is shown in Figure 4.19 in order to discuss the capsule-handling operation in general.

1. Rectification: The capsules are supplied in bulk containers. It is necessary for the machine to orient the capsules such that they are all pointing in the same direction, i.e., body first. For this, the capsules are loaded into the hopper (1) and from here they pass through tubes to a 'rectification' section (2). Here the capsules are held in tight fitting slots. A metal finger strikes them in the middle causing them to rotate. The body is more free as it has a smaller diameter than the cap and therefore the capsules rotate with the body facing the direction of motion.

2. Separation of caps and bodies: The capsules enter into the two-piece hold-ing rings (3A and 3B) from the rectifier. Both the rings contain the same number of holders as capsules. The diameters of the holders are so designed that the body can pass through the upper ring, but the cap cannot. The transfer is usual-ly assisted by vacuum. When the two rings are separated, they retain caps and bodies respectively, thus causing their separation.

3. Filling: When all the rows in the ring assembly are filled with capsules, the top ring, filled with caps only, is removed and set aside. The lower ring now contains the body halves, ready for filling. The drug hopper is swung over the lower ring which is now rotating. The powder is filled in the cavities and when one revolution of the ring is complete the hopper is swung aside. The cap holding ring is placed over the body holding ring and the assembly is ready for joining.

4. Rejoining: Capsule holding ring assembly is placed over the joiner and the joiner plate is swung down into position to hold the capsules in the ring. The pins in the peg ring enter the holes of the body holding ring and are tapped in place by the air cylinder pushing the body halves back into the cap halves.

5. Ejection: The holding ring assembly is pushed back onto the peg ring, away from the joiner plate, pushing the capsule out into the collector.

Types of Industrial capsule filling Machines:

There are various types of industrial scale machines in use for capsule manufacturing. They are discussed below.

i) Semi-automatic machines

In these machines, some operations are carried out by hand, while some operations are performed automatically. Operations like loading of capsules in the hopper, separation of cap and body rings are carried out manually, while the rest of the operations are carried out automatically. They claim to have an output of 58,000 capsules/hour.

ii) Automatic machines

These machines perform each step in the capsule filling operation automatically and hence obviously have better output. They are further classified as Intermittent and Continuous motion automatic machines.

A. Intermittent motion machines

In these machines, capsules are moved by carrier mechanism which move rapidly, usually by rotation around the axis and then stop while the separation or filling mechanism takes place at a fixed station.

B. Continuous motion machines

In these machines, capsules are transported by some flexible conveyor and the separation and filling is carried out while they are moving.

Table 4.6: Examples of hand-operated. Semi-automatic and automatic machines.

Type	Example
Hand operated	Feton, Chemipharm, Zuma
Semi automatic	Pendini model 21B LAF Multifill Cotton 8
Automatic-intermittent motion	Zanasi LZ-64, AZ-60
	Macofar- MT-13//
	Hofliger and karg - GKF series
Automatic-continuous motion	Harro Hofliger - KFM III MG2 - G36

FINISHING OF CAPSULES

Finished capsules sometimes require some sort of dusting and polishing, for which following methods are used-

1. *Pan polishing:* Tablet coating pans may be used for this purpose. Accela Cota may be used with a polyurethane or cheese cloth liner, which traps the dust and imparts a gloss.

2. *Cloth dusting:* Bulk filled capsules are rubbed with a cloth manually. The cloth may or may not be impregnated with some inert oil.

3. *Brushing:* In this procedure, capsule cores are fed under rotating soft brushes, which removes the dust. The operation must be assisted by vacuum to remove the dust.

WEIGHING AND SORTING

Finally the capsules are weighed after the filling and dusting process and batches are sorted. Those that show a wider weight variation are not acceptable and are separated. They are likely to be rejected.

many commercially available capsule-finishing equipment can also perform several finishing operations concurrenly.

1. *Erweka capsule de-dusting and polishing machine :* It moves capsules between soft plastic tassels against a perforated plastic sleeve, which may or may not be under vacuum.

2. *Seidender PM 60 Capsule Polishing Machine :* It offers two units that may be used separately or in combination - a conveyor belt for visual inspection and a cleaning and polishing machine consisting of two lamb wool belts moving in opposite directions. Capsules are carried on the belt that may be supplied with vacuum.

3. *Rotosort :* A mechanical device to remove loose powder, unfilled closed capsules, filled and unfilled bodies and loose caps.

4. *Elanco Rotoweigh:* Capsules are gravity fed onto vacuum pins which presents them to a unique weight detection system. It measures the reflectance or back scatter of a x-ray beam which is directed onto capsules. The reflectance is proportional to the capsule weight.

5. *Vericap 1,200 weight analyser :* Filled capsules are propelled at high speed by compressed air between two charged plates. The change in capacitance is measured as a function of capsule weight.

FORMULATION

Following factors must be considered while formulating materials for encapsulation:

1. The size of shell should be chosen by considering the bulk density of the material.

---

2. The colours used in the shell must be different to provide product identification.

3. The flow properties of powders should be adequate for that particular method of filling. The powder bed from which the dose of mixture is measured must be homogenous, to have uniformity of fill weight.

For low dose drugs, ample space is available in the capsule shell for the addition of excipients. Flow properties of low dose drugs may be modified by using free flowing diluents like maize starch. For high dose drugs, flow modifiers, which are effective in low concentration, like glidants, (e.g. fumed silicon dioxide) or lubricants, (e.g. magnesium stearate), may be used.

4. In encapsulation machines that fill fixed doses of powders in the form of slugs, the powder must have sufficient cohesiveness to retain its slug form during delivery into the capsules. Thus if a drug is to be encapsulated on a machine working on auger principle, magnesium stearate can be the excipient of choice. Whereas, if it is to be filled on a machine working on dosing disc and tamping finger principle, a compactable excipient like microcrystalline cellulose can be an excipient of choice. Sometimes small concentrations of oils, such as mineral oil, can also be incorporated in the latter case as a binder.

5. Chances of drug-excipient incompatibilities must be anticipated. Reactions should be studied at elevated temperatures and pressures.

6. The particle size of drug must be reduced to improve the rate of dissolution. Insoluble drugs must be mixed with soluble excipients to render the mixture more hydrophilic. Soluble drugs should be mixed with insoluble excipients to avoid competition for solution.

QUALITY CONTROL AND OFFICIAL STANDARDS :

Quality control is an important criterion during every step of the manufacturing process. Official standards have been set by the governments to ensure the good quality of all pharmaceutical products.

Weight Variation Test

Weight variation test according to I.P.

Weigh intact capsule. Open the capsules and remove the contents as completely as possible. For soft gelatin capsules, wash the shell with solvent ether and allow the shell to stand at room temperature until the odour of the solvent is no longer perceived. Weigh the shell. The difference in the two weights gives the weight of contents. Repeat the procedure for 19 more capsules.

Determine the average weight of contents. Not more than two individual weights should deviate from the average by more than the percentage of deviation shown in table and none should deviate by more than twice of the allowed percent deviation.

Average weight of content	deviation (%)
< 300 mg	+ 10 per cent
> 300 mg	+ 7.5 per cent

If more than two, but less than six, weights deviate from the average by the percentage deviation shown in table and none deviate by twice the percentage, determine weight of contents of additional 40 capsules. Find out average weight of 60 capsules. If not more than six individual weights deviate from the average by more than the percentage of deviation shown in the table, and none deviates by more than twice that percentage, capsules pass the test.

Weight variation test according to U.S.P.

Stage 1 : Same as stage one of weight variation test I.P.

Stage 2 : Not more than two individual weights vary by more than + 10 per cent and in no case the difference is more than 25 per cent, capsules pass the test. If more than two, but less than six, capsules deviate from average weight between 10-25 per cent and none deviates by more than 25 per cent, retest contents of 40 more capsules. Find the average of weight of the 60 capsules. If not more than 6 (1/10th of total sample) out of 60 capsules deviate by more than 10 per cent and none deviates by more than 25 per cent, capsules pass the test.

Disintegration Time

As per I.P. : The procedure is same as that for Disintegration Test for Tablets as per I.P.

Limits :
Hard gelatin capsules: 30 minutes
Soft gelatin capsules: 60 minutes
Enteric coated capsules:
Same as for enteric coated tablets

As per U.S.P. :

Limits:

Hard and soft gelatin capsules : As per monograph

Enteric coated capsules : Same as for enteric-coated tablets.

Test for content of active ingredients

- The test for capsules is same as for tablets.

Test for content uniformity

- This test for capsules is same as for tablets.

SOFT GELATIN CAPSULES

Soft gelatin capsules are also referred to as soft elastic gelatin capsules or soft gels. The shell consists of continuous units of gelatin and a plasticiser surrounding a liquid-filled material. They are formed, filled and sealed in one operation and are available in various sizes and shapes as shown in figure 4.20.

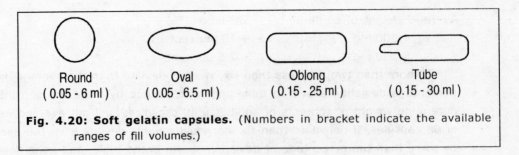

Fig. 4.20: Soft gelatin capsules. (Numbers in bracket indicate the available ranges of fill volumes.)

| Round (0.05 - 6 ml) | Oval (0.05 - 6.5 ml) | Oblong (0.15 - 25 ml) | Tube (0.15 - 30 ml) |

APPLICATIONS OF SOFT GELATIN CAPSULES :

Soft gelatin capsules, because of their special characteristics and advantages, have the following applications in the pharmaceutical industry-

i) As an oral dosage form, being particularly useful for filling liquids.

ii) As a speciality package in tube form, for single dose application of topical, ophthalmic and nasal preparations.

iii) As a suppository dosage form for rectal and vaginal use.

iv) Speciality package for breath fresheners, perfumes, bath oils and skin creams.

ADVANTAGES -

1. Poorly compressible drugs can be presented in their solid dosage form by filling in soft capsules.

2. Useful for drugs showing poor content uniformity. The drug is dissolved or dispersed in a liquid and then dose is volumetrically filled in the capsules.

3. Drugs sensitive to oxidation or hydrolysis can be protected by dissolution or dispersion in oil and subsequent encapsulation by gelatin shell.

4. The drugs show good bioavailability as they are present in solution, suspension or emulsion forms.

NATURE OF THE CAPSULE SHELL

The shell is similar to hard gelatin capsules, but in addition contains a plasticiser in larger concentrations. Other ingredients, such as preservatives, colours, opacifiers, flavours, sugars and acids may also be present.

Gelatin having bloom strength* between 150 and 250 gm and viscosity between 25 and 45 millipoise, may be used. Low viscosity (25 to 32 millipoise), high-bloom (180-250 g) gelatins are used for encapsulation of hygroscopic materials and solids. Iron content of gelatin should not be more than 15 ppm to avoid its effect on dyes used in the shell and its possible colour reactions with organic compounds.

Glycerin and sorbitol are the two most commonly used plasticisers.

* (Refer page 183).

The ratio of dry plasticiser to dry gelatin by weight, governs the hardness of the capsule shell. Table lists typical plasticiser/gelatin ratios.

Table 4.9: Typical plasticiser/gelatin ratios and corresponding shell hardness.

Hardness	Ratio of dry glycerin/dry gelatin
Hard	0.4/1
Medium	0.6/1
Soft	0.8/1

The water content of the gelatin solution ranges between 0.7 and 1.3 parts of water to each part of dry gelatin, but the most commonly used ratio is 1:1.

Preservatives may be added to prevent growth of microorganisms in gelatin solution. Potassium sorbitate and methyl, ethyl and propyl parabens are most commonly used.

A wide variety of colours may be incorporated in the shell, like synthetic and vegetable water-soluble dyes, insoluble organic and inorganic pigments and lakes. Titanium dioxide may be incorporated as opacifier.

NATURE OF THE CAPSULE CONTENTS :

A very wide range of liquid materials can be filled in soft gelatin capsules, including suspensions, pastes, oily solutions, self emulsifying oils and water miscible liquids. However, the liquids that can be encapsulated have following limitations-

i) High concentrations of water or gelatin solvents must be avoided.

ii) Emulsions should not be filled in capsules as they crack due to loss of water through the shell.

iii) pH below 2.5 must be avoided as it hydrolyses gelatin.

iv) pH above 7.5 has a tanning effect on the shell.

v) Aldehydes have tanning action on shells.

Following types of solutions or suspensions can be incorporated-

1. Solutions in water-immiscible oils, like fixed and aromatic oils, aliphatic, aromatic and chlorinated hydrocarbons, liquid ethers and esters.

2. Solutions in water-miscible liquids like polyethylene glycols (400-600 mol. wt.), alcohols, polyols, triacetin, glyceryl esters, sorbitan esters, sugar esters and polyglyceryl esters.

3. Suspensions: Insoluble drugs suspended in above vehicles and contain ing suspending agents and surfactant as wetting agents. Particle size of suspended drug must be reduced to below 180 micron (μ).

The choice of the vehicle for a suspension should be such that the smallest possible size of capsules can be produced. A guideline is provided to formulators for selection of a suitable base by two values, namely 'Base Absorption' (B/A) and Minims/gram (M/G) factors. These factors have been worked out for some commonly used drugs with some commonly used bases.

Base absorption factor is the number of grams of liquid base required to produce a mix that can be filled in a capsule, with 1 gram of the solid. The value of B/A depends on particle size and shape, density, moisture content and hydrophobicity and hydrophilicity of the solid in question.

The minim/gram (M/G) is defined as the volume in minims of 1 gram of the solid plus weight of the liquid base required for a mix that can be filled in a capsule. It is calculated by the following formula-

$$M/G = \frac{(B/A+s)\times V}{D}$$

Where,

B/A - Base Absorption factor

S - 1 gram of the solid

V- unit volume in cubic centimeters

D - weight of the mixture per cubic centimeter.

The B/A factor determination : A small amount of solid is weighed in a tared beaker and the liquid in another tared beaker. The liquid base is added to the solid in small amounts with the help of a spatula, ensuring that the base gets mixed uniformly with the solid. The liquid addition is continued till the mixture flows steadily from the spatula blade when held at a 45° angle above the mixture. The flow should be even and continuous, and not in globs. The nature of the cut off quality of the mixture should be observed. As the mixture stops flowing from the spatula, a proper cut off is observed, where the stream contracts rapidly upwards, rather than stringing out in intermediate flow. The weight of the base so needed, divided by the weight of the solid gives the B/A factor.

PRODUCTION OF SOFT GELATIN CAPSULES:

The soft gelatin capsules are formed, filled and sealed in a single process, unlike the hard capsules. Different methods are used for their production.

PLATE METHOD :

This process was developed by Upjohn. A set of molds is used for this method. A warm sheet of gelatin is placed over the lower plate. The liquid to be encapsulated is poured on it. Another sheet of gelatin is placed over it. The top plate of the mold is placed over this. Pressure is applied to it to form the capsule. The capsules are then washed with some organic solvent to remove traces of oil from the exterior of the shell.

THE ROTARY DIE PROCESS :

This process was developed by R.P. Scherer in
1933. It improved the accuracy and dose
uniformity of the soft gelatin capsules. Figure below illustrates the principle of rotary die elastic filler.

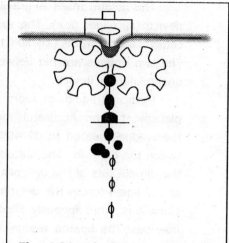

Two continuous gelatin ribbons,
formed by the machine are made to converge between a pair of revolving dies. At
the same time, a metered liquid feed is
injected between the ribbons, precisely at
the moment the dies form pockets of the
gelatin ribbons. These pockets containing
the fill are then sealed by pressure and
heat and cut off from the ribbon.

Fig. 4.21 Principle of rotary die elastic capsule machine

Usually, two tanks for feeding the liquid material to the machine are present.
One contains molten gelatin at 60°C and the other contains the liquid core material at 20°C. If a two-coloured shell is required, two tanks containing gelatin with
different colours are required.

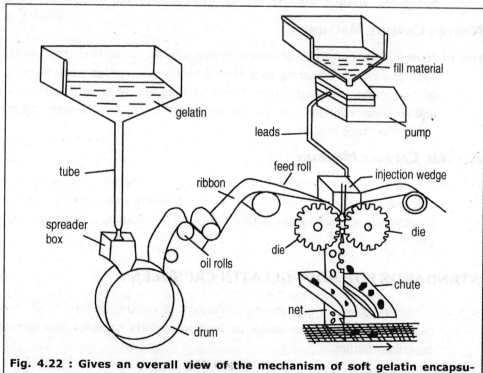

**Fig. 4.22 : Gives an overall view of the mechanism of soft gelatin encapsu-
lation on a rotary die process.**

The gelatin mass is gravitationally fed through heated pipes to a metering device (spreader box). The spreader box feeds the material onto two large air-cooled casting drums (16-20ºC). Gelatin ribbons of controlled thickness are formed. The two ribbons are fed between mineral oil lubricated rollers and then into the encapsulation device.

Medicinal liquid, at room temperature, flows by gravity into a positive displacement pump. Accurately metered volumes of the liquid fill are injected through the wedge (heated to 37-40ºC) between the gelatin ribbons as they pass between the die rolls. The bottom of the wedge contains small orifices lined up with the die pockets of the die rolls. The capsule is about half filled when the injection of the liquid forces the gelatin to expand into the pockets of the dies. Here, the capsule is simultaneously filled and shaped hermetically. The ribbon continues to flow past the heated wedge and pressed between the die rolls where the capsule halves are sealed together by the application of heat and pressure. The capsules are cut out automatically from the gelatin ribbons by the dies. The capsules are then passed through a naphtha wash to remove the surface oil. They, then are passed through a rotating basket through on infra-red dryer and then spread onto trays to complete the drying process in a tunnel corridor and air-dried using air at relative humidity of 20 per cent. The capsules are inspected for quality, washed again in naptha, graded according to size and packaged.

NORTON CAPSULE MACHINE :

This machine passes two films of gelatin between a set of verticle dies. As these dies open and close alternately, they form a continuous verticle plate forming rows of pockets cross the gelatin film. These pockets are filled with the medicaments, and as they progress through the dies, they are sealed, shaped and cut out of the film as capsules.

ACCOGEL CAPSULE MACHINE :

This process was developed by Lederle. It also used a system of rotary dies. It is the only machine that can successfully fill dry powders into a soft gelatin capsule. It is extremely versatile and can fill mixtures of two liquids, a liquid and a powder or tablets.

STANDARDS FOR SOFT GELATIN CAPSULES :

Tests like content of active ingredients, uniformity of weight, uniformity of content and disintegration tests are similar as for hard gelatin capsules and carried out as described earlier.

◆◆◆◆◆

Pharmaceutical Semisolids

INTRODUCTION

Pharmaceutical semisolid dosage forms include ointments, creams, pastes, gels and rigid foams. Most of these preparations serve as vehicles for some drugs for topical application. Majority of the semisolid preparations are applied to the skin for the following purposes-

1. Surface effects like cleansing, cosmetic, protective, sunscreen or antimicrobial action.
2. Effects on the stratum corneum like protective or keratolytic action.
3. Effects on the viable epidermis or dermis, like anti-inflammatory, anesthetic and antihistaminic actions.
4. Systemic effects produced by drugs like scopolamine, nitroglycerine, clonidine, estradiol.
5. Some effects on the skin, as depilation, exfoliation, antimicrobial effects and antiperspirant effects.
   Some semisolid preparations are meant for application to vaginal, rectal, nasal, buccal or urethral mucosa, cornea and external ear.

THE HUMAN SKIN :

It is essential to study the anatomy and physiology of the human skin to understand the mechanism of drug delivery from semisolid dosage forms, since majority of them are applied to the skin.

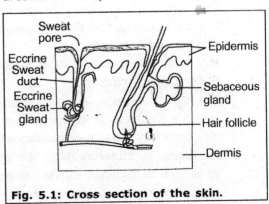

Fig. 5.1: Cross section of the skin.

The skin is the largest single organ of the body, with an average surface area of about 2 m². It separates the internal body structures from the external environment.

ANATOMY OF HUMAN SKIN:

Human skin may be anatomically described to consist of three distinct tissue layers the epidermis, the dermis and the subcutaneous fat.

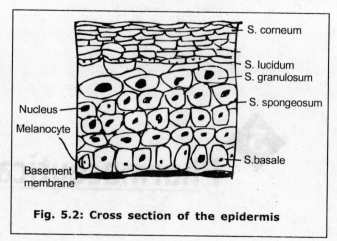

Fig. 5.2: Cross section of the epidermis

The epidermis varies in thickness, depending on the cell size and number of cell layers, ranging from about 0.8 mm on the palms to 0.06 mm on the eyelids. There are five individual layers of the epidermis-

1. Stratum basale (stratum germinativum):

It consists of large, columnar, nucleated cells arranged with their axes perpendicular to the skin surface. These cells continuously undergo mitosis to form new cells that travel upwards and are continuously lost as dead cells from the skin surface. The cells also contain melanin.

2. Stratum spongeosum:

As the cells of the basal layer move upwards, they alter morphologically and histochemically. Cells flatten and their nuclei shrink. These cells are interconnected by fine prickles. Each prickle encloses an extension of the cytoplasm, and the opposing tips of the prickles of adjacent cells adhere to form intercellular bridges, called the desmosomes.

3. Stratum granulosum:

Keratocytes manufacture the basic staining particles as they approach this layer. The particles are called keratohyaline granules. A dynamic operation involving intense biochemical activity manufactures keratin.

4. Stratum lucidum :

This is an anatomically distinct, poorly staining hyaline zone on palms and soles.

5. Stratum corneum :

This is the outermost layer of the epidermis. The ability of man to survive in non-aqueous environment is mainly due to almost impermeable nature of the stratum corneum. This layer consists of vertical columns of flattened, keratinised, dead cells, 10-15 layers thick. The layer is as thin as 10 µm when dry, but swells up several times when exposed to water. The dead cells are continuously lost as horny flakes with an average daily loss of 0.5-1 gm. Passage through the stratum corneum becomes the rate limiting step in drug absorption through the skin, because of the impermeable nature of this layer.

Below the epidermis lies the dermis (corium) – 4-5 mm thick, comprising mainly of protein embedded in mucopolysachharide ground substance. Below the dermis lies the subcutaneous layer. This area is supplied with blood capillaries and nerve endings.

THE SKIN APPENDAGES:

The Eccrine sweat glands: They produce sweat (pH 4.0-6.8) and may also secrete proteins and antibodies. Out of the total skin surface, around 10^{-5}th area is occupied by the eccrine sweat glands. The gland arises as a secretary coil in the lower dermis or the subcutaneous tissue, a duct arises through the dermis and it opens on the skin through a pore invisible to the naked eye. It manufactures a watery solution from plasma, called as sweat, which has an output of about 1lit/day.

The Apocrine sweat glands: They are present in adults only in the axila, breast areolar tissue and perianal region. They secrete a small quantity of milky, oily fluid which is acted upon by skin bacteria to produce a characteristic body odour. The glands play no role in temperature control. Most of the ducts open into the neck of hair follicles, while some open on the skin surface.

Hair follicles: They are present all over the skin except the lips, the palm and soles and parts of the sex organs. Hairs grow from the follicle present in superficial epidermis. The follicles extend into the dermis. One or more sebaceous glands, and in some body regions, apocrine glands, open into the follicle above the arrector pili muscle that attaches the follicle to the dermoepidermal junction. The hair shaft consists of keratin.

Sebaceous glands: They are most numerous on the face, forehead, in the ear, on the midline of the back and on anogenital surfaces. These are flask shaped glands producing sebum from cell disintegration. Their ducts usually open into the necks of hair follicles, the entire unit being called pilosebaceous apparatus.

FUNCTIONS OF THE SKIN -

1. To contains body fluids and tissues.
2. To protect from potentially harmful external environment containing chemicals, radiations, mechanical shocks, heat, electrical shocks and microorganisms.
3. To mediate sensations, i.e., pressure, temperature, pain, etc.
4. To regulate body temperature.
5. To synthesise and metabolise compounds.
6. To dispose off chemical wastes.
7. To provide identification by skin variation.
8. To regulate blood pressure.

TOPICAL TREATMENT OF SKIN :

A topical dosage form is formulated for either of the three reasons.

1. To manipulate the barrier function of the skin, e.g. sunscreens and emollients.
2. To direct the drugs to the viable skin tissues without using oral, systemic or other routes.
3. To deliver the drug systemically.

Table 5.1: Main target regions for topical treatment and medications used

Target Area	Type of treatment	Examples
Skin surface	1. Camouflage or Cosmetic application	Make up
	2. Protective application	Protective Sunscreens
	3. Attacking bacteria and fungi	Topical antibiotics, antiseptics, deodorants
Stratum corneum	1. To improve water content	Emollients, humectants
	2. To stimulate keratosis	Keratolytics
Skin appendages	1. To reduce hyperhydrosis of sweat glands	Antiperspirants
	2. Treatment of acne	Topical exfoliating antibiotics
	3. Chemical removal of hair	Depilatories
	4. Treatment of fungal disease of hair	Topical antifungals
Viable epidermis and dermis	1. To treat inflammation	Topical steroids and NSAIDs
	2. To anaesthetise a small area	Topical anaesthetics
	3. To treat premalignant skin tumours	5-fluorouracil Methotrexate
Systemic treatment	1. Motion sickness	Scopolamine
	2. Angina	Nitroglycerin
	3. Hypertension	Clonidine

PRINCIPLE OF DIFFUSION THROUGH SKIN :

Skin is a multilayered tissue. In percutaneous absorption, the concentration gradient develops over several levels. Each layer contributes to the resistance to diffusion, R, which is directly proportional to the layer thickness, h, and is inversely proportional to the product of the diffusivity, D, and the partition coefficient, K. The skin is considered as a three-ply membrane (stratum corneum, viable epidermis and dermis). The total diffusion resistance of all the three layers is given as,

$$R_T = \frac{1}{P_T} = \frac{h_1}{D_1 K_1} + \frac{h_2}{D_2 K_2} + \frac{h_3}{D_3 k_3}$$

Where,

R_T = total diffusion resistance

P_T = thickness weighted permeability coefficient

The numerals refer to the separate skin layers.

Hair follicles and sweat glands are shunts and pores that pierce through the human skin. This is considered in a simplified manner as a diffusion medium consisting of two or more diffusion pathways linked in parallel. Then the total diffusion flux per unit area, F_T is the sum of the individual fluxes through the separate routes,

Thus,

$$\mathcal{I}_T = f_1 \mathcal{I}_1 + f_2 \mathcal{I}_2 + \ldots\ldots$$

Where,

f_1, f_2, etc., denote the fractional areas for each diffusion route. In general,

$$F_T = C_o (f_1 P_1 + f_2 P_2 + \ldots\ldots)$$

Where,

P_1, P_2, —— represent the thickness weighted permeability coefficients

FACTORS AFFECTING DIFFUSION :

The physicochemical properties of the solute and the skin affect the process of diffusion.

Diffusant solubility : The flux of the solute through the skin is directly proportional to the concentration gradient across the entire skin. Therefore, if the donor solution is saturated, the flux is maximum. The saturated solution of the drug in the formulation should be obtained by choosing a correct blend of solvents.

Partition coefficient : In percutaneous absorption, diffusion of the drug through the stratum corneum is often a rate limiting step, due to impermeability of the stratum corneum. In order to establish high initial concentration of the diffusant in the first layer of the membrane, stratum corneum-to-vehicle partition coefficient is critically important.

---

pH : Only unionised molecules pass readily across lipid membranes. Most of the drug molecules are weak acids or bases. The proportion of the unionised drug in the applied phase depends on pH of the preparation and pK_a/pK_b of the drug.

Co-solvents : Polar co-solvents like propylene glycol may be used to solubilise the drug, in order to achieve saturated solutions. But as the solubility of the drug in the vehicle goes on increasing, the partition coefficient of the drug between the skin and the solvent mixture falls. Hence, the drug should not be over solubilised in the formulation, but should only be at or near saturation.

Surface activity and micellisation: If the drug is surface active, it may micellise and thus there is dramatic increase in its solubility. But if the micelles are too large to cross the membrane, then this solubilisation hardly has any positive effect on permeation. If a surfactant is present along with the drug, they are able to lower interfacial tension in hair follicles and change the protein conformation in the stratum corneum. This enhances the diffusion rate.

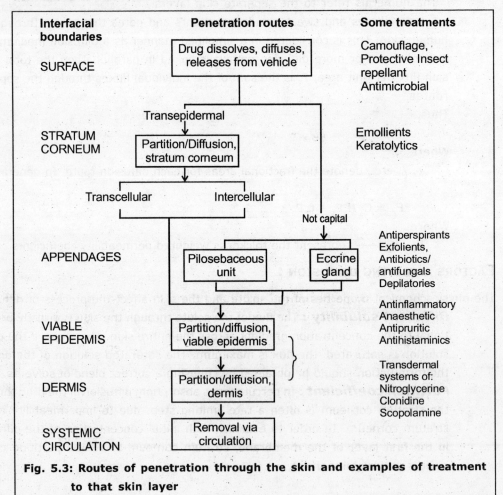

Fig. 5.3: Routes of penetration through the skin and examples of treatment to that skin layer

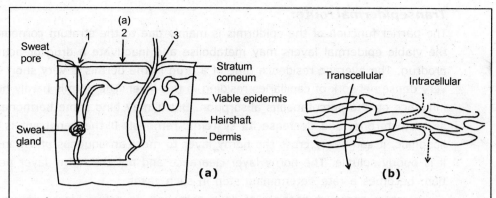

Fig. 5.4: Routes of drug penetration a) Route (1) via sweat ducts (2) via intact stratum corneum (3) via pilosebaceous unit b) Two possible routes of penetration via intact stratum corneum (transepidermal route)

PERCUTANEOUS ABSORPTION AND ROUTES OF PENETRATION :

Skin acts as a very effective and and selective penetration barrier. Epidermis provides the major barrier element. Many small, water soluble non-electrolytes would have diffused much more rapidly through the skin if the epidermis had not been there.

ROUTES OF PENETRATION :

When a molecule reaches intact skin, it comes in contact with cellular debris, microorganisms, sebum and other materials. The layer of the sebum mixed with sweat, bacteria and dead cells is thin, irregular and discontinuous. It hardly affects percutaneous absorption. The diffusant then has three potential entry routes to the viable tissue (fig. 5.4) i.e., through the hair follicles and associated sebaceous glands; through the sweat ducts (transeppendageal route) and through the stratum corneum (transepidermal route).

Transappendageal routes:

The fractional area available for absorption through the skin appendages, viz., hair follicles, sebaceous glands and sweat glands is very small. Therefore, this route cannot contribute appreciably in percutaneous absorption. But this route is important for ions and large polar molecules, which cross the stratum corneum intact, though with difficulty. The actual pathway through the pilosebaceous apparatus could be through hair fiber itself, or through the outer root sheath of the hair into the sebaceous gland. The route through the sweat duct may be either through the lumen or through the walls. Dense capillary network closely envelops the bases of the sweat ducts and hair follicles, into which the drug may finally get absorbed.

Transepidermal route:

The barrier function of the epidermis is mainly due to the stratum corneum. But the viable epidermal layers may metabolise and inactivate a drug or activate a prodrug. The average residence time of a drug in the dermis is very short due to very dense network of capillaries residing in this layer. The dermis hardly has any influence on the percutaneous absorption. But it may bind some hormones such as testosterone, and decrease its systemic removal. If the penetrant is highly lipophilic, it can easily cross the horny layer to meet an aqueous phase in which it is poorly soluble. The horny layer clearance and not the horny layer penetration, becomes a rate determining step in such cases.

Stratum corneum consists of dead cells and no active transport processes exist in this layer. It is assumed therefore, that there are no fundamental differences between *in vivo* and *in vitro* permeation through this layer, though some differences may arise due to manipulation done with the skin, to insert it into the diffusion apparatus.

The transport of substance through the transepidermal route is quite rapid. This is because, though the rate of permeation is slower compared to the transappendageal route the area available for permeation is very large. Therefore, the amount of drug absorbed is more. The molecules permeate either intercellularly or transcellularly. Lipid is segregated between protein filaments in the intercellular material. Again, the rate of transcellular absorption is more than intercellular absorption, because the area occupied by intercellular spaces is quite small as compared to the area of the entire epidermis.

The stratum corneum presents a relatively impermeable barrier, which provides the rate limiting step in percutaneous absorption. No drug passes readily through this membrane, but almost all drugs penetrate to some extent. The membrane provides a mosaic of polar and non-polar regions through which substances dissolve and diffuse according to their chemical affinities. The intercellular region, containing neutral lipids, provides an alternative pathway.

The particular route a substance may take, is decided by the physicochemical properties of the drug, the time scale of observation, the site and condition of skin and the vehicle components. Electrolytes and large molecules with low diffusion coefficients may take transappendageal route as the main entry route, e.g., polar steroids and antibiotics.

Once past the stratum corneum, the drug permeates rapidly through the living tissues and enters the systemic circulation. The systemic circulation acts as a sink or reservoir for the drug. Drug is then diluted and distributed rapidly.

METHODS FOR STUDYING PERCUTANEOUS ABSORPTION :

Experiments can be designed to study the percutaneous absorption for finding out what is the flux of the drug through the skin, the dominant route of penetration through the skin, drug-binding rate, limiting step in percutaneous absorption, factors affecting effect of vehicle on release rate, etc.

In vitro Methods:

This technique involves use of excised skin to study percutaneous absorption. *In vitro* methods are valuable for screening procedure. But the disadvantage is, these methods do not exactly duplicate the behavior of the tissue. Any suitable assay technique may be used to measure the penetrant, like UV, GC or HPLC.

A. *Release methods without a rate limiting membrane:*

These procedures record the kinetics of drug release from a formulation to a

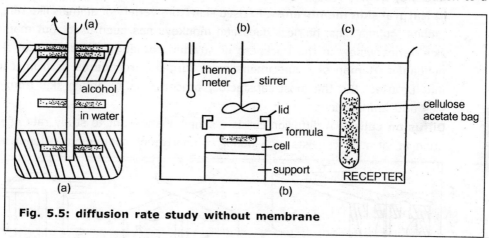

Fig. 5.5: diffusion rate study without membrane

simple immiscible phase, which is supposed to correspond in properties with human skin. But such methods cannot match the complexity of human skin. They are valuable to study drug vehicle interactions and the release characteristics of the formulation, but they have little relevance to the process of percutaneous absorption. Solvents which have been used include simple aqueous media such as water, agar and gelatin and isopropyl myristate, an organic solvent with a blend of polar and non-polar groups, which makes it more like skin.

Arrangement (a) includes an ointment floating on aqueous alcohol (representing skin) on top of a chloroform sink (simulating blood supply), a stirrer with three vanes agitates the layers and the amount of drug delivered to the chloroform is measured as a function of time.

Arrangement (b) has an open-neck glass vessel filled with a formulation, exposed to the environment, to a stirred immiscible receptor phase. A filter paper or a similar material may hold the product in place. A simple dialysis membrane, such as cellulose acetate, can be used to close the receptacle, or a bag of the membrane itself can be used, as shown in arrangement (c).

The drug release may be given by-

$$M \cong 2c_0 \left(\frac{D_v t}{\pi} \right)^{1/2}$$

M = amount of drug released/unit area of application

C_o = initial concentration of penetrating solute in vehicle

D_v = differential coefficient of drug

t = time

B. Diffusion methods with a rate-controlling membrane:

i) Simulated skin membranes: Because human skin may be difficult to obtain, many workers use other materials to simulate it, e.g. cellulose acetate membrane, egg membrane, silicones, etc. But most of the times these membranes merely bind to the penetrant as it diffuses through fluid filled channels; therefore they do not exactly simulate human skin.

ii) Natural skin membranes: Excised skin from variety of animals like rats, mice, rabbits, guinea pigs, hairless dogs and monkeys has been used. But mammalian skin varies widely in the thickness of stratum corneum and density of skin appendages. Human skin specimens from surgical procedures or from cadavers may be used. But the most satisfactory procedure is to obtain skin from autopsies and amputations.

Diffusion cells : A diffusion cell is a simple instrument to study rate of permeation in vitro. It consists of a donor compartment containing a donor solution

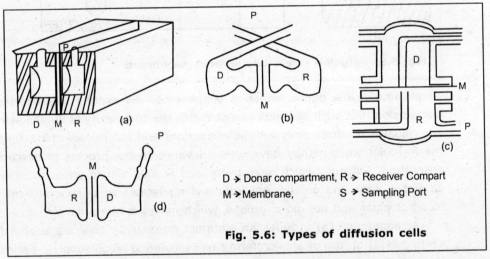

D → Donar compartment, R → Receiver Compart
M → Membrane,   S → Sampling Port

Fig. 5.6: Types of diffusion cells

that continuously delivers penetrant across the membrane to be received by an agitated sink reciever liquid, which simulates blood supply in skin. The reciever fluid can be water, saline, buffer or alcohol-water mixture. The compartment can be placed horizontally or vertically. The concentration of drug reaching the receiver compartment is measured by withdrawing samples through the sampling port and analysing them with suitable techniques like UV, HPLC, GC or radioactive measurement. Cells are made up of suitable material like glass, Stainless steel, perspex.

In vivo methods:

Animal models are valuable for studying the anatomy, physiology and biochemistry of skin, for screening topical agents, for detecting possible hazards and for biopharmaceutical investigation. However, animal studies cannot substitute human studies as most animals differ from man in the thickness of their stratum corneum, the density of hair follicles and sweat glands and the nature of the blood supply.

The major *in vivo* techniques include - observation of pharmacological or physiological response, changes in physical properties of the skin, analysis of body tissues or fluids, surface loss, histological techniques and bioassays and use of tracers.

The drug may stimulate a reaction in the viable tissue, which can be used to determine the penetration kinetics. Certain physiological responses induced by topically applied agents, such as sweat secretion, vasoconstriction, vasodilatation, pigmentation, sebaceous gland activity, vascular permeability, epidermal permeability and keratinisation, can be recorded and considered as a measure of the amount of the drug absorbed.

The drug may change certain physical properties of the skin, viz., transepidermal water loss, skin temperature and mechanical properties. These may be studied by spectral analysis, photoacoustic and electrical studies and use of ultrasound and considered as measure of the amount of the drug absorbed.

Analysis of body fluids like urine, blood and faeces may be done to measure the amount of drug penetrating the skin. Urine analysis is a frequently used method. The recovered drug in urine is analysed. But caution is indicated, since the recovered agent will not necessarily indicate the recovered drug. Some of the drug may have gone elsewhere other than the urine.

The flux of the drug into the skin may also be determined from rate of loss of the drug from the vehicle. But the decrease in drug may merely reflect deposition on the skin surface or combination with the stratum corneum, rather than penetration to the systemic circulation.

Tracers like dyes, fluorescent or radioactive materials, can be used to locate the skin penetration routes. Histological techniques may be used to determine the concentration of the tracer reaching a particular tissue. Histochemical techniques have been used for those few compounds which produce coloured end products after a chemical reaction. A few compounds fluoresce, making their identification by microscopy possible, e.g. vitamin A and tetracycline.

Many special bioassays may be used to screen topical formulations, including those for antibacterials, antiperspirants, autibiotics, sunscreens, anaesthetics and topical corticosteroids.

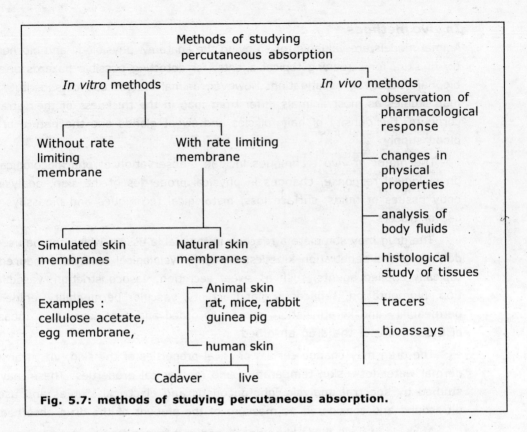

Fig. 5.7: methods of studying percutaneous absorption.

FACTORS AFFECTING PERCUTANEOUS ABSORPTION:

Biological factors :

Figure 5.8 shows the complex process of percutaneous absorption. The process is further complicated by various factors related to skin drug and vehicle.

a. **Skin age:** Skins of foetus, young and elderly are more permeable than adult tissue.

b. **Skin condition:** Certain irritant chemicals, or disease may degenerate the stratum corneum, thus increasing the permeability of skin to almost any substance. Stripping off stratum corneum with adhesive tape increases skin permeability.

c. **Regional skin sites:** The skin permeation varies depending on the variation in epidermal thickness, number of skin appendages, nature of epidermis.

d. **Skin metabolism:** Human skin may store and metabolise certain hormones, and such metabolism may prove a critical determinant of therapeutic efficacy of topically applied drugs.

e. **Species differences:** Mammalian skin from different species exhibits vast differences in thickness of stratum corneum and number of skin appendages, which in turn affects rate of percutaneous absorption.

Physicochemical factors: The principal physicochemical factors that govern passive diffusion of the solute, are the molecular properties of the diffusant, the vehicle and the skin. We can identify four possible interactions - drug-skin, vehicle-skin, drug-vehicle and drug-vehicle-skin, interactions that are likely to affect the percutaneous absorption.

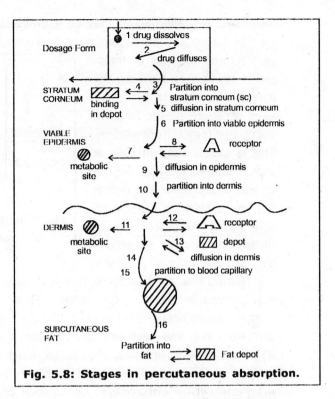

Fig. 5.8: Stages in percutaneous absorption.

A. Drug-skin interactions:

i) Skin hydration: When water saturates skin, the skin softens, swells and its permeability dramatically increases. Some drugs that can rapidly penetrate the skin to yield tissue concentrations that are high enough to exert an osmotic effect may increase skin hydration. A compound that efficiently hydrates the skin may significantly improve the treatment of dry skin. A hypothetical substance, which is naturally present in skin, is called as Natural Moisturising Factor (NMF). A compound called as pyrrolidone carboxylic acid is found to resemble NMF and may be used for treatment of dry skin.

ii) Drug-skin binding: Many penetrants may bind in part to skin proteins, thus making it unavailable to reach the systemic circulation.

B. Vehicle-skin interactions:

The pharmaceutical vehicles, when applied to skin, may change the physical state of the integument, thus changing its permeability. This alteration in the permeability might be due to solvent action on stratum corneum, a hydration effect or effect on skin temperature.

i) Vehicle effect on skin hydration : The NMF is necessary to maintain moisture content of stratum corneum above 20 per cent, which makes the skin is soft and pliable. With increase in hydration of skin, the permeation rate of penetrant increases. Two approaches may be followed to increase hydration status of skin, viz., occlusion and humectancy. In occlusion, the oleaginous vehicle applied on skin retards the loss of moisture from skin by blocking the sweat pores. This principle uses occlusive plastic films to cover the topical formulation. This is mainly used in case of topical steroid therapy. Another way to increase skin hydration by occlusion is to incorporate some oleaginous hydrophobic material as vehicle in the formulation, e.g. paraffins, lanolin.

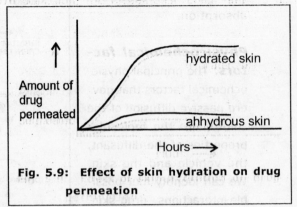

Fig. 5.9: Effect of skin hydration on drug permeation

Humectants are the hydrophilic materials having very high affinity for water, e.g. glycerin, proylene glycol, sorbitol. These materials absorb moisture from atmosphere and deliver it to skin. But many times these materials withdraw moisture from skin and decrease its hydration, thus retarding rate of permeation.

ii) Effect of temperature: Skin temperature increases under occlusive dressings or in diseased state. This slightly increases permeability of the penetrant.

iii) Penetration enhancers: Penetration enhancers are the substances which can temporarily diminish impermeability of skin. If these materials are non-toxic and safe, they can be used in dermatological vehicles to enhance permeability of drugs. Ideal features of penetration enhancers are-

- It should be pharmacologically inert.
- It should be non-toxic, non-irritant and non-allergenic.
- Onset of penetration enhancement should be immediate on application.
- The penetration enhancement should be reversible.
- The barrier function of skin should reduce in one direction only.
- It should be physically and chemically compatible with a wide range of drugs and adjuvants.
- It should be an excellent solvent for drugs.
- It should easily spread on skin and should be cosmetically elegant.
- Formulation of the substance into various types, viz., lotion, cream, ointment and suspension should be possible.
- It should be inexpensive, odourless, tasteless and colourless.

Some pentetration enhancers increase the percutaneous adsorption of the penetrant by increasing its thermodynamic activity, thus increasing its escaping tendency and concentration gradient of the diffusing species. Some have a direct effect on skin permeability, e.g. solvents, surfactants, urea, DMSO, 2-Me-pyrrolidone. The mechanical action is complex since they also increase penetrant solubility. But the predominant effect of these enhancers on stratum corneum is either to increase its degree of hydration or to disrupt its lipoprotein matrix. Water also affects skin permeability by increasing hydration of stratum corneum. It is a factor even in anhydrous delivery system due to their occlusivity. Due to its safety and efficacy, it has been described as ultimate penetration enhancer. Other solvents include DMSO, DMF, DMAC, etc. But DMSO is now of limited utility because of its potential ocular and dermal toxicity, objectionable taste and odour and need of concentration in excess of 70 per cent to promote absorption. Other solvents, like laurocapram, act in quite low concentrations (=5%). Azone effect persists long.

Surfactants are recognised for their ability to alter membrane structure and function and can have substantial effect on permeability. However, surfactants applied chronically have irritation potential.

Solvents : Water, alcohols, MeOH, EtOH, IPA, Alkyl Me sulfoxides, DMSO, Decylmethyl SO, Tetradecyl methyl SO.

Pyrrolidones : 2-pyrrolidones, N-methyl-2-pyrrolidone, N-(2-hydroxyethyl) pyriolidone, laurocupram

Miscellanous : Acetone, DMAC, DMF, Amphiphiles 1-α amino acids, Clofibric acid amides, Hexamethylene lauramide, Proteolytic enzymes, Terpenes, sesquiterpenes, d-limonene, Urea, N,N-diethyl-m-toluamide

Such materials appear to increase skin permeability by increasing the diffusion resistance of stratum corneum, by reversibly damaging the stratum corneum or by altering its physicochemical nature.

The penetration enhancers are also called as accelerants or sorption promoters. The term is limited only to materials, which significantly increase the drug permeation, but do not severely damage the skin.

Examples of penetration enhancers:

Dimethyl Sulfoxide	N, N dimethyl acetamide	N, N dimethyl formamide	2-pyrrolidone	1 methyl, 2-pyrrolidone

5-methyl 2-pyrrolidone	1,5-dimethyl 2-pyrrolidone	1-ethyl 2-pyrrolidone	2-pyrrolidone 5- carboxylic acid

Dimethl Sulphoxide (DMSO): This is a nearly odourless, water-white, dipolar solvent. It enables low molecular weight substances to penetrate quickly into deeper layers of the skin. But it does not abolish the skin barrier, nor does it allow penetration of macromolecules. It produces local irritation on skin, but it diminishes with continued application.

Some other agents used are-

1. Dimethyl acetamide/ Dimethyl formamide

Sonophoresis and Iontophoresis : In addition to chemical methods, there are some physical methods being used to enhance transepidermal drug delivery and penetration viz., iontophoresis and sonophoresis.

Iontophoresis involves the delivery of charged chemical compounds across the skin membrane using an applied electrical field

e.g. Lidocaine, dexamethasone, amino acids/peptides.

Sonophoresis or high frequency ultrasound is also being investigated to enhance percutaneous absorption. It is thought that high frequency ultrasound can affect integrity of stratum corneum and thus affect its penetrability.

C. Drug-vehicle interactions:

a. Vehicle-skin partition coefficient of drug: The release of substance is favoured by the selection of vehicles that have a low affinity for penetrant, or in which the drug is least soluble. The rate of release is governed by drug's vehicle stratum corneum partition co-effficient.

b. Transdermal drug delivery systems: These are the topical devices for delivery of the drug to surface of the skin at controlled rate. The device controls drug release rate and the rate at which the drug passes into the circulation. It is used for providing systemic therapy for acute or chronic conditions, e.g. nitroglycerine in angina and scopolamine in motion sickness.

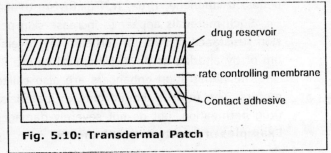

Fig. 5.10: Transdermal Patch

The device is a multilayer laminate. It contains a drug reservoir held in a polymeric gel, sandwiched between a backing sheet and the controlling microporous membrane. Above this is placed a contact adhesive which sticks the device to skin.

D. Drug-vehicle-skin interactions :

The vehicle may sometimes get control on the diffusion flux of the drug through the skin under certain assumptions. The diffusion model of simple zero-order flux is used to explain this & is given by :

$$\frac{dm}{dt} = \frac{KC_v D}{h}$$

Where,

dm/dt - steady state flux of penetrant/unit area of membrane

K   -   Parfition Coefficient of drug between stratum corneum and vehicle

C_v -   Concentration of drug in vehicle

D   -   diffusion coefficient of drug in stratum corneum

h   -   thickness of stratum corneum.

FORMULATION OF DERMATOLOGICAL VEHICLES

In the past, the dermatological vehicles were formulated in terms of stability, compatibility and patient acceptance. It is only in recent years, that the importance of dermatological vehicles in bioavailability and release of drug has been understood. Ideally, a pharmacist would want to formulate a single component vehicle to avoid problems due to interaction of components. But the dermatologists prefer that in addition to the requirement of releasing the drug at optimum rate, the vehicle should perform following functions-

i)   Anti-inflammatory effects in acute inflammation -vasoconstriction, cooling, astringent.

ii) Symptomatic relief of pain and itch.

iii) Protection from mechanical, microbiological, thermal and chemical irritation.

iv) Cleansing - removal of dirt, exudates, previous applications.

v)   Lubricant and emollient effects.

The dermatological vehicle should promote healing and do no further damage, as it has to help in application of a therapeutic agent. Pharmaceutically, the vehicle should be aesthetically acceptable, should have ease of application and must be odourless, non-staining and homogenous.

The three main components of a dermatological vehicle are an aqueous phase, oil and powder. Different types of formulations may be obtained by permutation and combination of these three components.

RAW MATERIALS

A wide range of materials is available and the proper material should be selected after thoroughly studying stability, compatibility and aesthetic appeal of the vehicle with drug.

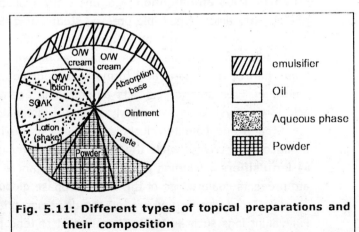

Fig. 5.11: Different types of topical preparations and their composition

i) Hydrocarbons: Petrolatum and mineral oil are the most widely used raw materials after water. Both are obtained from petroleum. Petrolatum is a complex mixture of semisolid hydrocarbons, containing aliphatic, cyclic, saturated, unsaturated, branched and unbranched substances in variable proportions. Broad variation in density, melting point and chemical composition is permissible in compendia. It is available in two varieties - long fiber and short fiber, the former being preferred for occlusive dressings, as it forms a continuous film.

Mineral oil is obtained from petroleum by collection of a particular viscosity-controlled fraction. Lower viscosity grades are preferred.

ii) Hydrocarbon waxes: They are mainly incorporated to increase viscosity of mineral oil in order to prevent its oozing from ointment. They prevent oozing by forming a matrix-like structure in which the oily phase is retained.

e.g. Ozokerite - melting point $65-75^0c$ - mixture of saturated hydrocarbons ranging in carbon carbon chain length from 35 to 55.

Paraffin wax – melting point $35-75^0c$.

Ceresin - mixture of ozokerite and paraffin wax.

Synthetic waxes are also developed from vegetable oils by hydrogenation and catalytic splitting. They are chemically closely related to naturally occurring waxes, e.g. Synchrowaxes. They have unique gelling characteristics.

iii) Oleaginous substances: Vegetable oils, viz. peanut oil, almond oil, sesame oil and olive oil are mono-, di- and tri- glycerides of mixtures of unsaturated and saturated fatty acids. Presence of trace metals in oils initiate oxidation of oleaginous substances. This can be avoided by addition of anti-oxidants like butylated hydroxy anisole (BHA), butylated hydroxy toluene (BHT), propyl gallate or chelating agents like EDTA. Vegetable oils also vary in their chemical composition depending on their source. Therefore, nowadays the trend is towards isolating and synthesizing chemically pure ingredients of the vegetable oils.

iv) Fatty acids and alcohols: Commercially available fatty acids are mixtures of related fatty acids, e.g. triple pressed stearic acid. Stearic and palmitic acids are mainly present along with other fatty acids. Stearic acid is mainly used in water-removable type of bases as emulsifier, along with NaOH/KOH/triethanol amine. Some part of the stearic acid forms sodium or potassium soap which acts as an emulsifier. Free stearic acid acts as stiffening agent for the preparation. Stearic acid forms crystals on skin slowly, giving a luster upon ageing.

Stearyl and palmityl alcohols are used as auxiliary emulsifiers. The former produces stiff cream, while the latter forms softer creams

v) Emulsifiers : Addition of fatty polar substances such as glyceryl monostearate prevents coalescence of the internal phase globules and stabilises the cream. The interfacial film formed around the dispersed phase globule is generally solid. Polyvalent ions such as Mg^{++}, Ca^{++} and Al^{+++} tend to stabilise w/o emulsions by cross-linking polar groups of the fatty materials.

A soluble surfactant is adsorbed at the interface and forms a film. Oil-soluble polar substances react with the surfactant at the interface making it more complex.

Cationic and non-ionic surfactants are preferred for drugs requiring acidic pH and non-ionics are suitable to most of the drugs.

vi) Polyols: Glycerin and propylene glycol/sorbitol are many times added as humectants. They prevent the cream from drying out and also improve texture and feel of the product. They also act as emollients on skin to some extent.

vii) Insoluble powders: Many times drugs are present in insoluble powder form. It must be finely divided (< 74 μ or 200 mesh USP) to avoid grittiness. Milling allow more surface area of the drug to come in contact with skin.

Table 5.2: Raw materials for semisolid preparations.

Category	Examples
Hydrocarbons	Petrolatum, mineral oil
Hydrocarbon waxes	Ozokerite, paraffin wax, Ceresin, synchrowaxes
Oleaginous substances	Peanut oil, almond oil, sesame oil, olive oil
Fatty acids & alcohols	Stearic acid, Palmitic acid,
	Stearyl alcohol, Cetostearyl alcohol
Emulsifiers	Anionics: Alyl sulfates, soaps, phosphate esters, monoglycerite sulfates
	Cationics : Quaternary ammonium compounds, Alkoxyalkyl amines
	Non-ionics:Tweens, Spans, Promulgens
Polyols	Glycerin, Propylene glycol, Sorbitol
Insoluble powders	Drug powders

TYPES OF DERMATOLOGICAL PREPARATIONS:

OINTMENTS:

Ointments are greasy semisolid preparations, often anhydrous and containing dissolved or dispersed medicaments.

Types of ointment bases :

i) Hydrocarbon bases : Usually consist of soft paraffin or its mixtures with soft paraffin. Paraffins form a greasy film on skin, inhibiting water loss, thus hydrating skin. Because of their hydrating effect on skin, ointments are very effective in improving its hydration status.

Examples of this type of base are petrolatum and white ointment.

Plastibases are a series of hydrocarbons containing polyethylene. They are soft, smooth, homogenous, neutral, colourless, odourless, non-irritating, stable vehicles.

Hydrocarbons are difficult to wash off the skin, they stain cloth and give a feeling of discomfort. Very little water can be incorporated into these greasy bases without the addition of other substances.

Examples of hydrocarbon base-

1. Petrolatum, U.S.P.
2. White petrolatum, U.S.P.
3. Yellow ointment, U.S.P. :

Yellow Wax	- - -	50 gm
Petrolatum	- - -	950 gm

4. White ointment, U.S.P.

White Wax	- - -	50 gm
White petrolatum	- - -	950 gm

ii) Absorption bases: These bases soak up water to form w/o emulsions, while retaining their semisolid consistency. The maximum amount of water that can be added to 100 gm of such a base, at a given temperature, is called as water number. Substance which act as a w/o emulsifiers, e.g. lanolin, lanolin isolates, cholesterol, lanosterol, partial esters of polyhydric alcohols, e.g. sorbitan monostearate may be added to these bases.

These bases deposit an oily layer on skin, similar to hydrocarbon bases, but the suppression of transepidermal water loss is low as compared to hydrocarbon bases.

Examples of anhydrous absorption base-

1. **Hydrophilic petrolatum, U.S.P.**

Cholesterol	- - -	30 gm
Stearyl alcohol	- - -	30 gm
White Wax	- - -	80 gm
White petrolatum	- - -	860 gm

2. **Wool fat or anhydrous lanolin**

Examples of hydrous absorption base-

1. **Lanolin, U.S.P.**
2. **Cold Cream**

Mineral oil	- - -	40 % w/w
White Wax	- - -	6
Polyglyceryl 5-trioleate	- - -	8
Isopropyl palmitate	- - -	3
Sorbital monostearate	- - -	3.5

Polysorbate 60	- - -	2.5
Propylene glycol	- - -	4.0
Water	- - -	33.0
Preservative, qs.		

Synthetic waxes (Water removable bases): They are commonly referred to as creams and are most widely used.

iii) Emulsifying bases: They are miscible with water and are washable or self-emulsifying. Depending on the ionic nature of the emulsifier there are three types, anionic (emulsifying ointment, BP), cationic (cetrimide ointment, BP) or non-ionic (Cetomacrogo emulsifying ointment, BP). As they contain surfactants, these bases bring the drug in more intimate contact with the skin. They can be readily washed off and hence have good patient acceptance.

The o/w vehicle tends to absorb exudates from skin lesion. They are used for wet dressing.

Example of water removable base

1. Hydrophilic ointment U.S.P.

Methyl paraben	- - -	0.25 gm
Propyl paraben	- - -	0.15 gm
Sodium lauryl sulfate	- - -	10 gm
Propylene glycol	- - -	120 gm
Stearyl alcohol	- - -	250 gm
White petrolatum	- - -	250 gm
Purified water	- - -	370 gm

2. Vanishing Cream

Part A

Mineral oil, light	5% $\frac{w}{w}$
Stearic acid	2.5
White wax	1.5
Cetyl alcohol	6.5
Stearyl alcohol	5.0

Part B

Propylene glycol	5.0
Triethanolamine	2.0
Water	72.5
Preservative, q.s.	

iv) Water-soluble bases : They are prepared from mixtures of high and low molecular weight Polyethylene glycols (PEGs) having general formula $HOCH_2$ $(CH_2OCH_2)_n CH_2OH$. The low molecular weight glycols are liquids, moderately high molecular weight glycols are greasy liquids and high molecular weight are solids. Suitable combination of high and low molecular weight PEGs yield products having an ointment-like consistency, which soften or melt when applied to skin. No water is required for their preparation. They are water-soluble because of the presence of many water-soluble polar groups. They are much less occlusive than w/o emulsions and can be removed easily with water.

Table 5.3: Expected effects of common vehicles on skin hydration and permeability

Vehicle	Constituent/ Example	Effect on skin hydration	Effect on skin permeability
Occlusive dressing	plastic film	prevents water loss full hydration	marked increase
Lipophilic	paraffins, oils fats, waxes, silicones	prevent water loss may produce full hydration	marked increase
Absorption base	lanolin, hydrophilic petrolatum	prevents water loss, marked hydration	marked increase
Emulsifying base w/o emulsion	hydrophilic ointment	marked hydration	marked increase
	oily creams	retard water loss, raised hydration	increase
O/W emulsion	aqueous cream	may donate water, slight hydration	slight increase and
Humectant	water soluble base, glycerol	may withdraw water, decrease hydration	can decrease or act as penetration enhancer
Powder	clays, organics, inorganics	aid water evaporation	little effect on permeability

PASTES :

Pastes are ointments that contain high proportion of powder (as much as 50 per cent) dispersed in a fatty base. Typical powder ingredients include Zinc oxide, starch, calcium carbonate, talc, salicylic acid. Pastes are stiffer than the parent ointments. They were originally formulated with the concept that the high solid content absorbs skin exudates. But afterwards it was found out that a powder coated with a hydrocarbon cannot absorb any aqueous exudates. Because of their consistency, pastes are useful for localising the action of irritant chemicals like coal tar.

Pastes lay down a thick, unbroken, impermeable film on the skin that can be opaque and act as a sun filter. Pastes have dilatant rheology.

CREAMS :

Pharmaceutical creams are semisolid emulsions of o/w or w/o type containing medicinal agents dissolved or dispersed in internal or external phase. They may be classified as o/w or w/o creams. Many pharmaceutical creams are classified as water removable bases and are described under ointments.

In addition to ointment bases, creams include variety of cosmetic preparations. Creams of o/w type are called vanishing creams. Examples of this type are shaving creams, hand creams and foundation creams. W/o creams include cold creams and emollient creams.

GELS AND JELLIES :

A. Definition :

A gel is a semisolid two-phase system consisting of a condensed three dimensional network enclosing and interpenetrated by a continuous phase. The dispersed phase particles link together to form an interlaced network thus imparting rigidity to the structure. The continuous phase is held within the meshes.

A gel may be called as 'jelly' if the water content is relatively high. If such liquid from the gel is removed, only the three dimensional network remains. Such a gel is called as xerogels. Xerogels can be converted to gels by contact with water, e.g. acacia tears, sheet gelatin and tragacanth flakes.

B. Classification of gels :

The gels may be classified depending on following different criteria :

i) Depending on structure: Small organic partides such as aluminium hydroxide form a floccule-like structure throughout the gel. The inorganic particles being insoluble in the continuous phase, the system is a true two-phase system. If the inorganic particles are slightly bigger in size, the gel is called as magma, e.g. bentonite magma.

Large organic molecules tend to exist in solution as randomly coiled flexible chains. These molecules are either synthetic or natural polymers that tend to entangle each other due to their random motion. These systems are actually single phase systems as the molecules exist in solution. However, the unique behavior of long molecules in solution, leading to fairly high viscosities and gel structure, makes it possible to consider these systems as two phase systems, e.g. tragacanth gel.

ii) Depending on nature of the gel forming phase: When the gel forming phase is inorganic, the gel is called as inorganic gel and when it is organic, the gel is called as organic gel. Most of the inorganic gels are two phase systems and organic gels are single phase systems.

iii) Depending on nature of the solvent : When the solvent is aqueous the gel is called as hydro gel, e.g. gelatin; and if it is organic, the gel is called as organo gel, e.g. polyethylenes in mineral oil.

Uses of gels :

Gels are becoming popular as pharmaceutical dosage forms because a drug that is dissolved in the continuous phase is relatively free. The pores allow relatively free diffusion of molecules, which are not too large. Therefore, release of medicament from a gel is very quick.

Gels are used as delivery systems for oral administration as gels proper, or as capsule sheets made from gelatin for topical drugs applied to skin, mucous membranes or eye and for long acting forms of drugs injected intramuscularly.

Gelling agents are useful as binders in tablet granulation, protective colloids in suspensions, thickeners in oral liquids.

Gels are used in wide variety of cosmetics including shampoos, dentifrices and skin and hair care preparations.

Advantages :

i)   Quick release of medicament.

ii) The thixotropic properties of gels make their removal from the containers easy. The shear force generated during topical application reduces their viscosity, making their application easy.

iii) A very low concentration of gelling agent produces fairly firm gel. Thus they are cost effective.

Disadvantages:

i)   Some anionic gel formers are incompatible with cationic drug preservatives or surfactants and inactivation of the drug or its precipitation may occur, e.g. sodium alginate decreases concentration of cations.

ii) Many gels, especially of polysaccharide nature, are susceptible to microbial degradation and subsequent loss of gel characteristics.

Characteristics of gels:

i)   Swelling and imbibition : Gels can take up liquids, thus increasing in volume. This is called as swelling of gels. A solvent penetrates the gel matrix and the gel-gel interactions are replaced by gel-sol interactions. Some gels may also take up liquid without increase in their volume and this is called as imbibition.

ii) Syneresis : Many gels shrink naturally upon standing and some of its liquid is pressed out. This phenomenon is known as syneresis. This is probably because of the continued coarsening of the

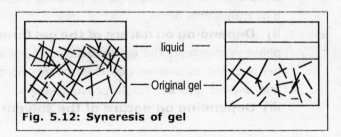

Fig. 5.12: Syneresis of gel

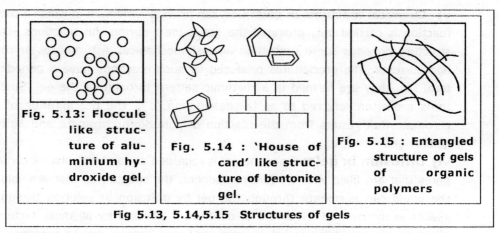

Fig. 5.13: Floccule like structure of aluminium hydroxide gel.

Fig. 5.14 : 'House of card' like structure of bentonite gel.

Fig. 5.15 : Entangled structure of gels of organic polymers

Fig 5.13, 5.14, 5.15 Structures of gels

matrix or fibrous structure, i.e., continued particle-particle linkages of the gelling agent with a consequent squeezing out effect.

iii) Structure :

a)   Some inorganic substances like aluminium hydroxide form a gel that can be looked upon like a continuous floccule. The forces holding the molecular particles together are weak Van der Waals forces.

b)   Montmorillonite clays such as bentonite and kaolin are hydrated aluminium magnesium silicates. Their crystals have a flat lamellar disc-like structure. The flat part on the face of the crystal carriers a net negative charge due to atoms and the edge carries a net positive charge due to oxygen atoms. As a result of electrostatic attraction between the negatively charged face and positively charged edge, these crystals form a house-of-cards-like structure. The particles are held together by weak electrostatic attraction.

c)   Organic macromolecules such as tragacanth and methyl cellulose form gels in different manner. They exist as twisted matted chains. The chains are extended in good solvents due to hydrogen bond formation between water and -OH groups on the gelling agent. Each sequence of the dissolved molecule is in continuous random motion. Due to the motion, the chains get entangled forming a gel matrix.

d)   The cross-linking of macromolecules by primary valency bonds provides a further mechanism for formation of gel matrix. The gelling process here is irreversible. Silisic acid molecules in silica gel network are linked by Si-O-Si covalent bonds forming a rigid gel. Some gels are elastic in nature and they do not deform on application of stress, e.g. Carrageenan gel.

iv) Adsorption by xerogels: The porous nature of xerogels provides a large surface area for the adsorption of vapours. The porosity also provides possibility of uptake of water vapour by capillary action. Xerogels, especially, silica gel is used as drying agent.

v) Chemical reactions in gels: Gels can provide a medium in which a chemical reaction is carried out, provided the gel is inert during the reactions. The gel structure provides some protection against mechanical disturbances or convection currents. The precipitates produced by such reactions have a periodic pattern, i.e., they are formed in a rhythmic pattern throughout the gel. Such patterns are often referred to as Leisegang ring, e.g. the precipitation of silver chromate that results from the reaction of potassium chromate and $AgNO_3$ in gelatin gel.

vi) Diffusion in gels: Since the gel is regarded as random network containing pores that are filled with a liquid component, the substances that are soluble in the liquid can permeate through the gel by diffusion in solution through the spaces in the network. The rate of diffusion is affected by all those factors that affect the normal diffusion, plus some additional factors, due to presence of the gel matrix. Diffusion is spontaneous transfer of solute from region of higher concentration to region of lower concentration, till equilibrium is achieved.

$$\frac{dm}{dt} = \frac{-DAdc}{dx}$$

Where,

dm - amount of solute transferred in time dt, across area A, under the influence of concentration gradient, dc/dx. D - diffusion coefficient, which is constant.

dc/dx is negative because diffusion occurs in the opposite direction to that of increasing concentration.

vii) Sieve effect : The rates of diffusion of small molecules and ions through gels are same as their rates of diffusion in simple solution. However, as the size of the particle becomes comparable to the pore diameter of the gel network, diffusion is retarded considerably. The diffusion ceases when particles are larger than the widest pores in the gel. This is known as sieve effect of the gel and considered as a normal filtration process.

The area through which the diffusion can take place is not the total surface area of the gel, but the combined surface area of the pores. The sieve effect of the gel is determined by concentration of the gelling agent and age of the gel.

Preparation of Gel :

i) Temperature effect : Solubility of most lyophobic colloids like agar and gelatin is decreased on lowering the temperature, so that cooling a concentrated hot solution will produce a gel.

ii) Flocculation with salts and non-solvents : Gelation is produced by adding just sufficient precipitant to produce gel, but insufficient to produce a precipitate, e.g. addition of non-solvent-like petroleum ether to solution of ethyl cellulose, polystyrene in benzene.

Addition of salts to hydrophobic solutions usually causes coagulation and gelation is rarely observed. But addition of salt to a moderately hydrophilic solution will cause gelation, e.g. addition of salt to solutions of aluminium hydroxide, ferric hydroxide and bentonite. Usually, addition of about half the amount of electrolyte needed for complete precipitation is adequate. With positively charged hydroxide solutions, divalent ions such as SO_4^{-2} are more effective than univalent ions such as Cl^-

iii) Chemical Reaction : In preparation of gels by precipitation from solution, e.g. aluminium hydroxide gel prepared by interaction of aqueous solution of an aluminium salt and sodium carbonate.

Clear jelly base :

Sodium alginate	3 gm
Methylparaben	0.2 gm
Sodium hexamide phosphate	0.5 gm.
Glycerin	10.0 gm
Purified water	

Dissolve methyl paraben in glycerin by heating. Dissolve Na-hexametaphosphate in this solution. Add Na-alginate with rapid continuous stirring.

GEL FORMING AGENTS:

A) Natural gums : Most of the natural gums used as gelling agents, are anionic and very few are non-ionic, e.g. guar gums, because of their natural origin, are prone to microbial attack and need to be preserved. Also, anionic gums have a tendancy to react with cationic preservatives, e.g. sodium alginate reacts with quaternary amino compounds. As most of the gums are obtained from plants, they may differ in their properties·depending upon the regional variations in plant species.

i) Alginates: Alginates are natural polysachharides mainly containing various proportions of D-mannose and L-guluronic acid. They are obtained from brown seaweeds in the form of monovalent and divalent salts.

The most popularly used salt is sodium alginate. Gelation occurs by acidic pH or presence of divalent cation, e.g. Ca^{++}. At acidic pH, the carboxylate ions are converted to carboxylic groups. This decreases hydration and repulsion between the polysaccharide chains. Some amount of Ca^{++} must be present for gelation, usually contributed by the alginate itself.

At neutral pH, the alginates gel in presence of divalent cations, especially with Ca^{++}. Calcium ions react preferentially with polyguluronate residues, forming a crosslink between the polymers and bringing about gelation. The pH at which gelation occurs is inversely proportional to calcium ion concentration.

The calcium ions first react with the surface polymer, diffuse down through the gel formed on the surface, and the reaction proceeds. More the concentration of Ca^{++} ions, stiffer is the gel. But as the structure becomes 'tight' and the Ca^{++} ions diffuse slowly through it, the reaction becomes slow. Slightly soluble calcium salts or sequestering agents are used. The gel strength and other properties such as brittleness are functions of chemical make up of alginate, while gelation rate is function of Ca^{++} concentration.

ii) Carrageenan : It is sodium, magnesium, calcium, ammonium and potassium sulphate esters of polymerised galactose and 3,6-anhydrogalactose. The main copolymer types are labelled as kappa, iota and lambda. Kappa and iota carrageenans form thermo-reversible gels. This is attributed to temperature sensitive polymer arrangement. At high temperatures the polymer chains are coiled randomly, cooling results in formulation of double helix which act as a crosslink. Kappa-carrageenan gels are brittle, while iota gels are elastic.

Ephedrine Sulphate jelly:

Ephedrine sulphate	10 gm
Tragacanth	10 gm
Methyl-salicylate	0.1 gm.
Eucalyptol	1 ml
Pine needle oil	0.1 ml
Glycerin	150 gm.
Purified Water	830 ml.

Dissolve Ephedrine SO_4 in purified H_2O, add glycerin, tragacanth and then remaining ingredients, mix well and keep in closed container for 1 week.

iii)Tragacanth : Tragacanth is a gummy exudation from *Astragallus gummifer*, Fam. Leguminosae, and other Asiatic species of *Astragallus*. It is composed chiefly of an acidic polysaccharide tragacanthic acid containing Ca, Mg, K and a smaller amount of natural polysaccharide tragacanthin. The gum swells in water, and concentrations of 2 per cent and above produce a gel. Hydration takes place over a long period of time and gel formation is slow.

iv) Pectin : It is a polysaccharide obtained from inner rind of citrus fruits and apple pomace. Gel is formed in acidic pH in aqueous solution containing calcium and possibly another agent that dehydrates the polymer. Gel formulation is more effective in pectin with low methoxyl content.

v) Xanthan gum: It is produced by bacterial fermentation. Therefore its quality is not subject to many of the uncertainties that affect other natural products. At 0.5 per cent concentration, it is used as stabiliser of suspension and emulsion. At 1 per cent concentration it acts as gelling agent. Thermo-reversible gels are formed by combination with guar gum and locust bean gum.

vi) Other gums: Gelatin used as bodying agent and gel former in food industry. Agar is used as culture media. Gellan gum is a newer material produced by fermentation that has been proposed as substitute for agar.

B) Carbomer : Carbomer 934 P is an official name given to one member of a group of acrylic polymers cross-linked with a polyalkenyl ether. The carbomer forms gel at concentrations as low as 0.5 per cent. They are available as free acids. They are first dispersed uniformly in aqueous media. Entrapped air is removed and then the dispersion is neutralised with a suitable base. Introduction of negative charges around the polymer cause it to uncoil and expand. Bases such as sodium hydroxide, potassium hydroxide, ammonium hydroxide or salts such as sodium carbonate can be used for neutralisation. Organic bases such as triethanolamine make the carbomer compatible with semi-polar solvents.

Zinc oxide gel	% by weight	Sunscreen gel	% by weight
Water	76	Ethanol	53.0
Carbomer 934 p	0.8	Carbomer 940	1.0
Sodium hydroxide 10% solution	3.2	Monoisopropanolamine	0.09
Zinc oxide	20.0	Water	52.91

C) Cellulose derivatives : Many synthetic derivatives are prepared from natural cellulose by breaking down the backbone structure or replacing some -OH groups in cellulose. The factors affecting their rheology are degree of substitution, nature of substitution and molecular weight of resultant polymer. Cellulose derivatives are prone to depolymerisation by microbial attack. Their formulations should be protected by sterilisation or addition of preservative. e.g. methyl cellulose, sodium carboxy methyl cellulose, hydroxyethyl cellulose, hydroxypropyl cellulose.

D) Polyethylenes : They are used to gel hydrophobic liquids to form soft, spreadable semisolid, hydrophobic film on skin. Polyethylene is a gelling agent for simple aliphatic hydrocarbons. It is incompatible with many other oils. Acrylic acid and vinyl acetate copolymers of polyethylene are therefore prepared. Polymers are dispersed in oil at elevated temperatures and shock cooled to form a gel.

Mineral oil gel	% by weight
Polyethylene (A-C 617)	10
Mineral oil	90

E) Solids in colloidal dispersions : Microcrystalline silica can be used as gelling agent in various liquids. Network formed is due to attraction of particles by polar-forces, principally, hydrogen-bonding. It gels at low concentration in non-polar liquids, but high concentrations are required in polar liquids due to competition of the medium for hydrogen binding sites.

Montmorillonite clays form gels due to electrostatic forces of attraction between particles. These gels are therefore affected by presence of electrolytes.

Colloidal cellulose can also be used effectively as gelling agent.

F) Surfactants : Clear gels are produced by combination of mineral oil, water and high percentage of (20-40 per cent) certain non-ionic surfactants. These gels are mainly used in hair grooming products.

OINTMENT BASES :

Table 5.4: Some differences in properties of ointment bases

Hydrocarbon bases (Oleaginous)	Absorption bases (anhydrous)
Example white ointment	Example hydrophilic petrolatum, Anhydrous lanolin
Emollient	Emollient
Occlusive	Occlusive
Non-water washable	Absorb water
Hydrophobic	Anhydrous
Greasy	Greasy

Absorption Bases w/o	Water-Removable o/w	Water-soluble
e.g. Cold cream	e.g. Vanishing cream	e.g. Polyethyleve glycol ointment
Emollient	Water Washable	Usually anhydrous
Occlusive	Non-greasy	Water-soluble & washable
Contain water	Can be diluted with water	Non-greasy
Some may absorb water	Non-occlusive	Non-occlusive
Greasy		

Absorption bases :

Absorption bases are hydrophilic, anhydrous materials, or hydrous bases that have ability to absorb additional water. The former are anhydrous substances that can absorb water to form w/o emulsions. The latter are w/o emulsions which can farther absorb water. Both types of bases are exemplified by anhydrous lanolin (wool fat) and lanolin (hydrous wool fat). The former is converted to the latter by absorbing 30 per cent water. The latter further absorbs water.

Hydrophilic petrolatum, U.S.P., is anhydrous absorption base. It contain :

Cholesterol   Stearyl alcohol

White wax   White petrolatum

Emulsion base :

The emulsion base is composed of oil phase (internal), the emulsifier and the aqueous phase (external). The medicinal agent may be included in any of the three phases. The oily phase, is typically made up of petrolatum or/and liquid petrolatum together with one or more high molecular weight alcohols, such as cetyl or stearyl alcohol. The aqueous phase may contain preservatives, stabilisers, antioxidants, emulsifiers, etc.

i) Anionic emulsifiers : Sodium lauryl sulphate is a typical example of this class. The active portion of the emulsifier is anion (SO_4^{-2}). Other emulsifiers from this class are soaps such as triethanolamine stearate. Sodium lauryl sulphate and other anionic surfactants of this class are more acid-stable and permit adjustment of emulsion pH to the desirable acid range of 4.5-6.5. Anionic emulsifiers may cause irritation to skin in certain situations. They may sometimes act as penetration enhancers.

ii) Cationic emulsifiers : They are highly surface active, but are not used very frequently as emulsifiers. The cation portion is usually a quaternary ammonium salt with a fatty acid derivative. They may cause irritation to skin and eyes and are incompatible with anionic materials.

iii) Non-ionic emulsifiers : They have excellent pH and electrolyte compatibility. They are both hydrophilic and lipophilic and may be used in combination by making use of the HLB scale. Emulsions made with non-ionic substances are usually low in irritation potential, are stable and compatible.

Table 5.5 : Surfactants for semisolid emulsions

Anionic	Cationic	Non-ionic
Alkyl sulfates Soaps	Quaternary ammonium compounds	Polyoxyethylene alkyl-aryl ethers Polyoxy propylene akyl aryl ethers
Dodecyl benzenesulfonates		Polyoxyethylene fatty acid esters
Lactylates	Alkoxyalkyl amines	Polyoxyethylene sorbitan esters
Sulfosuccinates		Sorbitan fatty acid esters
Monoglycerite sulfates Phosphate esters Silicones Sarcosinates Taurates		Glyceryl fatty acid esters Sucrose fatty acid esters

PRESERVATION OF DERMATOLOGICALS

Dermatological vehicles often contain aqueous and oily phases, together with carbohydrates and proteins. Therefore they are prone to attack by bacteria and fungi. Microbial growth not only spoils the formulation, but is a source of infection, especially when the formulation is applied on broken skin.

SOURCES OF CONTAMINATION:

i) Raw materials, water ii) Manufacturing and filling equipment

iii) Personnel iv) Plant environment v) Final container

MICROORGANISMS IN DERMATOLOGICALS:

The three terms that are used to describe microorganisms associated with pharmaceutical products are - harmful, objectionable and opportunistic.

Harmful microorganisms:

These are the microorganisms or their toxins that are responsible for human diseases or infections, e.g. *Salmonella, E. coli, Pseudomonas, S. aureus.*

Objectionable microorganisms :

They may cause disease when ingested, or may interrupt the function of the drug, or lead to deterioration of the product.

Opportunistic microorganisms :

They produce disease or infection under special environmental conditions, when body resistance is low, e.g. in newborn and debilitated persons, aged people, or those undergoing excessive surgical or accidental trauma and compromised hosts. These sets of people are the ones who are on antibiotics, anticancer or immunosuppressive therapy. Recognised opportunistic pathogens are objectionable, e.g. *P. putida, P. multivorans, Proteus mirabilis, S. maltophilia, Serratia marcescens, Klebsiella* spp. and *Candida* spp.

The popular methods of sterilisation for dermatological products are moist heat sterilisation, dry heat sterilisation, ethylene oxide sterilisation. But once the sterile product is opened by the patient, there are always chances of contamination; therefore a better way of prevention of contamination is to add a preservative.

FACTORS INFLUENCING PRESERVATIVE EFFICACY:

1. Spectrum of activity : In a multidose container, the preservatives must have broad spectrum of activity covering gram-positive and gram-negative bacteria, together with yeast and fungi. Most of the preservatives have a limited spectrum and are therefore used in combination.

2. pH : Most of the preservatives are weak acids and bases. They are more active in non-ionic forms as they penetrate the bacterial cell wall easily. When pH of the product is equal to the pKa of the preservative, 50 per cent of preservative is unionised.

3. Temperature : Over a narrow range of temperature, activity of preservative increases with increase in temperature. This is calculated by Q_{10} value, which describes the effect of 10°C rise in temperature on the activity of a preservative.

$$Q_{10} = \frac{t_{(T)}}{t_{(T+10)}}$$

Where,

$t_{(T)}$ - death time at T°C

$t_{(T+10)}$ - death time at T+10°C

Effect of temperature on preservative is important in products recommended for refrigerated storage.

4. Stability: Some preservatives are unstable at certain pH or at certain temperatures.

5. Availability of preservative: Microorganisms grow only in the aqueous phase of the product and hence an adequate concentration of the preservative must be maintained in this phase. A number of factors affect the availability of the preservatives:

i) Solubility: For remaining in aqueous phase of the formulation, the preservative must have sufficient aqueous solubility and for passing through the bacterial cell wall, it must have sufficient lipophilicity. Thus, the partition coefficient of the preservative between the aqueous and oily phases of the given formulation is important. This problem can be overcome by using a combination of preservatives.

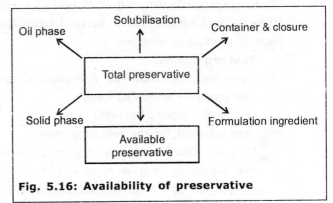

Fig. 5.16: Availability of preservative

ii) Solubilisation : Many cationic surfactants and some anionic ones are inherently bactericidal and have an additive effect on the preservative action. But there may be incompatibilities between cationic surfactants and anionic preservatives. Sometimes, the preservatives bind with the surfactant micelles and become unavailable.

iii) Oily phase : The preservative gets partitioned between oily, aqueous and micellar phase $C_W = \dfrac{C(\theta+1)}{K\theta + R}$

Where,

C_w - Concentration in aqueous phase

C - Total concentration

θ - o/w ratio

K - o/w partition co-efficient

R - Ratio of total v/s free preservative.

iv) Interaction with containers and closures : The preservative may partition or get adsorbed on surface of the container. The glass and plastic containers and rubber closures adsorb preservatives, making it unavailable in the formulation.

Testing of Preservative efficacy:

The minimum inhibitory concentration of preservative necessary to prevent microbial spoilage may be estimated by use of experimentally determined physico-chemical parameters, such as oil-water partition co-efficient, ultra-centrifugation and direct dialysis. The effective concentration of the preservative, however, may be reduced during shelf-life. The only reliable means of demonstrating adequate preservation of the product is the biological one, i.e., a preservative efficacy test.

Principle : It involves addition of known concentration of organisms to the manufactured product, removal of samples for viable counting at appropriate time intervals, and comparison of survival rates against the standard criteria for the class of product in question.

Test organisms:

Three bacteria - *S.aureus*, *P. aeruginosa* and *E. coli*

one yeast - *Candida albicans*

one mold - *Aspergillus niger*

They are selected for the following reasons-

- They are representatives of groups which are typical contaminants during manufacturing, e.g. *A. niger* spores are present in dust.

- They arise as contaminants during use: *S.aureus* and *C. albicans* from patient's skin.

- They have undemanding nutritional requirements or are commonly associated with preservative resistance, e.g. *P. aeruginosa*.

They have pathogenic potential.

Media and neutralisers : It is necessary to inactivate the preservative contained in the sample to avoid continued microbial action during dilution and recovery processes. This can be done by dilution to an ineffective concentration, by combination of lecithin and polysorbate 80 to inactivate parabens and quaternary ammonium compounds and by membrane filtration.

Preparation of inoculum : The pure or mixed cultures of microorganisms are added to finished preparation. The number of microorganisms initially present in the inoculum material is determined by plating aliquots of suitable dilution, e.g.

U.S.P. recommends dilution of 0.1 ml-20 ml and 1,00,000-1,000,000 cells/ml. Sampling is done on 7th, 14th, 21st and 28th days following inoculation.

Effectiveness : Vegetative cells – not more than 0.1 per cent of initial concentration by 14th day,

Concentration of viable yeasts and molds at or below initial concentration after 14th days,

Concentration of each test organism remains at or below these levels for 28th days.

A manufacturer may set his own specifications, e.g.-

Total aerobic count - not more than 5000 microarganisms/gram

Total molds -   not more than 100 molds/gram

Total yeasts -   not more than 100 yeasts/gram

Total coliforms   not more than 90 coliforms/gram

Estimation of D-value: Preservative efficacy can be tested within short time (48 hours for bacteria and 7 days for fungi) by estimation of D-value, or decimal reduction time.The death of a population of microorganisms in response to a lethal agent is often seen to conform to first order kinetics. Fig. 5.17 is a plot of log number of surviving microorganisms against time. It is always linear, and time required for 1 log cycle reduction in viable count is always constant, and is

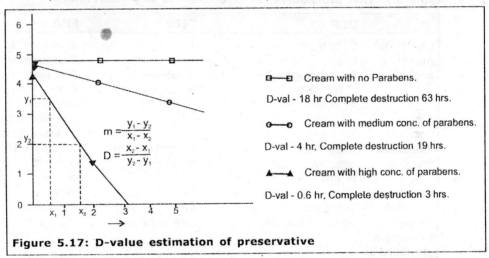

Figure 5.17: D-value estimation of preservative

called as D-value. It can be used to compare the rate of inactivation of different organisms in one or more products.

The product is inoculated with known number of microorganisms and sampled periodically to record population of each test microorganism and log of surviving microorganisms at each sample time is plotted. The slope of the line is determined by linear regression; and negative reciprocal of this slope is D-value. The time required for complete destruction of the microorganisms can be predicted from D-value, by linear estimate of 'X' intercept.

Commonly used preservatives :

Table 5.6: commonly used preservatives

Preservatives	Examples
Alcohols	Ethyl alcohol, isopropyl alcohol, chlorbutanol, B-phenoxyethyl
Acids	Benzoic acid, dihydroacetic acid, propionic acid, sorbic acid, cinnamic acid
Essential oils	Anethol, citronellol, eugenol, vanillates
Mercurials	Phenyl mercuric acetate, borate, Thiomersal
Phenols	Phenol, cresol, thymol, halogenated derivatives
hydroxy benzoates	Methyl, ethyl, propyl, butyl
Quaternary ammonium compounds	Benzalkonium chloride, cetyl pyridinium bromide cetrimide
Formaldehyde/formald-ehyde donors	Formaldehyde, Dowicil 200
Others	Chlorhexidine gluconate, chloroform, Imidazolidinyl urea, sugars, sulfites

Most widely used preservatives are pargshydroxybenzoate esters. They are usally used in combination. They are used at concentration levels approaching their maximum solubility in water. The propyl and butyl ethers are dissolved in fat phase and should

Table 5.7: Test procedures for effectiveness of preservatives.

	USP	CTFA	FDA
Challenge micro-organis	S. aureus E. coli P. aeruginosa C. albicans A. niger	P. latcum B. cereus B. subtilis	S. aureus, E. coli P. aeruginosa, P. putida, P. mutivorans Klebsiella S. marcescens, C. albicans, A.niger
Inoculum level	1×10^5-1×10^6 cells/ml or gm	1×10^6 cells/ml or gram	0.8-1.2 x 10^6 cells/ml or gm
Sampling schedule is one heading & standard is other	Days 0, 7, 14, 21, 28 Standard Bacteria < 0.1% Bacteria coil 14th day	Days 0, 1, 2, 7, 14, 28 Based on intended use	Weekly Veg. cells < 0.017 in 28 days
			C. albicans < 1.0 %
	Yeast & mold at or below initial conc. during frist 14 days. No increase in count for remaining of 28 days Bacteria live in front of wading 'standard'	0.1% survival in 28 days 0.1% survival in front of standard	A. niger < 1 % Re-challenge Vegetative cells in font of standard

be increased for vehicles with a high fat content. Their toxicity is low, are odourless, do not get discoloured and are non-irritating to skin. But they have low solubility in water and are ineffective against gram-negative bacteria. Combining them with phenoxyethanols or imidazolidinyl urea increases the spectrum of activity.

Table 5.8: Topical preservatives and their limitations

Preservative	Limitations
Quaternary ammonium compounds	Inactivated by anionic, non-ionic surfactants, proteins
Organic mercurial compounds	Potentially toxic & may sensitise skin Should not be used for ophthalmic products
Sorbic acid	Can be used below pH 6.5-7
Potassium sorbate	Photo discolouration
Benzoic acid	pH-dependent
Sodium benzoate	limited antimicrobial activity
Formaldehyde	Volatile, objectionable odour, irritant to skin, high chemical reactivity
Halogenated phenols Hexachlorophene p-chloro-m-cresol p-chloro-m-xylenol dichloro-m-xylenol	Objectionable odour Inactivated by non-ionic, anionic proteins Limited gram-negative antibacterial activity bacterial activity

RANCIDITY & ANTIOXIDANTS:

The drug itself, or the adjuvants, may get oxidised in presence of even small amounts of atmospheric oxygen. Most of the semisolids are emulsions, and the decomposition by oxidation may be more troublesome in these cases. This is because the emulsification introduces air into the product and also there is a high interfacial area of contact between water and oil. Also the fatty material present in the semisolid, on oxidation, develops a peculiar disagreeable odour called rancidity.

The decomposition process is usually auto-oxidation reaction. These are chain reactions catalysed by trace amounts of heavy metal ions. It forms highly reactive free radicals. This process can be inhibited in three different ways-

i) True antioxidants : They inhibit oxidation by reacting with free radicals blocking the chain reaction, e.g. tocopherols, BHA, BHT, nordihydroguaretic acid (NDGA).

ii) Reducing Agents : They have a lower redox potential than the chemical which they protect and are therefore more readily oxidised, e.g. ascorbic acid, isoascorbic acid, sodium and potassium salts of sulphurous acid.

iii) Antioxidant synergists : They are sequestering or chelating agents which possess little antioxidant effect themselves, but they enhance the action of the antioxidant by reacting with those heavy metal ions that catalyse oxidation, e.g. citric acid, tartaric acid, disodium edetate, lecithin and thiodipropionic acid.

MANUFACTURING OF DERMATOLOGICALS :

Aeration and rheological changes during manufacturing are the two challenges in ointment manufacturing. Aeration may lead to instability and variation in density within batch. Cause of aeration and remedies are-

Cause	Remedy
1. Splashing and streaming during the transfer of one phase to another	One phase should enter the mixing kettle below the surface of the other phase
2. Vortexing during mixing	Careful adjustment of mixing conditions
3. Processing in mixing kettle	Enclosed kettles operated under vacuum
4. Auger or worm device in hopper	Hopper must be full of product

Homogenisation increases viscosity of the product as it increases number of emulsified globules. The number of globule passing through the homogeniser, the pressure used in valve type homogeniser and the clearance between rotor and stator also influence the viscosity. Some creams are sensitive to agitation and stress and continuous rotation of auger during filling, can increase their viscosity. In such cases, the auger can be replaced by a gentler feeding device. Ointments are usually manufactured by mechanical incorporation or fusion. Fusion method is used for manufacturing of anhydrous ointments. Active substance is dissolved in molten fats and waxes or in one of the components of the vehicle and then mixed with the base.

PREPARATION OF OINTMENTS

Ointments are prepared by two general methods-

Incorporation:

In this method, the components are mixed until a uniform preparation is attained. On small scale, the incorporation is achieved by a pharmacist by the use of a spatula and an ointment tile. The finely powdered solid material is levigated thoroughly with a small quantity of base to form a concentrate. The concentrate is then diluted geometrically with the remainder of the base.

Liquids or drug solutions may be incorporated by use of a small amount of lanolin if the base is oleaginous. In all other types of bases, the capacity of the ointment base to accept the required volume should be considered. Alcoholic solutions of small volumes may be incorporated quite well to oleaginous vehicles or emulsion bases.

On large scale, the drug substances are incorporated by the use of mechanical mixers. Hobart mixers or pony mixers may be used. Finely divided drug substance is slowly sifted into the vehicle contained in a rotating mixer. The finished ointment may be further processed by the use of a triple roller mill.

Fusion:

In this method, all or some of the components are combined by melting together and cooling with constant stirring until congealed. Components that have not melted are added to the congealing mixture when it is being cooled by stirring. Heat labile and volatile components are also added at this stage.

Substances may be added to the congealing mixture as solution or insoluble powders. On large scale, the process is carried out in large steam jacketed kettles. Roller mills may be used to force coarsely formed ointments through stainless steel rollers to produce ointments that are uniform in composition.

MANUFACTURING OF EMULSIONS

Step I : Preparation of oily and aqueous phase

i) Oily phase : Components of oily phase are kept in a steam jacketed vessel melted and mixed. Petrolatum is inconvenient to handle unless it is in melted form. It is melted by immersing the heater coil in the drums in which it was supplied or by keeping in a hot room (65-70°C). It is then pumped through metal reinforced inert plastic hoses, with the help of a metering pump to a jacketed mixing kettle. Petrolatum is then passed through several layers of cheese cloth or filtered in case of an ophthalmic ointment. The kettle is preheated to melting point of the petrolatum to avoid congealing.

ii) Aqueous phase: Components of aqueous phase are dissolved in purified water and filtered. A soluble drug may be added to aqueous phase at this step, provided the high temperature does not degrade the drug or the emulsion is not adversely affected.

Step II : Mixing of the two phases :

Mixing is usually carried out at 65-70°C as intimate mixing can be achieved at this temperature. The phases may be mixed either by -

i)   Simultaneous mixing of two phases
ii) Addition of dispersed phase to continuous phase
iii) Addition of continuous phase to dispersed phase

The first method is used for continuous manufacturing process and it needs a metering pump. The second method is used when the volume of dispersed phase is too small compared to continuous phase. The third method is widely used for manufacturing of most of the emulsions. If an o/w emulsion is being processed, then to the entire volume of the oily phase a small volume of aqueous phase is added.

Step III : Cooling of the semisolid Emulsion :

The rate of cooling is usually kept slow to allow adequate mixing when the emulsion is still liquid. The temperature of the cooling medium should be decreased gradually, accompanied by scraping of the kettle walls to avoid formation of congealed masses. If perfume is to be added to a w/o emulsion, it has to

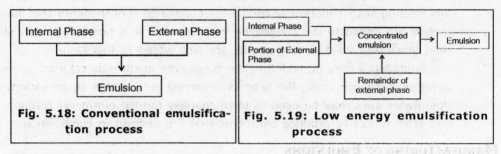

Fig. 5.18: Conventional emulsfica-tion process

Fig. 5.19: Low energy emulsfication process

be done at a temperature closer to room temperature, since the perfume has to dissolve in the external phase. But if the emulsion being made is o/w, the perfume should be added at 43-45°C to facilitate dissolution of the perfume oil in the still incompletely congealed internal phase, i.e., oil.

Low energy emulsification:

A lot of thermal energy is wasted in the conventional emulsification process, in the heating and cooling of the two phases. A lot of mechanical energy is also being spent as the phases have to be agitated while they are being heated and cooled. Low energy emulsification may be used to save this energy spent in emulsification. In this, the entire internal phase and only a small portion of the external phase are heated to form a concentrated emulsion. The remainder of the external phase is added at room temperature by diluting the concentrated emulsion. Thus, the energy required to heat the external phase and the mechanical energy of mixing during cooling is saved. Figure 5.18 & Figure 5.19 depict the conventional and low energy emulsification respectively.

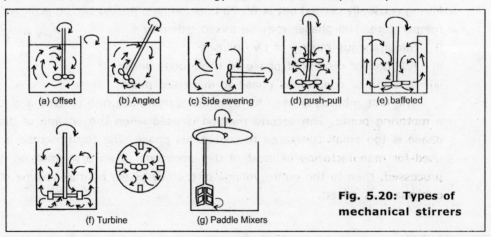

(a) Offset   (b) Angled   (c) Side ewering   (d) push-pull   (e) baffeled

(f) Turbine   (g) Paddle Mixers

Fig. 5.20: Types of mechanical stirrers

EQUIPMENTS USED FOR SEMISOLIDS PROCESSING :

i)   Jacketed kettles - Open or closed for vacuum operation.

ii) Mechanical stirrers

1) Propeller mixers:

Most widely used. The propeller is small and operates at high speed - 8000 rpm. They are not effective for liquids with very high viscosity. To avoid vortexing and aeration, the propeller should be deep in liquid and symmetry should be avoided. This can be done in a number of ways. The propeller shaft (fig. 5.20) can be offset from the centre or mounted at an angle (a,b) and enter the side of the vessel (c). Vortexing may also be avoided by using two propellers of opposite pitch (d) mounted on the same shaft. They rotate in opposite directions and nullify each other. The simplest method to avoid vortexing is to use one or more baffles, which are vertical strips attached to walls of vessels (e).

2) Turbine mixers:

They use a circular disc impeller (f) to which are attached a number of short vertical blades, which may be straight or curved.

Paddle mixers: They use an agitator consisting, usually, of flat blades attached to a vertical shaft and rotating at low speed. For more viscous range of liquids, is planetary motion mixer, which has a smaller paddle that rotates on its own axis, and also travels also in a circular path round the mixer vessel (g). The agitator scrapes the sides of the vessel to avoid dead spots.

3) Triple Roller Mill : It is mainly used for ointments containing powdered

solids. It consists of three rolls composed of abbrasion resistant material like porcelain or metal. They are arranged close to each other and rotated at different speeds. Material coming in between the rolls is sheared, depending upon the gap, and is also sheared by the difference in rates of movement of the two surfaces. The material passes

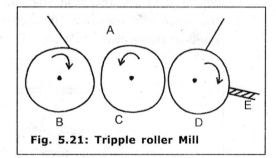

Fig. 5.21: Tripple roller Mill

from hopper A, between rolls B and C and decreases in size. The gap between C and D is usually less than that between B and C which further shears the mixture. Scraper, E, continuously removes the mixed material from D.

4) Ultrasonifiers/Ultrasonic homogenisers/Sonicators :

Ultrasonic energy is used to create cell disruption and homogenisation. The ultrasonic is developed mechanically or electrically. The mechanically developed effect works on the principle of Pohlman liquid whistle. A pump forces the combined phases past a vane or blade which vibrates rapidly and produces an ultrasonic

note. This produces energy via
cavitation.

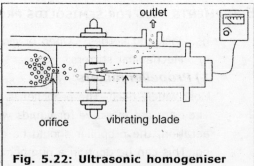

Fig. 5.22: Ultrasonic homogeniser

In electrical operations, an oscillator generator causes ultrasonic vibration in a peizoelectric crystal. A generator generates an electric current of high frequency. The output of the generator is supplied to the converter, i.e., peizoelectric cell, which converts this electrical energy to mechanical energy. The converter transmits this energy to a specially designed acoustic tool known as horn or probe. When the tip of the horn is immersed in a liquid, the ultrasonic vibrations cause cavitation, i.e., formation of microscopic bubbles within a liquid caused by rapid reduction in local pressure. The intensity of the vibrations is sufficient to reduce the absolute pressure of the liquid below its vapour pressure, resulting in local 'cold boiling' or cavitation. Cavitation creates millions of very small, powerful vapour bubbles. Their collapse produces shock waves of sufficient magnitude to do useful work. Cavitation intensity depends on the amplitude of the horn and the properties of the process medium. Ultrasonic cavitation provides fast, complete and controlled processing.

5) Homogenisers :

Homogenisers may be used to prepare the emulsion or to improve the quality of the crude emulsion prepared by using mechanical stirrers, like mortar & pestle. Homogenisation is a process in which the mixed phase is forced through a fine orifice valve under high pressure. The impact of the mixture, as it strikes the valve head, results in atomisation of droplets of fine size producing emulsion.

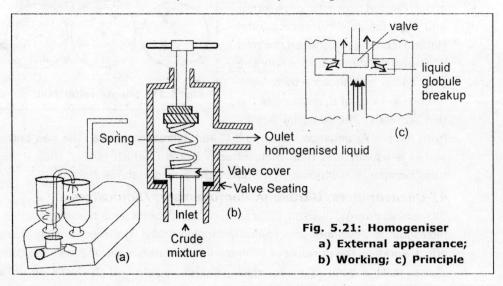

Fig. 5.21: Homogeniser
a) External appearance;
b) Working; c) Principle

The two phases are forced past one or two spring sealed valves through a small orifice at pump generated pressure. When the pressure builds up, the spring is compressed, storing energy and some of the dispersion escapes between the valve cover and the seat. Energy stored in the liquid is released at this instance, causing considerable turbulence and shear in the liquid and among the droplets and solid particles present. The crude emulsion is passed through the homogeniser several times. Laboratory hand-homogenisers with 0.5 liter capacity are also available.

6) Colloid mill : Operates on principle of high shear. The shear is generated between the rotor, having conical surfaces, and the stator of the mill. There is a small clearance in between, to which liquid is delivered and is sheared between the rotor and stator to bring about emulsification.

Advantages: High speed and large throughput

Disadvantage: Incorporates large amount of air in the system.

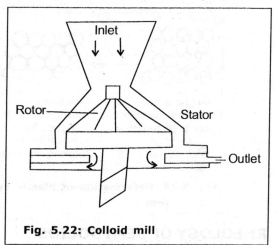

Fig. 5.22: Colloid mill

STORAGE OF SEMISOLIDS :

After the processing is complete, the semisolid is stored before packaging, till it is passed by quality control department. Some semisolids 'set up' on storage, i.e., increase in consistency, and therefore should not be stored for a longer time. The active substance may react with the storage container unless it is made up of stainless steel 316, which is highly resistant. Evaporation of water from a cream may be avoided by placing an inert plastic sheet in direct contact with the cream and closing with a tight fitting lid.

PACKAGING :

Ointments are usually packaged in ointment jars or metal or plastic tubes or straight sided, screw cap jars which are made up of clear, amber or opaque glass or high density polyethylene. Ointment tubes are made of tin or aluminium or of an increasing variety of plastic materials like polyethylene, polypropylene or other flexible heat sealable plastics.

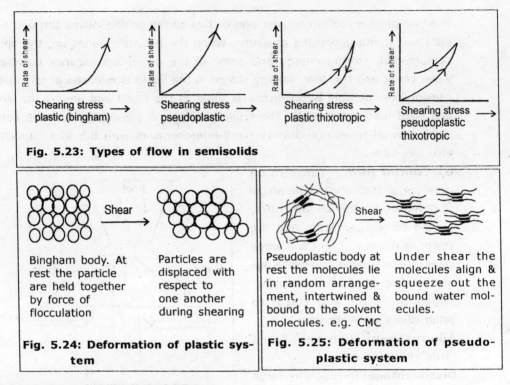

Fig. 5.23: Types of flow in semisolids

Bingham body. At rest the particle are held together by force of flocculation

Particles are displaced with respect to one another during shearing

Fig. 5.24: Deformation of plastic system

Pseudoplastic body at rest the molecules lie in random arrangement, intertwined & bound to the solvent molecules. e.g. CMC

Under shear the molecules align & squeeze out the bound water molecules.

Fig. 5.25: Deformation of pseudo-plastic system

RHEOLOGY OF SEMI SOLIDS

The flow of semisolids does not follow the simple Newtonian relationship, i.e., the graph of shearing stress v/s rate of shear is not a straight line passing through origin. They exhibit non-Newtonian flow either of plastic or pseudoplastic nature.

Thixotropy may be described as a reversible isothermal sol-gel transformation. Thixotropy arises from breakdown and build-up of floccules. Thixotropy may be observed in case of all the three types of non-Newtonian systems, i.e., plastic, pseudoplastic and dilatant. It is of particular importance in case of semisolids as it affects many properties, viz., spreadability, washability and extrudability.

MEASUREMENT OF VISCOSITY :

Viscosity $\eta = \dfrac{\text{Shearing stress (F)}}{\text{Rate of shear (G)}}$

In case of Newtonian systems and plastic systems, graph of F v/s G is a straight line, whereas, in case of a pseudoplastic system it is exponential, which means the viscosity of the system will not remain constant but vary depending on the changes in shearing stress.

A single point viscometer like Ostwald viscometer, can provide only one shearing stress. This means it provides only one point on the rheogram, which is of no use in case of non-Newtonian systems. Therefore, in order to study the rheology of semisolids, multipoint viscometers that can provide variable shearing stress values may be used, e.g. cup and bob viscometers and cone and plate viscometers.

DETERMINATION OF VISCOSITY :

Rotational viscometers are used to study rheology of semisolids. They measure the viscous drag exerted on a body when it is rotated in the semisolid. A wide range of shearing stresses can be applied and the rheogram may be obtained automatically. A number of instruments are available, but all are based on either of the two common designs - Cup and Bob (concentric cylinder) viscometers and Cone and Plate viscometers.

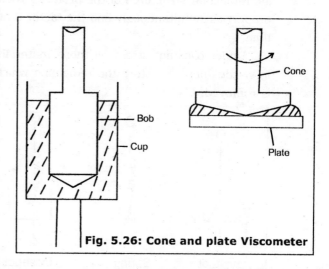

Fig. 5.26: Cone and plate Viscometer

Cup and Bob viscometers :

There are two coaxial cylinders of different diameters. The outer forms the cup containing the semisolid, in which, the inner cylinder or bob is positioned centrally.

The torque is set up either by revolution of the cup, e.g. McMichael viscometer, or by the revolution of the bob e.g. Searle type viscometer, Rotovisco viscometer and Stormer viscometer. The torque results because of the viscous drug of the system and is measured by a spring or a sensor in the drive.

In cone and plate viscometers, the sample is placed at the center of a plate, which is then raised in position below a cone. The cone is driven by a motor and the sample is sheared in the narrow gap between the plate and the cone. The rate of shear, i.e., rpm can be torque (shearing stress) produced on the cone.

A Brookfield viscometer may possess either a cup design or a cone and plate design or both.

VISCOELASTICITY :

A number of methods are used to measure the consistency of the cosmetic and pharmaceutical semisolid products. The rotational viscometers and continuous shear viscometers do not keep the material being tested in its rheologic ground state and causes gross deformation and alternation of the material during measurement.

The semisolids exhibit both viscous properties of liquid and elastic properties of solids and hence are said to be viscoelastic. Rotational viscometers yield large deformations and may produce false results. Creep and oscillatory methods to study viscoelastic materials use very low constant shears and hence are useful in studying molecular structures of the product. These materials display solid and liquid properties simultaneously and the factor that governs the actual behavior is the time.

Under constant stress all these materials will dissipate some of the energy in viscous flow and store the remaining which will be recovered when the stress is removed.

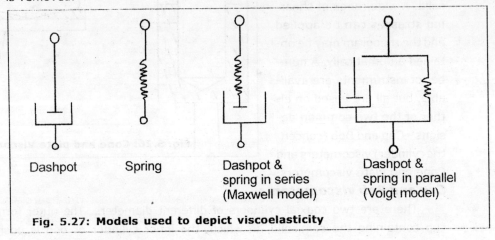

Dashpot   Spring   Dashpot & spring in series (Maxwell model)   Dashpot & spring in parallel (Voigt model)

Fig. 5.27: Models used to depict viscoelasticity

Using a mechanical model, a viscous fluid may be represented as movement of a piston in a cylinder filled with a liquid (dashpot). An elastic solid is modelled by a spring. The behaviour of semisolid as viscoelastic body may therefore be described by a combination of a dashpot and a spring.

Example: When a constant stress is applied to a 2 per cent gelatin gel and resultant change in shape i.e strain is measured and plotted versus time a following response may be observed.

In region AB initial elastic jump is observed followed by a curved region BC, when it tries to flow as a viscous fluid but being retarded by a solid nature of the material. At longer time intervals equilibrium is established and viscous flow predominates and curve becomes linear. When the stress is removed, only the stored energy can be recovered shown by an initial elastic recoil DE (equiva-

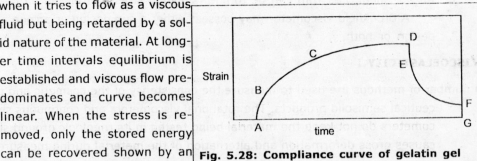

Fig. 5.28: Compliance curve of gelatin gel

ered shown by an initial elastic recoil DE (equivalent to AB) and retarded response EF (equivalent to BC). There is a displacement from the starting position FG and this is due to amount of energy lost in viscous flow.

Creep testing :

This phenomenon is known as Creep when the measured strain is divided by stress (which is constant), then a compliance (J) is produced. This compliance is

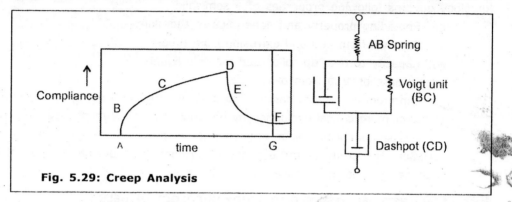

Fig. 5.29: Creep Analysis

then plotted versus time to obtain a compliance curve. The creep compliance curve will have the same shape as that of the original strain curve. The creep curve is analysed in terms of the mechanical models.

The example of such model is shown in the figure. The figure also indicates the regions on the curve, to which components of the model relate. The instantaneous jump is related to perfectly elastic spring. The viscous flow region CD is indicated by a dashpot to explain the region BC it is necessary to combine both these elements in parallel, i.e., the movement of the spring is retarded by a dashpot (Voigt model). The viscosity for the single dashpot can be calculated from the reciprocal of the slope of the linear part of the curve (CD). The viscosity would be several times greater than that obtained by the conventional techniques and may be considered as the viscosity of the rheological ground state. The compliance of the spring (J) may be measured by measuring height of the region AB and its reciprocal given elasticety ε_0. This value together with η_0 gives adequate characterisation of material.

The reverse of creep compliance test is stress relaxation test. The sample is subjected to a predetermined strain and stress required to maintain the strain is measured. Here, a spring and dashpot in series can be used. Initially the spring will extend and will then contract as the piston flows in the dashpot. The instrument used to carry out Creep's analysis is called Creep's viscometer. It consists of a rotational viscometer coup with a device to continuously record the Creep's compliance.

Another method to study viscoelasticity includes oscillatory analysis.

For an industrial pharmacist, it is more important to know how the rheology of a semisolid affects its spreadability and extrudability, instead of studying the detailed rheological data. And several empirical instruments are available to study these properties.

IMPORTANCE AND APPLICATIONS OF RHEOLOGY IN PHARMACEUTICAL SEMISOLIDS:

Rheology governs following properties of a semisolid-

    i)   Spreading property and adherence to the skin

    ii) Removal from jars and extrusion from tubes

    iii) Capacity to take up solids and miscible liquids

    iv) Release of drug from base

Ointments, creams, pastes and gels are the formulations subjected to a closer or more critical evaluation by the consumer. They must meet the criterion for feel, spreadability, colour, odour and other psychological and sensory characteristics. The study of these sensory parameters of dermatologicals that are affected by rheology is called psychorheology.

EMPIRICAL INSTRUMENTS USED TO STUDY RHEOLOGY OF GELS :

Penetrometer :

It measures relative hardness of the semisolid. Penetration is defined as the distance that a standard cone or needle penetrates a sample under known set of conditions of loading and time. Penetration tests are usually carried out at 25°C for 5 seconds, i.e., unit of penetration is expressed in 10th of millimeter.

A universal penetrometer consists of a dual angle cone, consisting of a small angled cone mounted on the top of a dual angle cone. A jar is placed below the apex of the cone resting on the surface of the sample. The plunger is released for 5 seconds, allowing the cone to penetrate into the sample. Penetration, in 10th of mm, is read from the scale. More the penetration, lesser is the consistency and hardness of the cream.

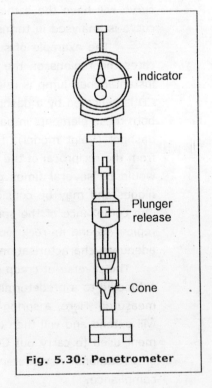

Fig. 5.30: Penetrometer

$$S_0 = \frac{K_1 mg}{P^n}$$

Where,

    S_0 - yield value (dynes/cm^2)

    K_1 - cos$^2\alpha$cos α (2α is cone angle)

n - material constant ≈ 2
g - gravitational acceleration
P - penetration depth
m - mass of cone and mobile parts

Spreadability test apparatus:

Parallel plate instruments are used to study spreadability of viscous semisolids. The measurement can be carried out by pulling plates apart, sliding one plate against the other, or rotating one plate with respect to the other.

Sliding box apparatus (fig 5.31): The ointment is placed in sample box, which has a narrow slit at the bottom. The box is covered with a lid. A weight is placed on the lid to exert pressure on the sample under test. The box is placed across a sheet of albanene paper (non-absorbent paper) on a temperature controlled plate by means of a pulley system. Weights are added to the pulley to increase driving force. During measurement, the antenna of the sliding box makes contact with the first switch and activates an electrical timer. Timer is turned off as the antenna touches the second switch. The time interval for the sample to travel between these two points is measured automatically. A consistency curve is made by plotting weights against time.

Sliding plate apparatus (fig 5.31): An excess of ointment is placed between two glass slides and a 1000 gm weight is placed on them for 5 minutes, to compress the sample to a uniform thickness. The bottom slide is anchored to the apparatus and weights are placed in the pan. The time in seconds needed to separate the two slides is taken as measure of spreadability. A shorter time interval indicates better spreadability.

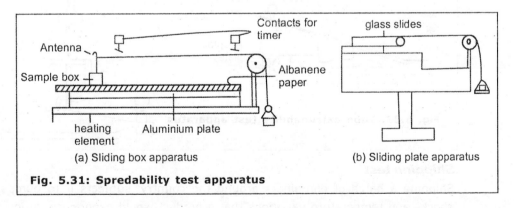

(a) Sliding box apparatus   (b) Sliding plate apparatus

Fig. 5.31: Spredability test apparatus

Apparatus to check tack/stickiness :

It measures the pull resistance of a semisolid by following procedure- A mechanical finger is pressed down on the sample on the plate. Weights are added to the lever arm connected to the mechanical finger. The time for the lever to rise and touch the set screw is taken as measure of tackiness or stickiness. Lesser the time, less is the tackiness of the sample.

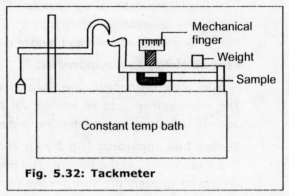

Fig. 5.32: Tackmeter

Tube Extrudability :

An extrusion rheometer extrudes the sample through an orifice under various pressures into tared container. The rate of flow is calculated from the weight and elapsed time of each extrusion. A modification of this instrument is done to check the extrudability of the sample directly from the sealed container. The figure shows two such modifications. The nozzle of the tube is screwed to an adapter plate. The sealed end of the tube is cut and the tube with the adapter is assembled into the rheometer above the capillary plate. Sample is extruded through the tube. Lesser the time required for the sample to pass through the tube, better is the extrudability.

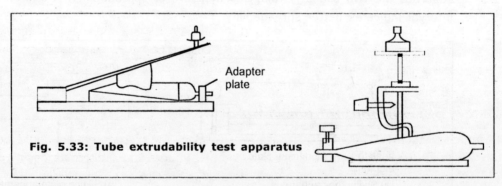

Fig. 5.33: Tube extrudability test apparatus

Shipping test :

Shipping a batch of containers around the country, subjects it to bumps and shocks and temperature variations that a product would experience during marketing. If it is still a good gel when it arrives back, the supply passes the test.

SAFETY, SAFETY TESTING AND TOXICITY:

Ointment bases may cause irritant or allergic reactions. Irritant reactions are more frequent and more important; therefore, a number of test procedures have been developed for testing in man and animals. The most common test is the Draize dermal irritation test in rabbits. The test material is applied repeatedly to the clipped skin on the rabbits back. The test material is compared with one or more control materials. Endpoints are dermal erythema or edema. Mathematical and statistical treatment of results is possible in humans, variety of tests are used to measure irritancy, sensitisation potential and phototoxicity.

TWENTY ONE DAY CUMULATIVE IRRITATION STUDY :

The test compound is applied daily to the same site on the back or forearm. Test materials are applied under occlusive tape, and scores are read daily. The test application and score are repeated daily for 21 days or until irritation produces a predetermined maximum score. Typical erythema scores are -

    0 = no visible reaction
    1 = mild erythema
    2 = intense erythema
    3 = intense erythema with edema
    4 = intense erythema and vesicular erosion
           Usually 24 subjects are tested.

KLIGMAN MAXIMISATION TEST :

This test is used to detect the contact sensitising potential of a product. Test material is applied under occlusion to the curve site for 48 hours periods. Prior to each exposure, the site may be pretreated with a solution of sodium lauryl under occlusion. Following a ten day interval the test material is again applied to a different site for 48 hours under occlusion. The ability to detect weaker allergens.

DRAIZE SHELANSKI REPEAT INSULT PATCH TEST :

Designed to measure potential to cause sensitisation. The test material is applied under occlusion to the same site for a period of 24 hours for 10 alternate days. Following a 7 day rest period the test material is applied again to a fresh site for 24 hours. The challenge sites are checked on removal of the patch and again after 24 hours, the 0-4 erythema scale is used. 100 individuals are used.

EVALUATION OF DERMATOLOGICAL SEMISOLIDS

The dermatological semisolids are either ointments or biphasic systems (emulsions or suspensions). The evaluation of biphasic systems has been discussed in detail elsewhere in the book (pg no 282-284, 308). Table 5.9 indicates the major evaluation parameters for dermatologicals based on their type.

Table 5.9: Evaluation parameters for semisolids.

		Ointment	Emulsion	Suspension
i	Sedimentation parameters			✓
ii.	Degree of flocculation		✓	
iii.	Ease of redispersibility		✓	
iv.	Rheological measurements	✓	✓	✓
v.	Zeta potential	•	✓	✓
vi.	Particle size analysis		✓	✓
vii.	Centrifugation			✓
viii.	pH -same drugs exhibit pH –sp	✓	✓	✓
ix.	Density :gives qualitative	✓	✓	✓
x.	Dissolution - Tab/Cap app	✓	✓	✓
xi.	Preservative efficacy •	✓	✓	✓
xii.	Safety	✓	✓	✓
xiii.	AST	✓	✓	✓

Dispersed Systems

A. GENERAL PRINCIPLES

INTRODUCTION:

Dispersion can be defined as a heterogeneous system in which one phase is dispersed with some degree of uniformity in the second phase.

CLASSIFICATION OF DISPERSED SYSTEMS:

The dispersed systems may be classified in different ways as follows-

1) Depending upon the nature of the dispersed and continuous phase, the dispersions may be classified as-

Table 6.1: Types of dispersed systems

Dispersed phase	Dispersion medium	Name	Example
Liquid	Gas	Liquid aerosol	Fog, mist, aerosols
Solid	Gas		Smoke, powder aerosols
Gas	Liquid	Foam	Foam on surfactant solutions
Liquid	Liquid	Emulsion	Milk, pharmaceutical emulsions
Solid	Liquid	Solid Suspension	Pharmaceutical suspension
Gas	Solid	Solid Foam	Expanded polystyrene
Liquid	Solid	Solid emulsion	Pearls, Opals
Solid	Solid	Solid Suspension	Pharmaceutical powders

2) Depending upon the particle size of the dispersed phase, the suspensions and emulsions are further classified as-

Table 6.2: Types of suspensions/emulsions based on particle size

Class of Suspensions	Particle/globule size
Molecular dispersion	Less than 1 nm
Colloidal dispersion	1 nm – 0.5 µm
Coarse dispersions	> 0.5 µm
Emulsions	
Microemulsions	
Macroemulsions	

3) Depending upon their use, the pharmaceutical dispersed systems may be classified as those meant for oral, topical or parenteral use.

Of the various pharmaceutical dosage forms, liquid dispersed systems are the most complex ones, because the method of manufacture, formulation approach, material selection and effect of environmental factors like temperature or holding time profoundly affect their stability.

PHYSICOCHEMICAL PRINCIPLES

FREE ENERGY CONSIDERATIONS:

Consider a beaker containing mixture of 50 ml water and 150 ml oil. They quickly form 2 layers, and the interface appears as a sharp discontinuity between the two phases, as it is actually a region of finite dimension. If the oil and water have densities of 0.9 and 1.0, gm/cc respectively, the density does not jump directly from 0.9 to 1.0 at the interface. Rather, there is a gradual change in density at the interfacial area, which has a definite thickness, d. Terms such as 'interface' or 'interfacial area' are often used to describe this region. The molecules at this interface are not locked in position, but are continuously in motion.

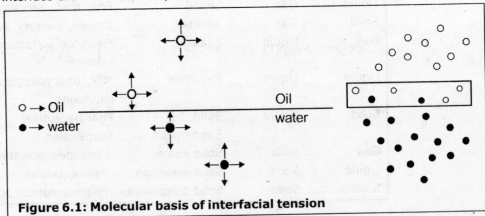

Figure 6.1: Molecular basis of interfacial tension

Thus the interfacial region of a suspension or an emulsion is a dynamic, clearly identifiable region that constitutes a large portion of the system, i.e., when particle size of suspension, or globule size of emulsion, is very small, properties of interfacial region largely affect properties of the system. In systems containing oil and water, oil molecules are located in the bulk of the system and are surrounded in all directions by the water molecules. Attractive intermolecular forces, e.g.hydrogen-bonding forces in case of water, exist between the molecules. Same is the case, with oil molecules located in the bulk of oil phase. However, the attractive forces here are Van der Waal's attractive forces. The water molecules that are located at the interface are not surrounded by water molecules in all directions; therefore they do not experience equal attractive forces in all direction. They are adjacent to oil molecules on one side, but the adhesive forces between water and oil molecules are not as strong as the cohesive forces between water-water molecules. This imbalance of the attractive forces exerts a net positive pull on water molecules at the interface towards the bulk of water, i.e., perpendicular to interface. This net attractive force results in a reduced number of molecules at the interface as compared to the bulk. Same kind of forces act on the oil molecules located at the interface. The molecules at interface are therefore in a higher energy state than the ones located in the bulk phase, and possess a positive free energy. The greater the preference of molecules for the bulk than for the interface, greater is the free energy of interface. This free energy of interface is given by Gibbs equation-

$$\Delta G = \gamma. \ \Delta A$$

Where,

ΔG = change in free energy of the system accompanied

ΔA = change in the interfacial area.

γ = interfacial tension

Since, this energy is always positive, the system always tends to minimise it in three ways.

1) By decreasing interfacial area, e.g. separation of oil and water layers in case of an emulsion and single large particle in case of suspension, is the thermodynamically more stable state. Although this thermodynamic stability is the fate of all dispersed systems, they may vary in the rate of this conversion. If a system undergoes only minor changes during the period of rest, i.e., shelf-life, it is viewed as a kinetically or pharmaceutically stable system, even though it may be unstable over a longer period of time.

   The job of a formulator is to retard the rate of conversion of a system, towards a thermodynamically stable state, i.e., to prepare a kinetically stable state rather than a thermodynamically stable system.

2) By arranging a surfactant, if present, at the interface and minimising the number of molecules, like water, at interface.

   This mechanism is advantageously used by the formulator, by introducing the materials that concentrate at the oil-water interface. This provides a mechanical barrier which delays the coalescence of internal phase.

3) It not only directs the surfactant molecules at the interface, but it orients them in the proper direction, i.e., non-polar ends towards the polar ends.

Surfactant molecules are never locked at interface, but are dynamic.

A system can be made kinetically more stable by different approaches-

i) By increasing free energy of system, i.e., mechanical work is done on the system to increase its free energy. This is a processing approach.

ii) By introducing the energy barrier, which the system has to cross for travelling towards the state of thermodynamic stability.

iii) By using stokes' approach to minimise particle size and increase the viscosity, of the enternal phase. So that the role of sedimention is decreased.

$$\varrho_s - \varrho_o$$

Despite the optimum manufacturing procedure and formulation, dispersed systems are still not be at thermodynamic equilibrium, but possess a free positive energy.

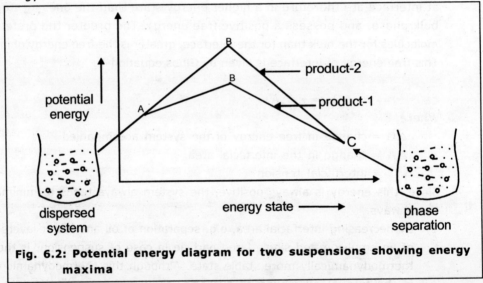

Fig. 6.2: Potential energy diagram for two suspensions showing energy maxima

Figure 6.2 represents hypothetical, interfacial free energy plots. A represents interfacial free energy of the product (low particle size will increase this value).

C represents the lowest free energy state attainable, i.e., complete coalescence of emulsion or caking of suspension.

Although it is known that reaching point C is the thermodynamic fate of a system, it is not known how much time it will take and what path it will follow to reach that point.

Curves for products 1 and 2 represent different pathways that can be imposed on a system by altering the formulation or processing variables.

Product stability can be increased by increasing the interfacial free energy, i.e., point A, but the most popular way is to introduce an energy barrier, i.e., point B. Product 2 is stabilised by a better formulation and processing approach and therefore enough energy barrier is created for the system to reach point C; and therefore, product 2 is kinetically more stable than product 1.

ORIGIN AND EFFECT OF SURFACE CHARGE

Most insoluble materials, either a solid or a liquid, develop a surface charge when dispersed in an aqueous medium. The surface charge arises by several mechanisms-

1) Ionisation of surface groups may produce a surface charge.

   eg Proteins contain COOH and NH_2 groups. At proper pH condition, COOH may ionise to form COO^-, or NH_2 may ionise to form NH^{3+}.

   The total charge on surface of protein molecule will be a summation of total positive and negative charges, which will depend upon pH of media.

2) Various colloids develop surface charge by adsorption or desorption of protons. An important property of the system is the point of zero charge (PZC), which represents the pH at which net surface charge is zero, e.g. for $Al(OH)_3$ gel, the surface hydroxyls may adsorb protons at low pH and become positively charged. At higher pH value, -OH may lose proton and become negatively charged. The pH at which hydroxyl neither adsorb nor donate a proton, but remain electrically neutral, is called the Point of Zero Charge (PZC).

3) Surface charge may also be created due to preferential adsorption of special ions on the surface. This is called as special adsorption, because the ion becomes as integral part of the solid phase. The ions that are specifically adsorbed are called as potential determining ions.

   If an electrolyte is present in solution, which provides cations or anions for specific adsorption, e.g. phosphate, silicate or carbonate ions. These ions are adsorbed. If the surface has both pH-dependent charge and charge due to adsorption, its PZC is different from its value than that with pH-dependent charge alone.

   Sometimes, charge arises due to adsorption of ions that are identical with those constituting the insolubilities, e.g. silver iodide particles in contact with solution containing Ag^+ and I^- ions. Adsorption of these ions depends on their concentration in bulk solution phase.

   Surface is positively charged when surface excess of Ag^+ ions is more than that of I^-. Charge may be created due to imperfections in the crystal structure. Many clays exhibit charge because of isomorphous substitution, e.g. In montamorillonite clays, Al^{3+} occupies site that is usually occupied by Mg^{2+}.

4) Oil globules of o/w emulsion exhibit a charge, if anionic emulsifier is used.

   The charged hydrophilic group forms outer surface of globule and therefore surface gets charged.

Presence of charge at interface has profound effect on the nature of interface, therefore, electrical double layer theory was developed by Gouy & Chapman and was modified by Stern.

ELECTRICAL DOUBLE LAYER:

Consider a solid surface in contact with polar solution containing ions, e.g. an electrolyte solution containing cations and anions (fig. 6.3). Suppose cations get preferentially adsorbed at surface, surface achieves net positive charge, as shown at interface aa'. The solution contains rest of the cations and all anions. These anions are attracted towards the positively charged surface by electrical forces that also tend to repel the approach of any further cations. In addition to these forces, thermal motion tends to produce equal distribution of all the ions in solution. As a result, equilibrium is set up, in which some of the excess anions approach the surface, while the remaining are distributed in increasing amount as one proceeds away from the charged surface. At a particular distance from surface, state of electrical neutrality prevails.

In fig. 6.3 aa' is the surface of solid, and the adsorbed ions that give the surface a positive charge, are termed as potential determining ions. Immediately adjacent to this surface layer is the region of negative ions tightly bound to the surface termed as 'stern layer' and is indicated by bb'. This layer is so tightly bound to the surface that if this surface is moved relative to the liquid, the plane bb' moves rather than the true surface aa'.

In the region bound by lines bb' and cc', there is an excess of negative ions. This region is called as 'diffused layer'. The potential at bb' is still positive as there are fewer anions in the stern layer as compared to cations on the solid surface. Beyond cc', there is uniform distribution of ions and electrical neutrality

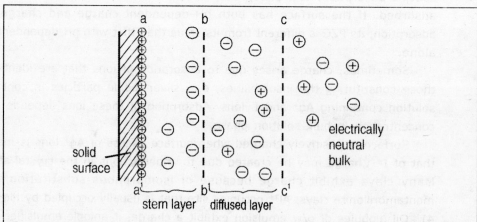

Fig. 6.3: Diffused double layer of a positively charged surface in aqueous medium

is obtained. Other than mentioned in the diagram, two situations may exist if cations are adsorbed as ions on the solid surface.

1) Anions in the stern layer equal the charge on the solid surface and electrical neutrality is obtained at bb' rather than cc'.

2) Anions in the stern layer are more than cations on the solid surface, so, the potential at bb' is negative and then becomes neutral at cc'. Similarly, three more situations exist if anions are adsorbed on solid surface and cations are present in stern layer.

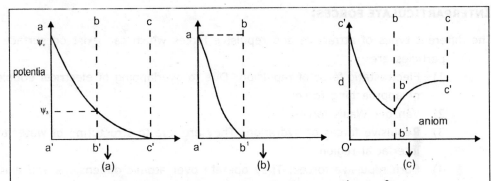

a) When anions in stern layer > cations on the surface
b) When anions in stern layer = cations on the surface
c) When anions in stern layer < cations on the surface

Fig. 6.4: Potential v/s interparticulate distribution plots, in diffused double layer of positively charged surface.

Potential of solid surface aa' due to adsorption of potential determining ions, is the potential, while the potential at stern layer bb' is Zeta potential. Nernst potential is the potential difference between actual solid surface and electrically neutral bulk.

The Zeta potential is the potential difference between stern layer and electrically neutral bulk. Because stern layer is tightly bound to the solid surface, it is difficult to measure the nernst potential. (Zeta potential measurement is more popular method of evaluation of dispersed system).

The potential at the true surface a' is reduced by stern layer bb' from ψ_o to ψ_δ. But the potential is completely neutralised by diffused layer. Both cations and anions are present in diffused layer, but the ions that are opposite in charge to the solid surface, predominate. The thickness of double layer is called the Debye length and is indicated by 1/k, which is given by formula,

Where,

$$\frac{1}{k} = \left(\frac{DKT}{2ne^2z^2}\right)^{\frac{1}{2}} = \sqrt{\frac{DKT}{2ne^2z^2}}$$

1/k	=	Debye Length
D	=	Dielectric const of medium
K	=	Boltzman const.
T	=	Temperature
n	=	Concentration of ions in bulk solution
e	=	Charge on the ions
z	=	Valency of the electrolyte

Therefore, electrolyte concentration of the solution and valency of the electrolyte largely affects the thickness of the double layer.

INTERPARTICULATE FORCES:

The different types of attractive and repulsive forces which can exist on surface of the particles are:

1) Electrostatic force of repulsion: Due to overlapping of electrical double layer of approaching forces.
2) Van der Waals forces.
3) Repulsive forces of hydration: They are due to structuring of water at the interfacial region.
4) Born repulsive forces: They operate over atomic dimensions and exist due to overlapping of orbitals.
5) Adhesive forces: Attractive forces between any two unlike molecules.
6) Stearic Repulsive forces: They depend on size, geometry and conformation of the molecules on which they are adsorbed, particularly, due to the tails of surfactants.

DLVO THEORY (Deryaguin, Landau, Verwey and Overbreak theory) :

Many observed properties of a dispersed system can be explained by the study of the net force of interaction between the particles. This is called as DLVO theory. The original statement of DLVO theory, considered only two types of forces,

1) Electrostatic repulsion
2) Van der Waals attraction

The figure indicates double layer repulsive forces and Van der Waals attractive forces at

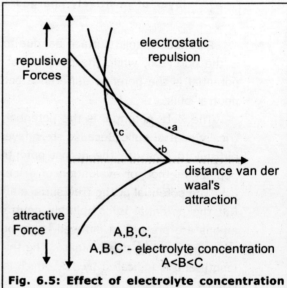

Fig. 6.5: Effect of electrolyte concentration on repulsive double layer forces and Van Der Waals attractive forces

three different electrolyte concentrations A, B and C. The repulsive forces predominate at low electrolyte concentrations, so that particles experience only repulsion upon approach. The particles remain independent and system is dispersed. At high electrolyte concentration, the double layer repulsive forces are greatly reduced and Van Der Waals forces predominate. These forces cause aggregation of particles and the system is said to be coagulated.

The DLVO theory explains the fact that addition of an electrolyte to a dispersed system, at increasing concentration, causes coagulation. The concentration of electrolyte required to collapse the repulsive film and permit coagulation is dependant on valency of the oppositely charged ion.

Table 6.3: Electrolyte concentration that coagulated a negative silver iodide colloid.

Valency	Electrolyte	Coagulation concentration (m mol/L)
1	$LiNO_3$	165
1	$NaNO_3$	140
1	KNO_3	136
2	$Ca(NO_3)_2$	2.6
2	$Mg(NO_3)_2$	2.4
3	$Al(NO_3)_3$	0.07

Table 6.4 : Thickness of double layer as a function of constant electrolyte concentration.

Concentration of ion having opposite charge to that of particles (m mole/L)	Thickness of double layer (nm)	
	Monovalent ion	Divalent ion
0.01	100	50
1.0	10	5
100	1	0.5

Concentrations of various electrolytes that coagulate suspension are given in the table 6.3, 6.4.

1) The coagulation concentration of all the silver iodide monovalent cations is almost same and maximum.
2) Coagulation concentration of different divalent cations is also almost the same but substantially low than coagulation concentration of monovalent cations.
3) Trivalent cations can induce coagulation at very low concentration.

The strong influence of valency of electrolyte on the double layer repulsive force is called as Schulze-Hardy rule.

For the electrolytes of same valency, there is a slight difference in their effect on double layer repulsion. The order of effectiveness is called the Hofmeister series.

$Cs^+ > Rb^+ > NH^{4+} > Na^+ > K^+ > Li^+$

$Mg^{+2} > Ca^{+2} > Ba^{+2}$

$F^- > Cl^- > Br^- > NO_3^-$

DLVO theory does not take into consideration, other types of repulsive and attractive forces and therefore it was further modified by taking into consideration the repulsive forces of hydration and born repulsive forces.

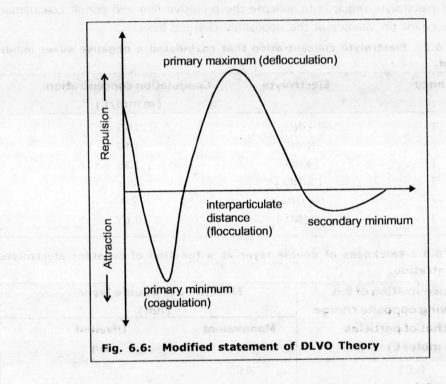

Fig. 6.6: Modified statement of DLVO Theory

When two particles approach each other in an aqueous medium proper electrolyte concentration, a weak attractive force exists beyond the range of the double layer repulsive forces. The region is called as secondary minimum and is responsible for particle interaction termed as flocculation. The particles form loose fluffy aggregates called floccules. Particles experience this weak force of attraction at significant interparticulate distance which is 10-20 nm. Secondary minimum is not observed when the repulsive forces extend further from the surface than the attractive forces. The Debye length can be so altered by adjusting the valency and concentration of the electrolyte that the repulsive forces do not extend beyond the range of these weak attractive forces and flocculation can be reduced.

REPULSIVE BARRIER:

A repulsive barrier, termed as primary maximum, separates secondary minimum, from primary minimum. When the interparticulate distance is in the range of Debye length, the particles experience strong repulsive forces indicated by primary maximum and the system is said to be dispersed. If the system can cross this energy barrier, then the particles are able to move closer together and encounter strong attraction due to primary minimum. These interactions give rise to coagulation of the system. Other types of energies, like centrifugation or freezing, forces the particles into the region of primary minimum and the system coagulates.

At low electrolyte concentration, the primary maximum is quite high and particle interactions are minimised, hence the system is said to be dispersed or peptised. If either the electrolyte concentration or valency increases, the primary maximum decreases and the system either flocculates or coagulates.

B. PHARMACEUTICAL SUSPENSIONS

GENERAL PRINCIPLES:

WETTING :

Wetting is the displacement of either liquid or gas, from the surface of a solid. When a drop of liquid is brought in contact with a flat solid surface, the solid and liquid surfaces develop cohesive forces between the molecules. The angle at the point where the drop and solid meet can be considered as a measure of degree of wetting of solid surface by the liquid. The angle made by the solid surface and the tangent to the liquid drop at point of contact, is called the contact angle. This angle is denoted by 'θ'.

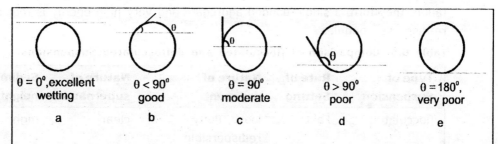

Fig. 6.7: A liquid droplet falling on a solid surface showing different contact angles.

CRYSTAL GROWTH:

Mechanism:

The size distribution of dispersed system may be altered during ageing due to three principle mechanisms-

1) Polymorphic transformation   2)Temperature cycling   3) Ostwald ripening

Ostwald Ripening :

Equilibrium solubility at given temperature will not be affected by the particle size, but the rate at which a substance dissolves is largely affected by its particle size. With decrease in the particle size, surface area of the particles available for dissolution increases, which in turn increases rate of dissolution. This means the solution, that is saturated with respect to small particles, will be supersaturated with respect to larger particles of the same substance. This condition causes crystal growth in a suspension as the solute diffuses from the saturated layer surrounding the larger particles. Crystalisation on the surface of larger particles occurs as the saturated layer becomes supersaturated, with respect to larger particles.

Polymorphic transformation :

Polymorphs exhibit differences in solubilities. Therefore, if the substance is present as a mixture of two or more polymorphs, or if polymorphic transformation takes places, then there are chances that the polymorph having less solubility will be crystallised out.

Floccules act as a single particle and start settling at a faster rate, forming high sediment. Floccules have open branched loose structures. For flocculation to occur, repulsive forces must be diminished to such an extent, that weak attractive forces predominate.

Floccules can be induced by addition of electrolytes, but concentration and valency of electrolyte should be controlled, to cause controlled flocculation, otherwise coagulation occurs. Coagules are strongly bonded particles. They are difficult to redisperse and settle to form closely packed sediment. Upon sedimentation, they form a single bonded aggregate and very high energy is required to re-disperse coagules.

Table 6.5: Comparison of flocculated and deflocculated Suspensions.

Type of Suspension	Rate of Setting	Nature of sediment	Nature of supernatant	Sediment height
flocculated	Fast	loose, fluffy redispersible	clear	high
deflocculated	Slow	hard, compact non-redispersible	cloudy	low

Deaggregated or deflocculated or dispersed or peptised suspension are the ones in which individual particles are dispersed as individual entities that separate slowly, achieve lowest possible sediment height and have very high potential to crystal bridging, if crystals are present on particle surface.

SEDIMENTATION:

Sedimentation rate is given by Stokes' equation.

$$V = \frac{2r^2 (d_1 - d_2) g}{g\eta}$$

Where,

V = Sedimentation rate

r = Radius of particle

d_1 and d_2 = densities of particle and liquid in gm/ml respectively

g = Gravitational constant

η = Viscosity of medium in poise

Dilute pharmaceutical suspensions, having concentration of solids less than 2 per cent w/v, confirm roughly to this equation. In dilute suspensions, particles do not interfere with settling of other particles and it is called as free settling. In case of concentrated suspensions, particles of different sizes are present, which interfere with settling of other particles. Therefore, it is called hindered settling. Stokes' equation is modified as-

$$V = \frac{K \; r^2 (d_1 - d_2) g}{\eta}$$

Where,

K - Experimental constant.

Experimental constant, K, helps to adjust different factors related to hindrance caused by adjacent particles. When settling of flocculated suspension is studied, it is seen that floccules have a tendency to stick together, producing a distinct boundary between sediment and suspension liquid. The sediment above is clear because even smaller particles get linked in the floccules. This is not the case with deflocculated system having a range of particle sizes where larger particles have settled and smaller particles are still in suspension. No clear boundary is found between the sediment and supernatant and the supernatant remains turbid. Therefore, clarity of supernatant is a good indicator of nature of system.

Sedimentation parameters

Sedimentation volume (F) = $\dfrac{\text{Final volume of Sediment (Vu)}}{\text{Original volume of suspension. (Vo)}}$

F is usually less than 1 because ultimate volume of sediment is less than orignial volume of suspension. If volume of sediment equals total volume of suspension, i.e., there is no settling, then F is equal to 1.

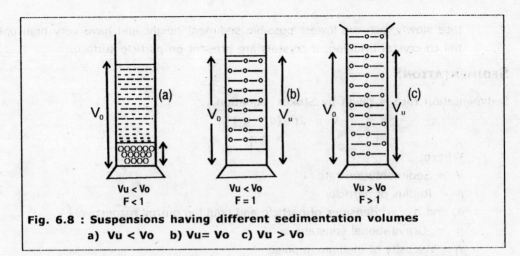

Fig. 6.8 : Suspensions having different sedimentation volumes
a) Vu < Vo   b) Vu= Vo   c) Vu > Vo

If volume of sediment exceeds volume of suspension due to formation of loose and fluffy aggregates, then F is greater than 1. This type of system is pharmaceutically acceptable.

More useful parameter is degree of sedimentation (β) In case of deflocculated suspension, ultimate volume of sediment is very small. If we call it as $V\infty$, then original equation becomes,

$$F_\infty = \frac{V_\infty}{V_o}$$

Degree of sedimentation is given as,

$$\beta = \frac{F}{F_\infty}$$

i.e. $\dfrac{V_u}{V_o} \times \dfrac{V_o}{V_\infty} = \dfrac{V_u}{V_\infty}$

Therefore, degree of sedimentation is equal to ultimate sedimentation volume of flocculated system divided by ultimate sedimentation volume of defloccu-lated suspension.

STABILIZATION OF SUSPENSIONS:

There are different approaches to produce a stable suspension-

BY CREATING ELECROSTATIC REPULSION :

This is achieved by repulsion due to large zeta potential and is best done by adsorption of an electrolyte or an ionic surfactant on the suspended particles because of which electrical double layers of adjacent particles overlap each other causing the particles to repel each other. e.g. moderate physical stability is achieved when Zeta Potential is between $\pm$ 30 mv and $\pm$ 60 mv.

Excellent stability is achieved when it is between $\pm$60 mv to $\pm$100 mv.

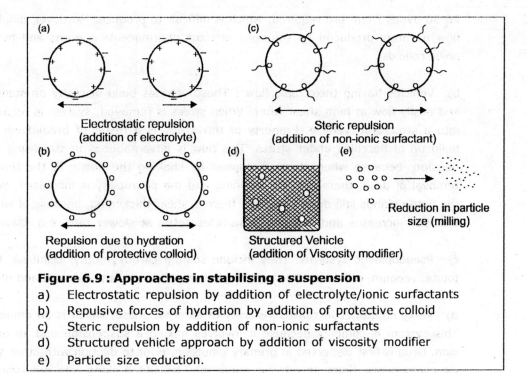

Figure 6.9 : Approaches in stabilising a suspension
a) Electrostatic repulsion by addition of electrolyte/ionic surfactants
b) Repulsive forces of hydration by addition of protective colloid
c) Steric repulsion by addition of non-ionic surfactants
d) Structured vehicle approach by addition of viscosity modifier
e) Particle size reduction.

BY ADDITION OF PROTECTIVE COLLOIDS :

When strongly hydrated hydrophilic protective colloid, like gelatin, is adsorbed on the surface of suspended particles, affinity of particles for water exceeds mutual attraction of adjacent particles. Protective colloids and hydrogen bonded water molecules form protective hydrated layer around each suspended particle.

BY STERIC REPULSION :

Steric hindrance due to adsorption of oriented non-ionic surfactant or polymer of sufficient chain length, creates stearic hindrance. This prevents protest adjacent suspended particles from coming close to join and form floccules. This is widely used in practise in stabilizing suspension.

STOKES' APPROACH : (STRUCTURED VEHICLE CONCEPT)

Many substances act as protective colloids in low concentrations (<0.2 %) and as viscosity building agents at higher concentrations. Structured vehicle concept can be used to stabilise suspensions, where viscosity under static condition of very low shear approaches infinity. Vehicle is said to behave in such a way that it is capable of maintaining particles in state of permanent suspension.

a) Vehicles used for this are polymers haring Bingham type plastic flow. These vehicles need to overcome a finite yield stress, before the flow starts. But for permanent suspension of any pharmaceutical product, yield values of around

20-50 dynes / cm^2 are required, which is difficult to produce. Moreover, bingham flow is rarely produced by solutions of most pharmaceutical gums and hydrophilic colloids.

b) Vehicles having thixotropic flow : These vehicles build viscosity on standing and easily flow at high shear rates. When stress is removed, system is reformed into a structured vehicle. Property of thixotropy is a result of breakdown and build up of floccules under stress. This flow is advantageous in stabilising suspension, because when shear is applied by shaking the bottle at the time of removal of dose, there is shear thinning and the pourability is increased. When the bottle stands still during storage, there is shear thickening, because of which, viscosity increases and suspended particles settle at slower rate. e.g. clays.

c) Pseudoplastic systems. They include sodium carboxymethyl cellulase, bentonite, veegum, cellulose, tragacanth, methylcellulose, propyl cellulose and HPMC.

d) Waxy emulsifier increases viscosity of external phase, which is an emulsion. This system is complex because it involves mixing a suspension and an emulsion. Drug is first dispersed in primary emulsion, prior to dilution with other vehicle components. Some thixotropic agent may be added along with emulsifier.

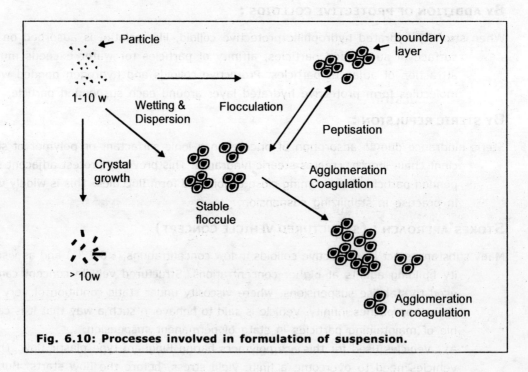

Fig. 6.10: Processes involved in formulation of suspension.

FORMULATION OF SUSPENSIONS

The ingredients of suspension formula are broadly divided into two categories as some are the components of the suspended phase and some are included in the continuous phase, e.g. drug particles, suspending agents are the components of suspended phase; while wetting agents, flocculating agents, preservatives, vehicles, sweeteners, colours, flavours or fragrances and buffers are the ingredients of continuous phase.

INGREDIENTS OF SUSPENDED PHASE:

Wetting Agents :

Certain solids are readily wetted by the liquid, whereas others are not.

Degree of wettability depends on affinity for water. Hydrophobic solids repel water. Majority of drugs in aqueous suspensions are hydrophobic. They are extremely difficult wet to and frequently float on the surface of water due to entrapped air.

Wetting agents are the surfactants that lower the interfacial tension and contact angle between the solid particles and liquid vehicle. If a wetting agent is present while adding powder to a liquid, penetration of the liquid phase into the powder will be sufficiently rapid to permit air to escape from the particles.

Table 6.6: Wetting agents for pharmaceutical suspensions

Name	HLB	Features
Non-ionic		
Polysorbate 65	10.5	Bitter
Octoxynol 9	12.2	Bitter
Nonoxynol 10	13.2	Bitter
Polysorbate 60	14.9	Bitter
Polysorbate 80	15	Bitter, most widely used
Polysorbate 40	15.6	Bitter, low toxicity
Poloxamer 235	16	Good taste & low toxicity
Polysorbate 20	16.7	Bitter
Anionics		
Docusate sodium	>24	Bitter, foaming agent
Sodium lauryl sulphate	40	Bitter, foaming agent

According to the HLB theory, the best HLB range for a non-ionic surfactant to act as a wetting agent is 7-10. Number of surfactants to act as a wetting agent may be used as wetting agents. Their concentration varies from 0.05-0.5 per cent.

Most of the surfactants, particularly anionic surfactants, are bitter in taste and they also act as foaming agents, e.g. sodium lauryl sulphate. The non-ionic surfactants that are used for this purpose are polysorbate 40, 60, 65 and 80. All of them are bitter in taste and need taste masking. Polysorbate 80 and 40 show lesser toxicity as compared to the others. Another popularly used surfactant is poloxamer, which is good in taste and shows low toxicity. Other two non-ionic surfactants are octoxynol and nonoxynol.

Use of surfactants at concentrations more than 5 per cent may solubilise ultrafine particles due to micellization and lead to crystal growth. If their concentration is reduced, they might show incomplete wetting.

Wetting agents having high HLB values are foaming agents, but foaming is undesired during wetting and hence sometimes antifoams are also added. Although, ionic surfactants are more effective than non-ionics as wetting agents, ionic surfactants are sensitive to pH changes and incompatible with many charged excipients.

Polysorbate 80 is widely used due to its low toxicity. If incorporated in oral suspension, it requires addition of strong flavouring agents and sweeteners. The degree of wetting is determined by placing a measured amount of powder on undistributed surface of water containing a wetting agent and noting the time required to completely wet and sink the powder.

Flocculated or deflocculated suspension

An important factor to be considered in deciding the formulation of the suspension is whether a flocculated or a deflocculated suspension is preferable. The relative magnitude of the attractive and repulsive forces on the particles decides whether the suspension would remain deflocculated or undergo flocculation. (fig. 6.10)
a) Flocculated with closed floccules   b) Flocculated with open network floccules
c) Deflocculated

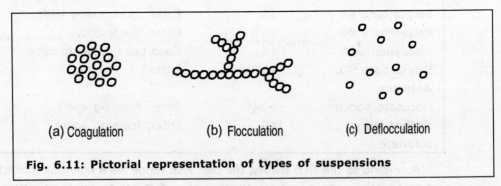

(a) Coagulation   (b) Flocculation   (c) Defloculation

Fig. 6.11: Pictorial representation of types of suspensions

If a suspension is deflocculated, the dispersed particles remain as discrete units and the rate of settling is slow. The slow rate of settling prevents the entrapment of liquid in the sediment and hence it becomes compact and very difficult to re-dis-

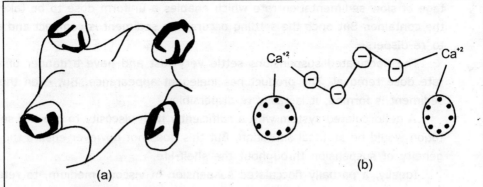

Fig. 6.12: Diagram of floccules formed by (a) polymer bridging; (b) polyelectrolyte bridging.

perse. This is called cementing/caking/claying or concreting of a suspension. It is the most serious problem encountered in suspension formulation.

Aggregation of particles in the form of loose floccules leads to a much rapid rate of settling, because each floccule now consists of many particles and is therefore larger. (Fig. 6.11)

The sediment of a flocculated suspension is different than that of a deflocculated suspension. Each floccule retains its structure even in the sediment and hence entraps a large amount of liquid phase. This makes the volume of the final sediment quite large and re-dispersing it is quite easy.

The supernatant of deflocculated system remains cloudy for a long period of time due to very slow settling rate. In a flocculated system, the supernatant quickly becomes clear as the floccules settle quickly. (Fig. 6.13)

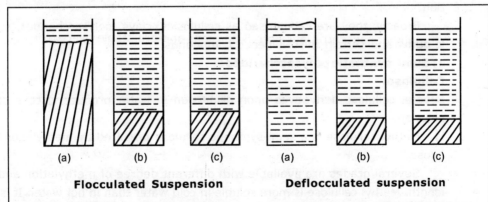

Flocculated Suspension   **Deflocculated suspension**

Fig. 6.13: Sedimentation behaviour of flocculated and deflocculated suspensions- (a) within a few minutes of manufacture; (b) after several hours; (c) after prolonged storage.

The deflocculated pharmaceutical suspensions therefore have the advantage of slow sedimentation rate which enables a uniform dose to be taken from the container. But once the settling occurs, the sediment is compact and difficult to re-disperse.

The flocculated suspensions settle very fast and have a danger of inaccurate dose removal. The product has inelegant appearance. But even though, a sediment is formed, it is easily re-dispersible.

A deflocculated system with a sufficiently high viscosity to prevent sedimentation would be an ideal situtation. But this does not however ensure the homogeneity of suspension throughout the shelf-life.

Ideally, a partially flocculated suspension in viscous medium, to retard the settling rate, is the right option. This is called controlled flocculation.

Table 6.7: Comparison of flocculated and deflocculated suspensions.

Flocculated Suspension	Deflocculated suspension
1. Rate of sedimentation is high	1. Rate of sedimentation is slow
2. The sediment is loose and porous	2. The sediment is compact
3. The sediment is easily redispersed	3. The sediment is difficult to re-disperse
4. The supernatant is clear	4. The supernatant is cloudy
5. It is a esthetically inelegant	5. It is aesthetically elegant

Viscosity modifiers and protective colloids

They are used to impart greater viscosity and retard sedimentation. They may be used alone or in combination. They act as protective colloids at lower concentration (may be less than 0.1 per cent) and as viscosity modifiers at high concentration.

Broadly, they are categorised as cellulosics, clays, polysaccharides, synthetic gums and certain miscellaneous compounds.

a) Semi-synthetic polysaccharides
Cellulose:

Several cellulose derivatives upon dispersion in water produce viscous colloidal solutions.

i) Methyl cellulose is a semi-synthetic cellulose prepared by methylation of cellulose.

Several grades are available with different degree of methylation and chain length. Methyl cellulose is more soluble in cold water than in hot water. It is often dispersed in hot water and then upon cooling by stirring, produce a clear viscous solution. Methyl cellulose is non-ionic and therefore stable over wide pH range.

ii) Hydroxy ethyl cellulose has –hydroxyethyl group instead of methyl group attached to the side chain. It has the advantage of being soluble in both hot and cold water. Otherwise, it exhibits same properties as that of methyl cellulose.

iii) Sodium carboxymethyl cellulose – Its viscosity depends on degree of poly-merisation. It produces clear solutions in hot as well as cold water. Being anionic, it is incompatible with cationic additives. It is widely used at concentrations upto 2 per cent in oral and external preparations.

iv) Avicel (Microcrystalline cellulose) - It contains crystals of cellulose having colloidal dimension, which disperse readily in water to produce thixotropic gel. It exhibits plastic thixotropic flow.

It is used often in combination with sodium-carboxymethyl cellulose. Rheologic properties can be further improved by incorporation of an additional hydrocolloid. Powdered cellulose and avicel are plastic in nature, while ethyl cellulose, propyl cellulose and hydroxy propy methyl cellulose exhibit pseudoplastic flow.

b) Inorganic Agents :

Clays :

There are four important materials in this class, namely bentonite, veegum, hectorite and colloidal silica. Silicates belong to the group of clays called as Montmorillonite clays.

They hydrate readily and absorb upto twelve times their weight of water, particularly at elevated temperatures and form thixotropic gels and therefore useful as suspending agent. They are naturally occurring substances and may be contaminated with microbial spores.

i) Bentonite : $Al_2O_3 \; 4SiO_2.H_2O$

It is used at concentrations upto 2-3 per cent, usually in preparations for external use, e.g.. Calamine lotion.

ii) Magnesium Aluminium silicate (veegum): Is is available as soluble clay which swells and disperses readily in water, forming thixotropic gel. Several grades are available, differing in their particle sizes and viscosities. It can be used internally as well as externally at concentrations upto 5 per cent and are stable over a pH range of 3-11.

i) Hectorite is used at concentrations between 1 and 2 per cent and is a thixotropic gel. Synthetic hectorite is called laponite and is used industrially in suspensions for external use.

c) Natural Polysaccharides

1) Acacia – It is often used as thickening agent for extemporaneous preparations. It is not a good thickening agent and its value as a suspending agent is because of its action as a protective colloid. It is not very satisfactory for suspending dense powder and therefore it is often combined with other suspending agents, e.g. compound tragacanth powder (acacia + tragacanth + starch + sucrose).

Acacia mucilage becomes acidic on standing due to enzyme activity as it contains oxidase enzyme, which may cause degradation of active drug. Because of stickiness of acacia mucilage, it is rarely used in colloid preparations.

2) Tragacanth – Viscous aqueous solution of tragacanth is pseudoplastic. It is thixotropic in nature, therefore, it is a better thickening agent than acacia and used for both internal and external preparations. It is stable over a pH range of 4-7.5. But it takes several days for complete hydration after dispersion in water. Its viscosity is affected by heating. Some other gums that are used apart from this are guar gum, locust bean gum, pectin and tamarind seed gum.

Guar gum produces high viscosity solution. Guar gum and locust bean gum are both non-ionic. Xanthan gum is a gum produced by microbial fermentation and therefore problems of batch to batch variation, as compared to other natural polysaccharides, are less.

3) Alginates - Alginic acid is a polymer of d-mannuronic acid obtained from seaweeds. Its salts have same suspending properties as that of tragacanth.

Alginate mucilage cannot be heated above 60°C as it undergoes depolymerisation.Sodium alginate is the most widely used material, but it is anionic and therefore incompatible with cationic substances.

Other polysaccharides of seaweed origin are agar and carrageenan.

4) Synthetic Gums - Carbopol is a synthctic gum popularly used as a viscosity modifier. It is a total synthetic polymer of acrylic acid. It is effective at concentrations upto 0.2-0.3 per cent. It is preferably used for external preparation although some grades can be taken internally when dispeersed in water. It forms an acidic, low viscosity solution that becomes extremely thick when the pH is adjusted between 6 and 10.

5) Miscellaneous Starch- It is rarely used alone as a suspending agent, but it is a component of compound tragacanth powder. It swells in water and hence, acts as viscosity modifier.

Sodium starch glycolate (Explotab) is a modified derivative of starch. It is also being evaluated for its use in suspension.

Gelatin can also be used as a suspending agent.

Table 6.8: Commonly used viscosity modifiers/Protective colloids.

Cellulosics	Clays	Natural gums	Synthetic gums	Miscellaneous
Methyl cellulose	Bentonite	Acacia	Carbopol	Starch
Hydroxyethyl cellulose	Hectorite	Tragacanth		Gelatin
	Veegum	Alginates		Lecithin
Sodium carboxy Methyl cellulose	Colloidal silica	Guar gum		PEGs
microcrysta- lline cellulose		Karaya gum		(3350,8000)
Hydroxypropyl cellulose	Attapulgite	Locust bean gum		
	Sepiolite	Agar		
Hydroxypropyl methyl cellulose		Carrageenan		
		Pectin		
		Xanthan gum		

Drug Particles :

The drug particles should lie between the particle size range of 1 and 15 µ. Commoly used methods for particle size reduction are dry grinding, micropulvarisation, spray drying and fluid energy grinding.

INGREDIENTS OF CONTINUOUS PHASE :

Flocculating agents:

In many cases, after addition of non-ionic wetting agent, suspension gets stabilised either due to reduction in interfacial tension or because of steric hindrance. Using an ionic surfactant to wet the solid, may produce either type of suspension. If charge on the particles is neutralised, flocculation will occur and if high charge density is imparted, deflocculation occurs. If it is necessary for a suspension to be converted from flocculated form to deflocculated form, flocculating agents are used. Flocculation is achieved either by the addition of an electrolyte or an ionic surfactant.

Addition of electrolyte to aqueous suspension alters the zeta potential of the dispersed particle; and if this value is lowered sufficiently, flocculation occurs.

The electrolytes in solution, that are capable of reducing the zeta potential, are primary flocculating agents.

Small concentrations of electrolyte, i.e., 0.01-0.1 per cent, such as NaCl and KCl, are often sufficient to induce flocculation for weakly charged drug particles, like steroids. For highly charged drug molecules, polyelectrolyte species at similar concentrations may be used. Divalent or trivalent soluble electrolytes like salts containing calcium (Ca^{+2}), Aluminium (Al^{+3}), sulphate (So_4^{-2}), citrate or phasphate (po_4^{-3}) my be used. Ionic surfactants may also cause flocculation by neutralising the charge on the particles.

Following are the examples of ionic surfactants which may act as flocculating agents

Anionic surfactants e.g. sodium laurlyl sulphate

Cationic surfactants e.g quaternary ammonium compounds.

pH control agents or buffers :

A Pharmaceutical suspension should be stable over a wide pH range. If a suspension shows optimum stability at a particular pH range, buffers are used. This is more important for drugs which possess ionisable acidic or basic groups. But careless use of salts and buffers should be avoided, because even small changes in electrolyte concentration affect suspension stability. Glutamate, citrate and phosphate buffers are popularly used.

Density modifiers :

If the dispersed and continuous phases have the same density, sedimentation does not occur. Minor modifications in the density of external phase can be done by incorporating glycerine, propylene glycol, sorbitol and sugar syrup.

Flavours and fragrances :

Use of a sweetener alone will not be sufficient to make a product containing bitter/unpleasant tasting drug palatable, and therefore flavours are included. This is particularly important in paediatric formulations, to increase patient compliance. Flavours and fragrances can be of natural or synthetic origin. The natural flavours are fruit juices, aromatic oils, herbs, spices and their distilled fractions like peppermint oil. They are available as concentrated extracts, alcoholic or aqueous solutions (tinctures) or syrups and spirits. Artificial flavours or perfumes are totally synthetic, they are economical more readily available, less variable in composition and are the most stable.

Synthetic flavours are available as aqueous or alcoholic solutions or powders. Choice of a suitable flavour can be made by subjective assessment.

GUILDELINES FOR FLAVOUR SELECTION :

Consumer preferences for flavours vary considerably, but general guidelines are given below. Certain flavours are particularly used for masking one or more basic tastes like, bitterness, saltiness, sweetness or sourness. These tastes are detected by sensory receptors on the tongue.

Table 6.9 : Guidelines for flavour selection

Taste	Flavour
Salty (e.g. KCl)	apricot, butterscotch liquorice, vanilla.
Bitter	Anise, chocolate, wild cherry
Sour (e.g. Aspirin)	Citrus, raspberry, liquorice
Sweet	Vanilla, rose, strawberry

- In some cases, there is a strong association between the use of products and its flavours. Antacids often have mint flavours.
- Personal preferences for flavours and fragrances often vary with age and sex.
- Children, in general, prefer fruity flavours and colours.
- Adults choose acidic taste and flowery odours.
- Certain other suitable materials for masking a bad taste are menthol, peppermint oil and chloroform. In addition to their good taste, they also act as desensitising agents by exerting a mild numbing action on the taste receptors.
- Flavour enhancers/adjuvants like monosodium glutamate are also widely used in liquid preparations.

Sweeteners :

Low molecular weight carbohydrates, particularly sucrose, are traditionally widely used. Sucrose is colourless, water soluble and stable over a wide pH range. It increases viscosity of the vehicle and leaves a pleasant feel and taste in the mouth and has a soothing effect on throat. For this reason, inspite of its high caloric value, sucrose is used.

Polyhydric alcohols like sorbitol, mannitol and glycerol have sweetening power and are used for diabetic preparation, but are expensive. Other substances which are sometimes used as sweeteners are glucose syrup, fructose, honey and liquorice.

Artificial sweeteners can be used, both in combination with sugar to enhance degree of sweetness or they are used on their own for patients who should restrict their sugar intake. They are called as intense sweeteners as they are 100-1000 times sweeter than sucrose and therefore are required in very low concentrations, e.g. sodium or potassium salts of saccharin, aspartame, cyclanate, acesulfame K and thoumarine. The main disadvantage of all of them is a bitter or metallic after taste. Therefore, they are often formulated with small concentration of sodium choloride or sugar.

Colours :

It is useful to choose a colour associated with the chosen flavour. Development of strongly coloured degradation products should also be masked by the incorporation of a proper colour. Natural as well as synthetic colours are available. Some examples of natural colours are carotenoids, chlorophyll & anthocyanins. Some examples of synthetic dyes give brighter colour and are more stable.

Humectants :

Glycerin and propylene glycol are often incorporated in external preparations. To some extent they act as emollients, but major use is the prevention of drying out of the product.

Preservatives :

Continuous microbial activity may reduce the zeta potential of a system and cause coagulation. Sweeteners, natural gums and cellulose derivatives are susceptible to microbial contamination and therefore addition of preservatives to suspension becomes important. Suspensions contain large amount of water and therefore provide good media for bacterial proliferation.

Table 6.10: Commonly used Preservatives for suspensions.

Preservative	Concentration (% w/w)	Use
Parabens (Methyl, Ethyl Propyl, Butyl parabens)	0.2	Dermatologicals
Sorbic acid	0.2	Orals
Thiomersal	0.01	Injectables
Quaternary ammonium Salts	0.01	Opthalmic
Benzyl alcohol	1.0	Injectables/topicals
Benzoic acid	0.2	Orals
Chlorhexidine gluconate	0.01	Opthalmic
Phenylethanol	1.0	Opthalmic, topicals

EVALUATION OF SUSPENSIONS :

PHOTO-MICROSCOPIC TECHNIQUES :

Microscope is used to detect the changes in particle size distribution and crystal growth. Its usefulness can be enhanced by use of Polaroid camera attached to the eye-piece of the microscope for rapid processing of photomicrograph, which can be used to distinguish between flocculated and deflocculated suspension and to determine changes in physical stability.

COULTER COUNTER :

It is an electronic particle counter and it measures the change in resistance caused by presence of particles in electrolyte solution. The size of particles of dilute suspension is measured.

SEDIMENTATION VOLUME :

Redispersibility is the major consideration in assessing suspension stability. The formed sediment should be redispersible; hence sedimentation volume and ease of redispersion are two major criteria in measuring suspension stability. Sedimentation volume is measured in graduated cylinders. V_u/V_o ratio should be plotted against time. The curve should be either horizontal or gradually sloping downwards to the right. A better formulation will produce lines that are horizontal or less steep.

RHEOLOGICAL METHODS:

They are used to determine setting behaviour of the particles. The most widely used instrument is Brookfield viscometer with Helipath stand. Helipath is a rotating T-bar spindle, which, while descending slowly into the suspension, encounters new undisturbed material as it rotates.

Rhoegrams can be taken at different time intervals. The technique is excellent for concentrated suspensions which possess high yield value.

SPECIFIC GRAVITY MEASUREMENT:

Specific gravity measurement provides information about the air entrapped in the preparation at various time intervals.

AGEING TESTS OR ACCELERATED STABILITY TESTING :

Subjecting the suspension to cyclic temperature change, i.e., to conditions of repeated freezing and thawing and exposing them to high temperatures for short periods of time is considered drastic. Exposing the suspension to elevated temperatures will cause a lot of suspended drug to go into the solution; and freezing causes the drug to re-precipitate. Thus, crystal growth during ageing test is of limited value, but if the suspension is able to withstand such drastic freeze-thaw cycle, it is assumed that it will have a good stability at ambient temperatures. On the other hand, failure of suspension to meet such stringent temperature conditions should not be considered as physical instability of suspension.

ZETA POTENTIAL MEASUREMENTS OR ELECTRO KINETIC TECHNIQUES :

Measuring the zeta potential of the particles in suspension, provides useful information about the sign and magnitude of the charge present on the particles, and its effect on the stability of suspension. Instrument used for zeta potential measurement is an electrophoretic cell. It consists of electrodes that are immersed in the dispersion, i.e., test suspension. Under the influence of potential, the particles migrate towards oppositely charged electrodes and rate of migration of the particles is the function of the charge on the particles. The cell is coupled with an electron microscope with the help of which the particle movements can be seen and the rate can be measured. This is called as microscopic electrophoretic technique. Zeta potential can be correlated to visually observed caking or flocculation or deflocculation of the suspension.

DRUG CONTENT UNIFORMITY :

This can be confirmed by using a unit of the used volume, i.e., usually 5 ml, and assaying the sample for drug content. The samples are removed from the bottom, middle and top of the container.

DISSOLUTION TESTING :

The favoured method is to submerge a small known amount of the test suspension in a secured membrane pouch of suitable porosity, (in a tea bag fashion) in a suitable dissolution medium using U.S.P. method-I

Some other tests which are carried out for the suspension are – assay, preservative efficacy testing, compatability testing with containers and closures, torque testing for closures.

METHODS OF PREPARATION OF SUSPENSION

The Suspensions may be prepared by dispersion method or precipitation method:

DISPERSION METHODS :

In this method, finely milled solid particles are dispersed in a suitable vehicle with the help of a mechanical agitator, a colloid mill or any other suitable equipment. The dispersion method may or may not cause size reduction of the solid particles. Even if the process reduces the particle size of the solids, the size reduction may not be uniform. So the solid particles may be micronised in advance in order to prepare a suspension with uniform and fine particle size.

Appropriate vehicle must be formulated so that the solid phase is easily wetted and dispersed. A surfactant may be incorporated if needed, to help uniform wetting of the solids.

PRECIPITATION METHODS :

The suspensions may be prepared by the precipitation method in either of the three ways, organic solvent precipitation, precipitation by change in pH or by double decomposition.

In organic solvent precipitation method, a water insoluble solvent is dissolved in some water miscible organic solvent and the solution is then added to distilled water to cause precipitation. Organic solvents like ethanol, methanol, propylene glycol and polyethylene glycols may be used, e.g. prednisolone is precipitated from aqueous methanol. Several factors that should be taken into consideration while using organic solvent precipitation method are : particle size of the precipitate, precipitation of the correct polymorph, toxicity due to solvent, possibilities of sterile processing, method of drying of precipitate, temperature control, volume ratios of organic to aqueous phase etc.

The method of precipitation by change in pH may be used only for those drugs that show pH-dependant solubility. For example, estradiol is freely soluble at alkaline pH. Its precipitation may be brought about by making the pH weakly acidic.

In precipitation by double decomposition method, two soluble reactants are chemically reacted in solution to form a product that has low solubility and precipitates out, e.g. white lotion consists of zinc polysulphide that is formed by mixing zinc sulphate and sulphated potash solution.

EQUIPMENTS FOR PRODUCING SUSPENSIONS

Different mixing and milling equipments are needed at different stages of processing (stage I, II and III) in the figure 6.14.

A) BLENDING OF MISCIBLE LIQUIDS:

In this stage all the miscible liquids are blended together to form a homogenous solution. The process is less demanding as it does not take a high level of shear to produce a homogenous mixture. The most widely used equipments for blending are pitched blade turbines or marine mixers (Fig. 6.15, 6.16). Propeller mixers are used for small batches. They can be placed vertically, with entry from top, or can enter through the side of the mixer, horizontally or angled, and with or without baffles.

B) MILLING OF SOLIDS :

Table 6.11 lists the equipments for medium, hard to soft pharmaceutical materials. Figure (6.17-6.22) gives the diagrammatic representation of these equipments. A detailed description of construction and working of these equipments has not been provided here.

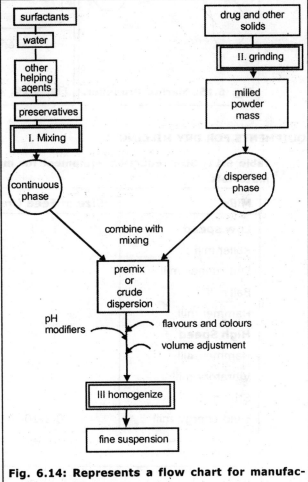

Fig. 6.14: Represents a flow chart for manufacturing a suspension.

C) HOMOGENISATION OF CRUDE SUSPENSION:

The commonly used equipments for this purpose are colloid mills, ultrasonifiers and homogenisers. The description of this may be found in chapter five.

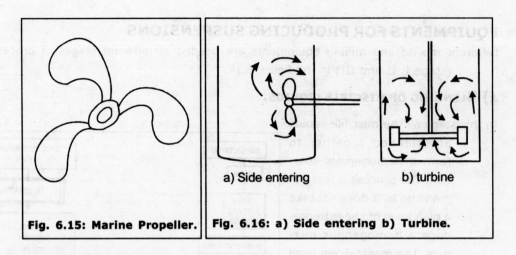

Fig. 6.15: Marine Propeller.

Fig. 6.16: a) Side entering b) Turbine.

EQUIPMENTS FOR DRY MILLING

Table 6.11: Size reduction equipment for medium, hard to soft pharmaceutical materials.

Mills	Size of Feed (mm)	Size of product (mm)
Low speed	1-10	0.1-1
Roller mill		
End runner mill		
Ball mill		
Hammer mill		
High Speed	1-10	0.01-0.1
Hammer mill		
Vibratory mill		
Stud mill		
Fluid energy mill	0.1-10	0.001-0-01

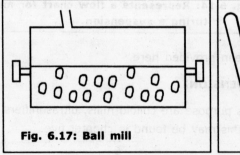

Fig. 6.17: Ball mill

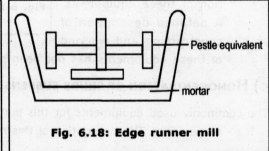

Fig. 6.18: Edge runner mill

Pestle equivalent

mortar

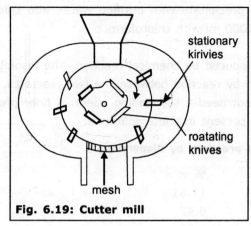

Fig. 6.19: Cutter mill

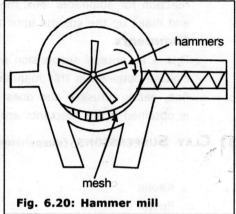

Fig. 6.20: Hammer mill

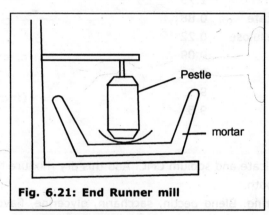

Fig. 6.21: End Runner mill

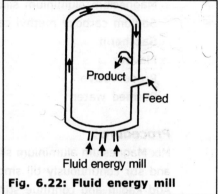

Fig. 6.22: Fluid energy mill

PRACTICAL EXAMPLES :

A) ANTACID SUSPENSIONS (suspension prepared by precipitation method)

Magnesium hydroxide suspension - BP

Magnesium sulphate	- 47.5 gm
Sodium hydroxide	- 15.0 gm
Light Magnesium Oxide	- 52.5 gm
Chloroform	- 2.5 ml.
Purified water	- 9.5.1000 ml.
(Freshly boiled and cooled)	

Procedure -

Dissolve sodium hydroxide in 160 ml water. Add magnesium hydroxide to this solution while stirring, to form a smooth cream. Add enough water to make the volume to 2500 ml. Pour this suspension, in a thin stream, into the water, stirring continuously during mixing. Allow the precipitate to subside and remove the supernatant. Wash the precipitate with purified water until it gives only a slight reaction for sulphates. Mix the precipitate with purified water, add chloroform and make up the volume upto 1000 ml with chloroform.

Comments

This is an antacid suspension produced by chemical reaction. The insoluble precipitate obtained in this manner, by reaction between the two reactants, is very fine, easily diffusible and does not need a suspending agent. A finer precipitate is obtained if the reactants are present in dilute solutions.

B) CLAY SUSPENSIONS (suspension prepared by dispersion)

	% w/w
Kaolin	17.51
Pectin	0.47
Glycerin	1.75
Magnesium aluminium silicate	0.88
Sodium carboxy methyl cellulose	0.22
Saccharin	0.09
Flavour	9.5
Preservative	9.5
Purified water	9.5

Procedure :

Mix Magnesium aluminium silicate and sodium CMC. Add this dry mixture to water and stir continuously till smooth.

Add kaolin and continue stirring. Blend pectin, saccharin, glycerine, flavour and preservative. Add this mixture to other components. Mix until smooth.

c) TOPICAL SUSPENSION

Aqueous calamine lotion

Calamine	15g.
Zinc oxide	5g.
Bentonite	3g.
Sodium citrate	0.5g
Liquefied phenol	0.5ml.
Glycerol	5ml.
Water	9.5.100ml.

Procedure :

Blend calamine, zinc oxide and bentonite together. Dissolve sodium citrate in a small quantity of water. Add this solution to the powder blend, stirring continuously. Add phenol and glycerol. Make up the volume with water.

d) RECONSTITUTED SUSPENSIONS

Ampicillin trihydrate dry	5.77 %
Sucrose	60 %
Sodium alginate	1.5 %
Sodium benzoate	0.2 %
Sodium citrate	0.125 %
Citric acid	0.051 %
Tween 80	0.08 %

Comments : Ampicillin trihydrate degradation products lower the pH of un-buffered vehicle. pH of maximum stability is 4.85. It is maintained by addition of citrate buffer.

C. PHARMACEUTICAL EMULSIONS

INTRODUCTION :

Dispersion of macro-droplets of one liquid in another immiscible liquid, with a droplet size distribution approximately in the range of 0.5-100 μm is called an emulsion.

Majority of emulsions consist only of two phases, but many emulsion formulations are more complicated. This has lead to formulation of new definition of emulsion. Emulsions are now defined as, "The dispersion of liquid droplet and liquid crystals in another immiscible liquid". In addition to this, almost all emulsions consist of solid particles which further complicate this situation.

An emulsion is formed when two immiscible liquids are mechanically agitated. During agitation, both liquids tend to form droplets, but when agitation ceases, droplets separate into two phases. If a stabilising compound, called as emulsifier, is added to the immiscible liquid, one phase usually becomes continuous and the other remains in droplet form. During agitation, droplets are formed by both the phases and continuous phase is actually obtained because its droplets are unstable, e.g. if water and oil are stirred together, both, oil droplets in water and water droplets in oil exist together during agitation and o/w emulsion is formed, because water droplets coalesce with each other faster than the oil droplets. When sufficient numbers of droplets have coalesced, this forms a continuous phase surrounding the oil droplets.

Process of formation of continuous phase is rapid and usually takes place within a few seconds and is not related with stability of emulsion. (Stability of an emulsion is a measure of duration of stability of dispersed phase droplets, which eventually coalesce together and emulsion exhibits phase separation). For formation of an emulsion, mechanical agitation is required. If one of the two phases is very viscous, or the emulsifier is solid at room temperature, heat is used for emulsification. The type of emulsifier is determined by the phase ratio.

If difference in the volume of the two phases is high, e.g. if 5 per cent water and 95 per cent oil is used, the emulsion will become w/o, unless extreme measures are taken to form o/w emulsion.

For moderate phase ratio, i.e., 1:10, type of emulsion is decided by combination of factors like order of addition and type of emulsifier. If one phase is slowly added to the other, it will usually result in last mentioned phase being the continuous phase.

Another factor is the solubility of the emulsifier. A phase in which emulsifier is soluble will usually become continuous phase.

TYPES OF EMULSIONS

An emulsion can be prepared from any two immiscible liquids, but in pharmaceutical emulsions, one of the two liquids is always water.

The o/w emulsion consists of oil droplets dispersed throughout an aqueous continuous phase; whereas, in w/o emulsions, water is dispersed throughout a continuous oil phase.

Table 6.12 Differences between o/w and w/o emulsions.

	o/w	w/o
Colour	Usually milky white	Affected by oil colour
Feel on skin	Initially non-greasy	Greasy
Dilution	Dilutes with water	Dilutes with oil
Electrical conductivity	Conducts	Very poor or non-conductive
Effects of dyes		
a) oil-soluble	Globules coloured	Continuous phase coloured
b) Water-soluble	Continuous phase coloured	Globules coloured
Drop on filter Paper	Rapid diffusion of water	Very slow diffusion of oil

It is also possible to form a multiple emulsion. e.g. a small water droplet can be enclosed in a larger oil droplet which is itself dispersed in water. This gives a multiple emulsion of water-in-oil-in-water type (w/o/w). The alternative to this is o/w/o emulsion.

If the dispersed globules are of colloidal dimensions (1 nm to 1 mm diameter) the preparation is called as microemulsion. It is often transparent.

TEST FOR IDENTIFICATION OF EMULSION TYPE:

There are several tests available for distinguishing o/w emulsions from w/o emulsions.

1. Miscibility tests with water: The emulsion will mix with water only if its continuous phase is water.
2. Conductivity measurements: Emulsions with aqueous continuous phases easily conduct electricity, while emulsions with oil as continuous phase are poor conductors of electricity.
3. Staining tests: Water soluble and oil soluble dyes are added to emulsion one of which will colour the continuous phase.

Table 6.13: Identification tests for emulsions.

o/w emulsions	w/o emulsions
Miscibility Test	
Miscible with water and immiscible with oil	Miscible with oil and immiscible with water
Staining test with oil Soluble dye	
When viewed micrscopically, coloured globules are seen on colourless background.	Colourless globules are seen on coloured background
Macroscopically, appear pale in colour than w/o emulsions.	Macroscopically appear more intense in colour than o/w emulsion.
Conductivity tests	
If two electrodes are placed in these with a battery & lamp in series will cause the lamp to glow	Do not conduct electricity. The lamp will not glow.

THEORIES OF EMULSIFICATION

The theory of emulsion should provide explanations for following phenomena: duality of emulsions, i.e., existence of both o/w and w/o emulsion type, inversion of phases, mode of action of the emulsifier and variation in consistency of emulsion even if closely related emulsifiers are used.

BANCROFT'S THEORY:

Donnan suggested that in emulsions containing soaps generated *in situ*, the soap molecules get adsorbed at the interface, the adsorbed layer being part of the aqueous phase.

Bancroft modified this theory by postulating that the interfacial adsorption gives rise to an interfacial film that constitutes the third phase separating the continuous phase from the dispersed phase. Thus there are two interfacial tensions - one operating between the film and the aqueous phase and the other between the film and the oily phase. Both the oily and aqueous phases are considered to be wetted by the film and are absorbed by it, so that the interfacial tensions on the two sides of the film are different. The side which has a greater interfacial tension will contract and cause the film to become concave on that side. The film will therefore tend to enclose the phase on the concave side and the phase on the outer side will become dispersed phase. Bancroft was probably the first to distinguish clearly between o/w and w/o emulsions. Thus, for o/w emulsions, $\gamma_{wf} < \gamma_{of}$ and for w/o emulsions, $\gamma_{of} < \gamma_{wf}$, where γ_{wf} and γ_{of} are the interfacial tensions between water and film and oil and film respectively. Thus when a hydrophilic surfactant is added, it reduces the interfacial tension on the water-side and therefore water becomes the continuous phase, i.e., forms o/w emulsion. Whereas, hydrophobic surfactants reduce the tension on oil-side of film, and oil becomes the continuous phase, i.e., forms w/o emulsion.

To act as an emulsifier, the substance must get adsorbed at the interface and must form a coherent film there.

Bancroft proposed that the type of emulsion formed depends upon the coherence and permanence of the film formed.

HARKINS ORIENTED WEDGE THEORY :

Harkins attempted to explain the types of emulsions formed using sodium and magnesium oleates. It was concluded that type of emulsion was intimately connected with the number of oleate radicals in the soap molecule. For stability, the adsorbed molecules must be closely packed at the interface and closed packing of both non-polar and polar ends is best achieved if the interface is curved. The direction of curvature will vary with the atomic volume of the metal combined in the soap and also with the valency of the metal, i.e., the number of non-polar groups attached to it.

The alkali metal soaps of sodium and potassium, having large ionic volumes and only one fatty acid attachment, favour o/w type emulsion; whereas, di-and tri-valent metals favour w/o type emulsions as their atomic volumes are small.

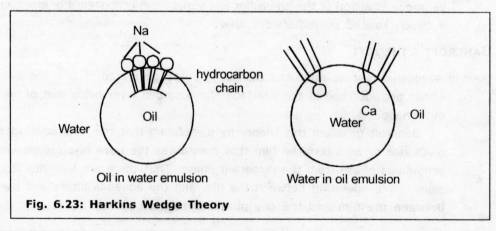

Fig. 6.23: Harkins Wedge Theory

EMULSION STABILISATION

A fine dispersion of oil-in-water requires a large area of interfacial contact and its production requires an amount of work done on the system, which is equal to the product of change in the interfacial area of the system and interfacial tension. This work is nothing but the interfacial free energy of the system. Whenever mechanical work is done on systems to reduce its globule size, there is gain in free energy of the system because of which it becomes thermodynamically unstable and therefore tries to reduce this energy in two ways-
1. Causing the droplets to take a spherical shape
2. Causing a droplet to coalesce
Final sign of emulsion in stability is separation in two layers. Steps involved in this are flocculation and coalescence.

In flocculation, two droplets become attached to each other, but are still separated by a thin liquid film. When more number of droplets come together, an aggregate is formed in which individual droplets cluster, but retain the thin liquid film between them. Coalescence is a final stage in which the thin liquid film between the globules is removed and they unite to form large droplets. There is a direct relation between the initial flocculation and coalescence and the final phase of separation into two layers. An emulsion containing only oil and water with no added stabiliser shows fast coalescence and hence, emulsion must be stabilised by addition of at least one substance, which is called a stabiliser.

I) VISCOSITY MODIFICATION: -

Change in viscosity from 0.01poise to 100 poise, by using thick syrup, reduces the flocculation rate by a factor of 10,000. But increase in viscosity of the external phase cannot be the only way of emulsion stabilisation. It is always combined with some other approach.

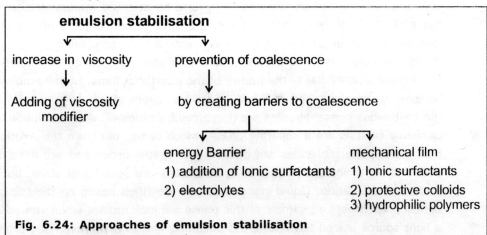

Fig. 6.24: Approaches of emulsion stabilisation

II) ENERGY BARRIERS: -

An energy barrier exists when droplets experience electrostatic repulsion on approaching each other. There are methods to create energy barriers. It is done by creating an electrical double layer by addition of electrolytes or ionic surfactants. The ionic surfactant gets adsorbed at the interface of the droplet. In proper orientation, the counter ions of the surfactant separate from the surfactant and form a diffused cloud, reaching out in the continuous phase. When these clouds of adjacent globules overlap, they experience the repulsive forces. This phenomenon is described in detail under the account of 'DLVO theory' at the begining of this chapter.

III) MECHANICAL FILM:

Polymers are adsorbed in the form of tails, loops or trains on the globule surface. Stabilising action of the protruding part of the polymer is extremely efficient to cause repulsion between the adjacent globules. The tails and loops are more efficient in preventing coalescence than the trains.

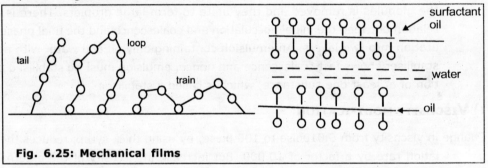

Fig. 6.25: Mechanical films

Formation of the film by an emulsifier on water surface or oil surface has been studied. Emulsifiers are known to form an oriented monomolecular film on the surface of internal phase. Emulsifiers tend to concentrate at the interface forming a mechanical barrier. If the concentration of emulsifier is high enough, the film is quite rigid and it inhibits adhesion and coalescence of droplets.

Recent studies clarify the nature of the interfacial films. Stable emulsions are believed to be comprised of liquid crystalline layers of emulsifying droplets and the continuous phase. Micelles are microscopic entities within the solution, whereas, liquid crystals are a separate phase, which comes out from the solution. In a true crystal, the molecules are packed in a spatial order and are fixed at their positions. In a liquid crystal, the hydrocarbons are in a liquid state, but with a preferred orientation. Liquid crystals can be identified based on their anisotropic optical properties, i.e., sample of this phase will look radiant when viewed against a light source placed between cross-polariser. This is a characteristic property of crystals. An isotropic substances looks black when viewed in this manner.

Emulsifiers interact with water and oil to form these three dimensional association structures. The classic theory of emulsions, which has two phase systems with a monomolecular layer of emulsifier at the interface, should be revised. Such emulsions should be considered as three phase systems containing oil, water and liquid crystals.

FORMULATION OF EMULSIONS: -

PHYSICAL PARAMETERS: -

Application of energy in the form of heat, mechanical agitation, ultrasonic vibration or electricity, is required to reduce the internal phase into small droplets.

1. *Heat :*

Approaches of emulsion stabilisation can break almost all the bonds between the molecules of a liquid; therefore, emulsion can be prepared by passing the vapours of a liquid into an external phase containing a suitable emulsifier. This is called as condensation method and can be used for materials having low vapour pressure (high boiling point).

Emulsification by dispersion method, which is more practical, is affected by heat or changes in temperature in a number of ways. It is impossible to predict whether rise in temperature will promote emulsification or coalescence. Increase in temperature decreases interfacial tension as well as viscosity; therefore usually, emulsification is favoured by increase in temperature. However, rise in temperature raises the kinetic energy of the droplets and thereby facilitates their coalescence. Change in temperature alters the distribution coefficient of an emulsifier between the two phases and causes emulsifier migration. Distribution of emulsifier, as a function of temperature, cannot be correlated directly with either emulsion formation or stability, because changes in surface tension and viscosity occur simultaneously.

Phase inversion temperature (PIT): - The most important influence that the temperature has on an emulsion is inversion. By increasing temperature, o/w emulsion can be inverted to w/o and vice versa. The temperature at which this occurs is called phase inversion temperature (PIT). This usually occurs during processing of an emulsion. As they are formed at high temperature and then allowed to cool, emulsions formed by inversion of temperature are usually more stable and contain finely divided particles.

PIT is generally considered to be the temperature at which hydrophillic and lipophilic properties of emulsifier are in balance and hence is also called HLB temperature.

An o/w emulsion, stabilised by a non-ionic polyoxyethylene derived surfactant, contains oil-swollen micelles of surfactant, as well as the emulsified oil. When the temperature is raised, the aqueous solubility of surfactant decreases. Water solubility of ether-type surfactant depends on the formation of hydrogen bond between water and oxygen atoms of ether. Surfactant solubility decreases when hydrogen bonds are broken by heat

As a result, micelles are broken and the size of emulsified oil droplets begins to increase. At the PIT, there is complete separation into oil, water and surfactant phases. Above the PIT, surfactant becomes oil-soluble, therefore forms w/o emulsion containing water swollen micelles of the emulsifier and emulsified water droplets.

The emulsion reverses back to o/w when the temperature is brought down to the ambient levels.

2. Time: - Timing exerts a profound influence on emulsification during the initial period of agitation, when droplets are formed. But as agitation continues, chances of collision between droplets become more frequent and coalescence can occur; therefore, excessive agitation after emulsification, should be avoided. The best way of forming emulsion by shaking together the contents, is by intermittent shaking. Reason for this could be the distribution of emulsifier between the phases or slow formulation of the barrier film around the droplets. The heating-cooling cycle and the cooling rate also affects emulsification.

Low energy emulsification: - If emulsification is done with the aid of heat, lot of thermal energy is wasted, as both the phases are being heated and then are being cooled. Moreover, lot of mechanical energy is wasted, as continuous stirring is required throughout the heating and cooling cycle. This wastage can be avoided by heating the entire internal phase and only a portion of the external phase to form a concentrated emulsion. This emulsion is then diluted with the remainder of continuous phase, which is at room temperature. The dilution is done during the cooling cycle. This process avoids wastage and thermal and mechanical energy and hence is called low energy emulsification.

3. Foaming :- Foaming occurs because the added surfactant (water soluble) reduces interfacial tension at the air-liquid interface, as well as at the liquid-liquid interface. Following remedies are used to avoid foaming :

1) Emulsification can be carried out in closed system
2) It can be carried out in vacuum
3) Mechanical stirring should be regulated to allow the entrapped air to rise.
4) Antifoams may be added (silicones, polyamides).

CHEMICAL PARAMETERS:

Choice of emulsion type

Fats or oils for oral administration, either as medicaments or as vehicles for oil-soluble drugs, are always formulated as o/w systems. They are formulated with a suitable flavour in the aqueous phase, which makes them palatable.

Emulsions for intravenous administration are always formulated as o/w type. Intramuscular injections can be sometimes formulated as w/o products, if a water soluble drug is incorporated as a depot.

Emulsions are most widely used for external application. Creams are semi-solid emulsions, lotions are fluid emulsions and liniments are fluid emulsions meant for massage into the skin. Both, o/w and w/o emulsions, may be used for topical application. W/o emulsions are occlusive as they inhibit evaporation of eccrine secretions. They are effectively used as cleansing creams. O/w emulsions are less efficient cleansers, but are more effective cosmetically as hand creams, moisturising creams and vanishing creams.

Emulsifiers are broadly classified as surfactants, hydrophillic colloids and finely divided solids.

Choice of surfactants:

Surfactants are cationic, anionic or non-ionic depending on the charge on the hydrophilic group.

Anionic Surfactants : These compounds dissociate in aqueous solutions to form negatively charged ions that are responsible for their emulsifying ability. They are economical, but are also toxic, hence used only in emulsions meant for external use.

Alkali metal and ammonium soaps: They are sodium, potassium or ammonium salts of long chain fatty acids such as stearic and oleic acid, e.g. sodium stearate $C_{17}H_{35}COO^-Na^+$.

They produce stable o/w emulsions, but may require an addition of auxiliary non-ionic emulsifier, for forming a mixed interfacial film. They are most efficient in basic medium. These emulsifiers can also be formed *in situ* during manufacturing, by reacting an alkali such as sodium, potassium or ammonium hydroxide with fatty acid. Fatty acids may be incorporated as such or as constituents of vegetable oil, e.g. oleic acid and ammonia are reacted together to form the soap responsible for stabilising White Liniment, B.P.

Soaps of divalent and trivalent metals : Many different divalent and trivalent salts of fatty acids exist, only calcium salts are commonly used. They are often formed *in situ* by interaction of the appropriate fatty acid with calcium hydroxide, e.g. oleic acid is reacted with calcium hydroxide to produce calcium oleate in Oily Calamine Lotion, B.P.

A number of amines form soaps with fatty acids. Most frequently used type is based on triethanolamine $N(CH_2CH_2OH)_3$, e.g. triethanolamine stearate forms stable o/w emulsions and is usually made *in situ*. These emulsifiers have neutral pH, but are still used only in external preparations.

Sulphated and sulphonated compounds : Alkyl sulphates have a general formula $ROSO_3^-M^+$, where R is hydrocarbon chain and M^+ is usually sodium or triethanolamine, e.g. sodium lauryl sulphate. It is widely used to form o/w emulsions, but is highly water-soluble and is unable to form condensed films. Hence it is often used in conjunction with non-ionic, oil-soluble emulsifying agents, e.g. it is used with cetostearyl alcohol to form emulsifying wax, B.P.

Sulphonated compounds are rarely used as emulgents, but are preferably used as wetting agents, e.g. sodium dioctylsulphosuccinate.

Cationic Surfactants : These materials form cations on dissociation, which provide the emulsifying properties. The most important cationic emulsifiers are quaternary ammonium compounds. Like the anionic surfactants, if used alone, they produce poor emulsions and are often combined with non-ionic, oil-soluble surfactants as auxiliary emulsifiers. They are toxic and are often used only for the formulation of antiseptic creams. They are incompatible with anionic emulsifiers and polyvalent ions and are unstable at high pH.

Cetrimide (cetyl trimethylammonium bromide) is the most effective of these surfactants. Cetrimide emulsifying wax, B.P.C., consists of 90 per cent cetostearyl alcohol and 10 per cent cetrimide.

Non-ionic surfactants : They range from water-soluble substances stabilising o/w emulsions to oil-soluble substances, stabilising w/o emulsions. Non-ionic surfactants have very low toxicity and irritancy and may be used in oral and parenteral emulsions. They have better compatibilities with other excipients and are less sensitive to pH changes. They, however, are more expensive. Most non-ionic surfactants are based on:

1. A fatty acid or alcohol (12-18 carbon chain length). The carbon chain length provides hydrophobic moiety.
2. An alcohol (-OH) and/or ethylene oxide grouping $\left(-\underset{}{CH}-\overset{O}{\underset{}{CH}}-\right)$ which provides the hydrophilic part.

The relative proportions of hydrophilic and hydrophobic groupings may be varied to obtain different products.

Glycol and glycerol esters : Glyceryl monostearate is a strongly hydrophobic material that produces weak w/o emulsions. Addition of small amounts of sodium, potassium or triethanolamine salts of suitable fatty acids, produce self-emulsifying glyceryl mono stearate, which is a useful o/w emulsifier.

Other polyhydric alcohol fatty acid esters are glyceryl monooleate, diethylene glycol monostearate and propylene glycol monooleate.

Sorbitan esters (Spans) : They are produced by esterification of one or more of the hydroxyl groups of sorbitan with louric, oleic, palmitic or stearic acid. e.g.,

They are lipophilic and form w/o emulsions. They are widely used with polysorbates to produce o/w or w/o emulsions.

Polysorbates (Tweens) : They are polyethylene glycol derivatives of sorbitan esters having general formula.

R-COOCH$_2$

HO$_Y$(OCH$_2$CH$_2$)

(CH$_2$CH$_2$O)$_w$OH

(CH$_2$CH$_2$O)$_X$OH

Where,

R = a fatty acid chain.

A range of products having variable oil and water solubilities may be obtained by varying carbon chain length and number of oxyethylene groups in the polyethylene glycol chain. Polysorbates are often used with the corresponding sorbitan ester to form a complex condensed film at the oil-water interface (See 'Formulation by HLB method').

Fatty alcohol polyglycol ethers: These are condensation products of polyethylene glycol and fatty alcohols, usually cetyl or cetostearyl alcohols.

ROH + (CH$_2$CH$_2$O)$_n$ → RO(CH$_2$CH$_2$O)$_n$ H

Where, R = Fatty alcohol chain

The most widely used surfactant of this type is cetomacrogol 1000, which is polyethylene glycol monocetyl ether.

Fatty acid polyglycol esters: These are the stearate esters or polyoxy stearates, e.g. Polyoxyethylene 40 stearate, Poloxalkols. Poloxalkols are polyoxyethylene/polyoxypropylene copolymers with the general formula

OH(C$_2$H$_4$O)$_a$ (C$_3$H$_6$O)$_b$ (C$_2$H$_4$O)$_a$.

Higher fatty alcohols: The hexadecyl (cetyl) and octadecyl (stearyl) members of the series of saturated aliphatic monohydric alcohols are useful auxiliary emulsifiers.

Fatty acid Lactylates: This series of emulsifiers consists of chemically bonded lactic acid with fatty acids. These acyl lactates are claimed to be mild and non-irritating on skin and eyes and are therefore useful in dermatological preparations. They can be used as w/o and o/w emulsifiers. Sodium salts are suggested to be used in o/w emulsions. Table below lists some available lactylates along with their HLB values.

Table 6.14: Some commercially available lactylates with their HLB values.

Type of Fatty acid	HLB
Stearic	6.5
Stearic/Palmitic	8.3
Lauric/Myristic	14.4
Capric/Lauric	11.3
Isostearic	5.9

Promulgens : This is a series of non-ionic emulsifiers composed of a mixture of fatty alcohols and their ethoxylates. Following table describes the two types available.

Table 6.15 : Two types of Promulgens.

	Promulgen D	Promulgen G
CTFA adopted name	Cetearyl alcohol And ceteareth-20	Stearyl alcohol & Ceteareth-20
Chemical description	Cetearyl alcohol & alcohol	Stearyl alcohol & ethoxylated cetearyl Alcohol
Melting point	47-55°C	55-63°C
Description	Forms creams	Forms liquid Emulsions

Amphoteric surfactants: They possess positively and negatively charged groups depending on pH of the system. They are cationic at low pH and anionic at higher pH, e.g. lecithin is used to stabilise intravenous fat emulsions.

Hydrophile-Lipophile balance (HLB) concept is used to determine the ratio of the surfactants in the mixed emulsifier system although it is an empirical method.

GUIDELINES IN CHOOSING PROPER SURFACTANT : -

1) HLB value of an emulsifier can be determined experimentally, or can be computed; but along with knowing the HLB value of emulsifier, HLB value required to emulsify a particular lipid in an o/w or w/o emulsion must be known. The HLB value of an ether based emulsifier is equal to the mole percentage of hydrophilic molecules divided by five.

For polyhydric alcohols, fatty acid ester: -

$$HLB = 20 \left(1 - \frac{S}{A}\right)$$ S - saponification number of ester.

A - acid number of fatty acid

HLB value for many other emulsifiers can be found out algebraically by adding the values assigned to a particular atomic grouping in the emulsifier molecule.

2) In general, molecules that are oil-soluble have low HLB values and favour formation of w/o emulsions, e.g. spans; whereas, water-soluble surfactants have high HLB values and favour formation of o/w emulsions, e.g. tweens.

3) HLB required for emulsifying a particular oil in water can be determined by trial

and error. This a called as required HLB (RHLB). RHLB values are readily available for different oily ingredients. RHLB to form an o/w emulsion and w/o emulsion with the same oil is different.

Table 6.16 : RHLB for some oily Components

Ingredient	in o/w emulsion	in w/o emulsion
Petrolatum	8	-
Beeswax	9	5
Paraffin wax	10	5
Mineral oil	10	5
Lanolin	12	8
Cetyl alcohol	15	-

4) A single emulsifier can yield a desired emulsion, but usually a combination is used, as this provides mixed interfacial films of high surface coverage, as well as sufficient viscosity.

Table 6.17 : RHLB values for a combination of oily ingredients can be determined by taking their weighted average.

Ingredient		Quality	RHLB
Beeswax		15 gm	2.7
Lanolin	Oily	10 gm	2.4
Paraffin wax	phase	20 gm	4
Cetyl alcohol		5 gm	1.5
		Total	**10.6**
Emulsifier		2 gm	
Preservative		0.2 gm.	
Colour		9.5	
Water, q.s.		100 gm	

Overall RHLB for an emulsion is found out by multiplying RHLB of each oil-like component with its weight fraction, which that component contributes to the oily phase.

For beeswax,   RHLB = 15/50 x 9   = 2.7

For lanolin,   RHLB = 10/50 x 12   = 2.4

For paraffin,   RHLB = 20/50 x 10   = 4.0

For cetyl alcohol, RHLB = 5/50 x 15   = 1.5

                  Total RHLB   = 10.6

So, overall RHLB for oily phase is 10.6. Now, the blend of emulsifier is chosen. One with a HLB value above, and other with a HLB value below RHLB, i.e., 10.6.

Almost any HLB value can be obtained by combination of any two surfactants, but blending surfactants of very low and very high HLB values do not produce very stable emulsions.

If we choose tween 80 (having HLB 15) and span 80 (having HLB 4.3), formula to calculate the weight percentage of surfactant having high HLB is,

$$\% \text{ surfactant } = \frac{\text{RHLB} - \text{HLB}_{low}}{\text{HLB}_{High} - \text{HLB}_{low}} \times 100$$

$$\text{Therefore, } \% \text{ tween } = \frac{10.6 - 4.3}{15 - 4.3} \times 100$$

$$= 58\%$$

2 gms of emulsifier has been estimated as proper protection.

$2 \times 0.58 = 1.16$ gms of tween 80

$2 - 1.16 = 0.84$ gms of span 80

Above calculated amounts should be chosen for 100 gms of emulsion.

5) Determination of surfactant mixture, of which least amount is required for optimum stability of emulsion, can be decided experimentally or calculate by using an empirical formula.

Experimental method:

10 gms of oily phase + surfactant is placed in a vial at a temperature at which the system is fluid. Water is added in 0.1 ml increments and mixture is shaken. Addition of water is continued till the system remains permanently turbid. If the initial lipid-surfactant mixture is turbid, it becomes clear on addition of water and then becomes cloudy again upon addition of further amount of water. This second cloud point is the end of titration. Usually, the most stable emulsion with the finest droplet size results at that lipid:surfactant ratio, which can tolerate largest quantity of water and will still remain clear.

6) The amount of surfactant can be found out by using an empirical formula.

$$Qs = \frac{6(\rho_s / \rho)}{10 - 0.5 \text{ RHLB}} + 4Q/1000$$

Where

$Qs \rightarrow$ minimum amount of surfactant mixture

$\rho_s \rightarrow$ density of surfactant mixture

$\rho \rightarrow$ density of internal phase

RHLB $\rightarrow$ HLB of oil phase in o/w or w/o emulsion

$Q \rightarrow$ Percentage of continuous phase

W/o emulsion containing 40 gms mixed oil phase and 60 gms water is to be formulated. Oil phase consists of 70 per cent paraffin and 30 per cent beeswax. Density of oil phase is 0.85 gms/cm³ and that of the aqueous phase is almost equal to 1 gm/cm³. Density of surfactant blend is 0.87 gm/cm³. RHLB of paraffin and bees wax is 4 and 5 respectively for w/o emulsion and sorbitan tristearate (HLB 2.1) and diethylene glycol monostearate (HLB 4.7) are chosen as surfactant.

$$\begin{aligned}
\text{RHLB} &= 4 \times 0.7 + 5 \times 0.3 \\
&= 2.8 + 1.5 \\
&= 4.3
\end{aligned}$$

$$Qs = \frac{6(0.87/1)}{10 - (0.5 \times 4.3)} + \frac{4 \times 40}{1000} = 0.82 \text{ gm}$$

There is no assurance that stable emulsion prepared by one chemical class of emulsifier at a particular HLB can be duplicated by another class of emulsifier having the same HLB.

7) It is believed that more hydrophilic emulsifiers promote formation of o/w emulsion. Usually emulsifiers of HLB 3.5-6.0 are used for o/w type of emulsions. This is because hydrophillic surfactant is present to a greater extent in aqueous phase and therefore promotes coalescence of aqueous phase globules during emulsion manufacturing; while the oil globules remain dispersed. Therefore, it forms an o/w emulsion.

8) A hydrophilic surfactant placed in aqueous phase prior to emulsification, usually migrates to oily phase as the temperature rises, until the equilibrium is reached. The second lipophilic emulsifier placed in the lipid phase retards establishment of this equation and decides rate of migration. If equilibrium can be established, then only can the inversion of emulsion from o/w to w/o take place.

b) Choice of auxiliary surfactants:

i) Naturally occurring polysachharides: Naturally occurring materials suffer from two disadvantages-

i) There is considerable batch to batch variation in composition.

ii) They are susceptible to bacterial or mould growth.

The most widely used polysaccharide is acacia. It stabilises o/w emulsion by forming a multimolecular film. It can also be used along with tragacanth and sodium alginate.

ii) Semisynthetic polysaccharides: Several grades of cellulosics are available (Refer page no.276 for details).

iii) Sterol containing substances: Beeswax, wool fat and wool alcohols are often used in emulsions for external use. Beeswax/borax systems are used as emulsifiers. Wool fat consists chiefly of normal fatty alcohols with fatty acid esters of cholesterol and sterols. It forms w/o emulsions. It is often used along with other emulsifiers, e.g., with calcium oleate in oily calamine lotion, B.P.; with beeswax in proflavine cream, B.P.C. and with cetostearyl alcohol in zinc cream, B.P.

The principal emulsifying agent in wool fat is wool alcohol. It consists of cholesterol with other sterols. It is an effective w/o emulsifier and it does not have a strong odour like wool fat.

iv) Finely divided solids: Finely divided solids which do not have any swelling properties, also behave as good auxiliary emulsifiers e.g. non-swelling clays and heavy metal hydroxides.

A polar solid without influence of surfactant will promote formulation of o/w emulsion and vice versa.

Montmorillonite clays (bentonite/aluminium magnesium silicate) and colloidal silicon dioxide are used in suspension for external use. Aluminium and magnesium hydroxides may be used internally.

v) Hydrophilic colloids: These are the swelling gums and clays like bentonite. As they are hydrophilic, they favour formation of o/w emulsion.

They also increase viscosity of external phase. The natural gums are extremely sensitive to pH and to presence of cations. Synthetic hydrocolloids like celluloses are extremely useful. Proteins are also useful auxiliary emulsifiers, particularly in oral emulsions.

Chemical stability : Prior to selection of emulsion additive, their chemical nature must be known, e.g. a soap cannot be added as an emulsifier to an emulsion which is required to have a pH of 4.0; alternatively, an easily hydrolysable ester should not be added to an emulsion having strongly acidic or basic pH. Some lipids have a tenancy to rancidity and their use should be avoided.

Chemical safety:

The safety and toxicological clearance of additives is extremely important; particularly for colorants, sweeteners and surfactants.

c) Choice of lipid phase:

All the pharmaceutical and cosmetic emulsions may contain variety of lipids. The drug should have sufficient solubility in both phases. For faster dissolution in GI contents, adequate aqueous solubility is required, whereas, for faster absorption, lipid solubility is essential. In case of topical emulsions, the feel of oily residue that an emulsion leaves on skin is of extreme importance. The ratio of lipid phase to the aqueous phase is usually determined by the solubility of drugs in both the phases and desired consistency. Also, higher is the percentage of internal phase more is the amount of emulsifier required.

d) Choice of preservative and antioxidants: -

A detailed account of preservatives & antioxidants used in emulsions can be found on pg no. 236 to 242.

e) Choice of emulsion consistency :

The texture and feel of the emulsion is also an important consideration. A w/o emulsion is greasy and often has more apparent viscosity than an o/w emulsion. O/w emulsions, however, feel less greasy or sticky on application to skin, are absorbed more readily and can be washed off easily.

Ideally, emulsions should be plastic or pseudoplastic in rheology with thixotropic nature. A high apparent viscosity at low rates of shear is essential on standing as it retards the movement of globules. It is important however that the products flow freely during agitation, and their removal from the container should be easy, i.e., they should have low apparent viscosity at these high rates of shear.

Dermatological emulsions may have different viscosities. Low viscosity lotions and liniments can be filled in flexible plastic containers via a nozzle. They require very light shearing to spread them on the skin, and this is particularly important for painful or inflamed skin conditions. But, they have a disadvantage of having increased tendencies of creaming.

High viscosity emulsions for external use are called creams and they are often packed in collapsible plastic or aluminium tubes.

Patient acceptability and aesthetic appeal are also very important criterion while formulating dermatological creams.

Rheological properties of emulsions may be altered in following ways-

i) Percentage of dispersed phase: As the concentration of dispersed phase increases, the viscosity of the emulsion increases. But the concentration should not exceed 60 per cent as this may cause phase inversion.

ii) Particle size of dispersed phase: The apparent viscosity of the emulsion maybe increased by decreasing the globule size and there are several postulated mechanisms to explain this.

iii) Viscosity of continuous phase: The increase in viscosity of continuous phase increases the viscosity of emulsion. Syrup and glycerol used as sweeteners in o/w emulsions for oral use, use of hydrocolloids as viscosity modifiers, and use of certain waxes in w/o emulsions thus increase emulsion viscosity.

iv) Viscosity of dispersed phase: The effect of viscosity of dispersed phase on viscosity of emulsion is not clearly understood. However, less viscous dispersed phase deforms easily during application of shear, which slightly increases the total interfacial area. This may alter double layer interactions and thus alter the viscosity.

v) Nature and concentration of emulsifier system: Hydrophilic colloid emulsifiers, while forming protective films on globule surfaces, also increase emulsion viscosities. Thus increase in their concentration increases viscosity of emulsion. Surfactants form condensed monomolecular films, influence the degree of flocculation by forming linkages in adjacent globules to form a gel-like structure. Thus increase in their concentration significantly increases viscosity.

STABILITY OF EMULSIONS :

A stable emulsion is the one that maintains the same number of globules of a particular size the dispersed phase per unit volume of the continuous phase. Accepted stability in pharmaceutical emulsion does not require thermodynamic stability. If an emulsion creams up (rises) or creams down (sediments), it is still pharmaceutically acceptable as long as it can be reconstituted by agitation. Kinetic stability of emulsion means that physico-chemical, properties do not change appreciably during shelf-life.

SYMPTOMS OF INSTABILITY:

Time and temperature dependant processes occur on emulsions to effect their separation. Instability is evidenced by creaming, reversible aggregation, i.e., flocculation and irreversible aggregation, i.e. coalescence.

1. Creaming :

Under the influence of gravity, suspended droplets rise or sediment depending upon the differences in specific gravities of the two phases. If creaming takes place, without aggregation, the emulsion can be reconstituted. Stokes' equation is useful in understanding process of creaming, although there is certain limitation.

1) The equation is based on spherical globules, whose settling is not influenced by settling of other globules, called free settling; whereas, especially in emulsions with high amount of internal phase, globules always interfere with settling of other globules (hindered setting).

2) If flocculation takes place, globules no longer remain spherical in shape, as the entire floccule behaves as a single globule while settling.

Yet, Stokes' Law can be applied in the following way to understand the be haviour of emulsions :

1) Rate of settling is inversely proportional to the square of the radius of globules; therefore larger globules cream more rapidly than the smaller ones.

2) Lesser the difference between the specific gravities of the two phases, slower is the rate of creaming. Therefore, adjusting the specific gravities of the internal and the external phase is the method of minimising creaming.

3) Rate of creaming is inversely proportional to viscosity; therefore, an increased viscosity of the external phase, increases the emulsion stability.

2. Flocculation :

Flocculation may take place before, during or after creaming. It is a reversible three dimensional aggregation of the droplets. It is influenced by charges on globules due to the effect of electrolytes or surfactants. In the absence of mechanical barrier on the globules, globules flocculate and coalesce more rapidly.

Flocculation can occur only when mechanical or electrical barrier is sufficient to prevent coalescence. In flocculation, the interfacial film and the droplets remain intact. Reversibility of this aggregation is determined by chemical nature of the emulsifier, phase volume ratio and concentration of dissolved substances.

Addition of small concentration of electrolyte or increasing concentration of ionic surfactant promotes flocculation.

3. Coalescence:

It is the growth process during which the emulsified globules join to form larger globules. When the smaller globules merge, it suggests that the emulsion will eventually separate completely. The major factor which prevents flocculated globule from coalescence is the strength of the mechanical barrier around the globules.

CHEMICAL INSTABILITY:

Following chemical problems may cause coalescence of an emulsion:

1. The emulgent has to be physically, and chemically, compatible with the emulsion ingredients, e.g. ionic surfactants are often incompatible with oppositely charged molecules.
2. Presence of electrolyte can alter emulsion stability by altering the interaction energy of the globules or by a salting-out effect.
3. Electrolyte addition may cause phase inversion, e.g. sodium soap is used to stabilise an o/w emulsion. Addition of divalent electrolytes, such as calcium chloride will form calcium soap, which will stabilise a w/o emulsion.
4. Addition of solvents in which the emulsifiers are insoluble may also cause chemical instability, e.g. precipitation of hydrophilic colloids by addition of alcohol.
5. Change in pH may lead to breaking of emulsion.
6. Oxidation: The oils and fats used in the emulsion are often of animal or vegetable origin. They are therefore susceptible to oxidation by atmospheric oxygen or due to microbial attack. Emulgents like wool fat or wool alcohols also undergo oxidation. The oxidation products have a very unpleasant odour, resulting in rancidity. Oxidation caused by atmospheric oxygen can be prevented by addition of antioxidant. Oxidation due to microbial action is prevented by addition of preservatives.

MICROBIOLOGICAL CONTAMINATION:

The contamination of emulsion by microorganisms may create problems such as gas production, changes in colour and odour, pH changes in aqueous phase, hydrolysis of oils and fats and breaking of emulsion. Even though there are no visible signs of contamination, the bacteria present may include pathogens and may constitute a health hazard. The fats, oils, emulgents and hydrophilic colloids may provide suitable medium for their growth. Water and the naturally occurring excipients like gums, may act as source of this contamination.

Improper storage conditions :

i) Increase in temperature decreases the apparent viscosity of the external phase, causing increase in the rate of creaming.
ii) Increase in temperature also causes increase in kinetic motion of the globules of external and internal phase. This increases number of collisions between

the globules. The increase in temperature also increases the motility of emulsifier molecules at the interface and also causes certain macromolecular emulsifiers to coagulate. The increased motion of the emulsifier molecules expands the mono layer at the interface, increasing coalescence.

iii) Freezing of aqueous phase produces ice crystals that exert pressure on the dispersed phase globules.

iv) If dissolved electrolytes are present they may concentrate in the unfrozen water, thus affecting the charged density on the globules. Certain emulsifiers may also participate at low temperatures.

v) Also, the effect of growth of microorganisms can cause deterioration of emulsions and hence should be protected against them.

ASSESSMENT OF EMULSION STABILITY:

Emulsions should maintain their stability, appearance and functionality throughout the shelf-life. Containers used for emulsions might also interact with them and extract the material from them or allow loss of water or other volatile ingredients. No quick and sensitive methods are available for predicting the shelf-life of an emulsion.

The formulator should put the emulsion under some kind of stress or use some sensitive method that can detect instability of emulsion, much before macroscopic examination.

1) *Stress condition:*

i) Ageing and temperature- The assumption that a 10° increase in the temperature doubles the rate of most chemical reactions, is not applicable to emulsions. It is based on the assumption that same chemical reactions take place at elevated temperatures but at a different rate. But in case of emulsions, changes in temperature bring about new reactions. Therefore, emulsions should not be exposed to unrealistically high temperatures for stability testing.

Usually, emulsions are stable at temperatures of 40-45°C. However, they become unstable at 55-60°C. Temperature affects viscosity, partitioning of the surfactant, inversion of phase and crystallisation of certain lipids; therefore, emulsion should not be exposed to temperatures above 50°C.

ii) Freeze-thaw cycle- It is an extremely important technique in evaluating emulsion stability, but extremes of temperature should be avoided. Usually, temperatures in the range of 40-45°C should be used. These temperatures approach realistic conditions, but yet place the emulsion under too much stress. With increase in temperature, rate of coalescence and creaming increases, due to decrease in viscosity. Freezing can damage an emulsion more than heating, since solubility of emulsifier in both the phases is more sensitive to freezing. Also, formation of ice crystals develops pressure that can deform spherical shape of the emulsion droplets.

iii) Centrifugation: - Stokes' law suggests that, with increase in gravity, separation is accelerated. Centrifugation at 3500 rpm for 5 hours is equivalent to effect of gravity for 1 year; whereas, effects of ultracentrifugation, (more than 25000 rpm) are not usually observed on normal ageing.

Ultra centrifugation causes the emulsion to separate into a top layer of coagulated oil, middle layer of coagulated emulsion and bottom layer of coagulated water. This take place only at high speeds, due to breaking of the adsorbed layer of emulsifier around the dispersed phase globules.

iv) Agitation: Coalescence takes place due to impingement of droplets upon each other as a result of the Brownian movement. Simple mechanical agitation can supply energy with which the droplets impinge upon each other.

Excessive agitation or homogenisation may interfere with formation of emulsion or sometimes break an emulsion.

2) *Physical parameters:*

Commonly used parameters for assessment of effect of stress conditions include phase separation, viscosity, electrophoretic properties, particle size analysis and particle count.

i) Phase separation: -

Whether phase separation is due to creaming or coalescence should be found out. A simple method of determining the cause of phase separation is by withdrawing a small specimen of emulsion from top and bottom of the preparation after some period of storage and comparing the compositions of the two samples by appropriate methods of analysis for water content, oil content or any other suitable constituent.

ii) Viscosity: - Changes in viscosity during ageing is an important parameter to measure stability. Multipoint viscosity measurement is usually done with instruments like Brookfield viscometer with helipath attachment. As a rule, globules in the w/o emulsions flocculate rapidly, with subsequent drop in viscosity for sometime,which then remains fairly constant. O/w emulsions behave differently. Flocculation causes immediate rise in viscosity. After this initial change, almost all emulsions show changes in consistency with time. Helipath attachment of Brookfield viscometer is used for detection of creaming and sedimentation before they become visibly apparent. Because of separation, the descending spindle encounters varying resistance and records it.

For example in fig 6.25, Lotion A contains suspended solids in an emulsion. High viscosity near the top is due to creaming and non-wetting of solids.

High viscosity at the lower level is due to sedimentation. Addition of a proper surfactant, along with a cellulosic viscosity modifier, will produce more uniform viscosity as shown for lotion B.

Best way of using viscosity determination for prediction of shelf-life is to relate them to changes in particle size. Decrease in viscosity with age, reflects increase of particle size due to coalescence, and is an indicator of poor shelf-life. Viscosity should be measured in undisturbed containers to avoid changes due to previous stress. Therefore, Helipath attachment is used. Also viscosity should be measured at different

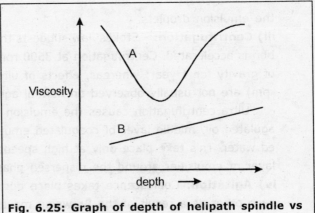

Fig. 6.25: Graph of depth of helipath spindle vs viscosity in two lotions A& B.

shear rates to obtain a clear picture of rheological behaviour.

EQUIPMENTS FOR MANUFACTURING EMULSIONS

The equipments used for emulsification have been discussed in detail in previous sections of this book (Page no. 245-247, 286-287).

Suppositories

INTRODUCTION

Suppositories are the most neglected dosage forms in medicine. The origin of the word 'suppository' is from the Latin word *Supponere*, meaning "to place under", as derived from *sup* (under) and *ponere* (to place). Thus, both linguistically and therapeutically, suppositories are the dosage forms to be placed under the body, i.e., into the rectum.

Although much work has been done in recent years, in Europe and U.S.A. there is a general rejection of rectal route as a route of drug administration. The use of rectal suppositories is still restricted to comatose patients, patients suffering from vomiting and nausea, paediatric and geriatric patients and patients requiring local therapeutic treatment.

In many countries, social conventions preclude greater use of suppositories. In addition to the above mentioned conditions, use of rectal and vaginal suppositories may prove beneficial in many other conditions, as would be discussed later.

DEFINITIONS

There are various ways in which suppositories may be described : They may be functionally defined as solid dosage forms used for rectal, vaginal, or urethral administration of drugs. They consist of a dispersion of active ingredients in an inert matrix containing solid and / or semisolid ingredients. The matrix should not ideally precipitate any chemical interaction between the drug and excipients. The dispersed phase may be a solid (powder) or liquid (aqueous, alcoholic or glycolic solutions, oils or extracts). The base may be natural in origin or synthetically derived and must have the ability to melt at the rectal or vaginal temperature to release the drug.

The suppositories are of various shapes and sizes. The size and shape of a suppository should be such that it can be easily inserted in the intended body cavity without causing undue distension, and once inserted, must remain in its place for the intended period of time.

APPLICATIONS OF SUPPOSITORIES

Suppositories were traditionally used for local applications and a wide range of drugs were incorporated in this form, e.g. local anaesthetics, laxatives, analgesics, antipyretics, sedative-hypnotics and antibiotics.

They are now being increasingly used for systemic drug delivery as well. Much ongoing research work is being targeted on insulin therapy via rectal route.

Advantages :

1. Rectal route of administration substantially reduces hepatic first pass metabolism, thereby enhancing bioavailability of the drug.
2. Some drugs are effectively absorbed from the rectal mucosa. For these types of drugs, suppositories are advantageous.

FACTORS AFFECTING DRUG ABSORPTION FROM RECTAL SUPPOSITORIES:

Various factors affect the absorption of drugs from rectal suppositories.

PHYSIOLOGICAL FACTORS

1. The lower and upper hemorrhoid veins are present surrounding the colon and rectum. The lower hemorrhoid veins enter inferior vena cava and thus bypass the liver. The upper hemorrhoid veins however connect with the portal vein and the drug absorbed through this vein enters the first pass circulation. The hepatic portal vein carries the drug from the small intestine if it is delivered by oral route. Liver modifies many drugs chemically and reduces their systemic effectiveness. If absorbed from the anorectal region, however, major portion of the drug bypasses the first effect and thus retains its therapeutic activity.

2. Rectal fluids have virtually no buffer capacity, and thus the dissolving drugs decide the pH in the rectal region. The barrier separating the colonic lumen from blood is preferentially permeable to unionised forms of drugs. Thus the absorption of the drug is enhanced, most likely, by a change in pH of rectal mucosa, as this change increases the proportion of unionised drug.

3. Drug absorption is also affected by the anorectal membrane. The membranous wall is covered with mucous, which can act as a barrier to its absorption.

4. The diffusivity of the rectal mucosa is influenced by nature of medicament, the hydrophilicity or lipophilicity of drug, presence of surfactant and physiological state of colon.

Physicochemical factors related to drug

The drug gets absorbed from the anorectal area in the following sequence:

Drug in vehicle

↓

Drug in anorectal fluids

↓

Absorption through rectal mucosa

Fig. 7.1: Drug absorption from anorectal area

The drug must be released from the suppository and get distributed by the surrounding fluids to the site of absorption. Following physicochemical characteristics of the drugs play an important role in absorption of the drug-

1. The lipid-water partition co-efficient :

If the suppository base is fats and the drug has a partition co-efficient favouring fat solubility, the drug is released slowly. A lipophilic drug present in low concentration in a fat-based suppository has lesser tendency to escape to the aqueous colorectal fluids, than a hydrophilic drug present in a fat base. Thus water soluble and oil insoluble salts are preferred in fat based suppositories.

The water-soluble suppository base releases the drug by itself getting dissolved. Thus it can release both water soluble and oil soluble drugs with equal efficiency. Thus more the concentration of the drug present in the base, more is the drug available for absorption. However, if the amount of the drug dissolved in the intestinal lumen is above a particular amount, the rate of absorption is not changed with further increase in the concentration of the drug.

2. Particle size :

For drugs suspended in a suppository, the drugs having smaller particle size dissolve faster and have better chances of getting absorbed.

3. Degree of ionisation :

After the release from the suppository base, on reaching the site of absorption on the lumen wall, undissociated lipid-soluble drug is the most readily absorbed form. Completely ionised drugs are poorly absorbed. Unionised, lipid-insoluble drugs are also poorly absorbed. Acids having pK_a values below 3.0 and bases above 10.0 indicate almost complete ionisation and negligible absorption rates. Drug absorption can be increased by use of buffers that can convert the pH of the anorectal rejoin to a value that decreases ionisation of the drug.

4. Surface properties :

When the drug is brought in contact with the vehicle, air has to be displaced from its surface. When this is not achieved, particles form agglomerates. This adversely affects content uniformity by an increased tendency to separate. If the wetting of the drug has been taken place by the vehicle, displacement by rectal fluid is needed to let the drug go into solution.

Table 7.1: Factors related to drug affecting drug absorption from suppositories.

Sr. No	Factors affecting drug absorption from suppositories
1.	Fat-water partition Co-efficient
2.	Surface properties
3.	Particle size
4.	pK$_a$

Physicochemical factors of the base and additives :

Various properties of suppository bases like melting range, hydroxyl value, molecular weight, etc., affect the drugs' effectiveness. The base can react physically or chemically with the drug to affect its absorption. If the base irritates the mucous membrane of the rectum, it can initiate colonic response which prompts a bowel movement, thus eliminating chances of complete drug release and absorption.

The additives can affect drug absorption by producing changes in rheologic properties of the base at body temperature, or by affecting properties of dissolution of the drug.

SUPPOSITORY BASES

The suppository base plays an important role in the release of the drug. Initially, the choice of suppository base was prompted by its availability. But now a number of physical and chemical parameters are being determined before choosing a suppository base. A few of these are listed below-

1. Origin and chemical composition :

Natural, synthetic or semi-synthetic origin of the base determines its chemical make up. Physical and/or chemical incompatibilities of the base with the formula ingredients may be predicted by knowing the chemical composition.

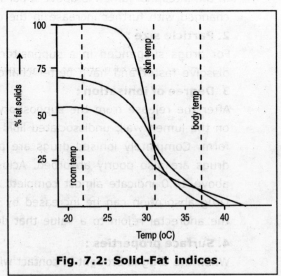

Fig. 7.2: Solid-Fat indices.

2. Melting range : Fatty suppository bases are mixtures and do not have sharp melting points. Melting range for such bases, is indicated by the temperature at which melting starts, to the temperature at which melting completes. Melting range is an important parameter to be considered, if the base releases the drug by melting.

3. Solid fat index (SFI) : The solidification and melting ranges of bases, along with the moulding characteristics and surface texture hardness, can be determined from the graph of percentage of solid fats versus temperature (Fig. 7.2). Solid content at room temperature is important in determining suppository hardness.

Suppositories having solid content above 30 per cent, at skin temperature (32°C), is dry to touch. A base with a sharp drop in solids content over a short span of temperature produces brittle suppositories if moulded quickly.

4. Hydroxyl value : It indicates the monoglyceride and diglyceride content of a fatty base, as it is a measure of un-esterified positions on glycerides.

5. Solidification point : It is useful for predicting the time required for solidification of suppository in the mould. If the difference between melting range and solidification point is more than 10°C, refrigeration is suggested, to shorten the solidification time.

6. Saponification value : It is an indication of the type and amount of glyceride used. It is the number of milligrams of KOH required to neutralise the free acids and saponify the esters contained in 1 gm of fat.

7. Iodine value : Number of milligrams of iodine that react with 100 gm of fat or other unsaturated material. Fats having higher iodine values have more chances of getting decomposed by moisture, acids and oxygen.

8. Water no. : It indicates the amount of water that can be incorporated in 100 gm of base. It is important to have an idea about the amount of aqueous liquids that can be incorporated in the suppository.

9. Acid value : The amount of KOH, in milligrams, required to neutralise free acid in 1 gm of substance. Good suppository bases have low acid values as free acids may react with other ingredients and complicate formulation.

CHARACTERISTICS OF IDEAL SUPPOSITORY BASE

1. A good suppository base should be physicochemically stable during storage as a bulk product and as a suppository.
2. It should not show any physical or chemical incompatibility with the drug.
3. It should be non-toxic and non-irritant to sensitive skin.
4. It should be compatible with broad variety of drugs.
5. The fatty bases should have a melting range lower than approximately 37°C (body temperature). The melting range should be small enough to give rapid

solidification after moulding. This prevents separation of suspended high density particles. On the other hand, the melting range should be large enough to facilitate manufacturing, which takes considerable amount of time.

6. High rates of solidification may result in fissures in a suppository. The base should exhibit enough volume contraction during solidification to ensure its ease of removal from the moulds.

7. It should have high water number to allow incorporation of high amount of water.

8. It should have wetting and emulsifying properties.

9. The molten base should have low enough viscosity to easily flow into the moulds. Low viscosity values are also beneficial for ensuring easy transport of the drug to the absorbing surfaces after the suppository melts at body temperature. But high viscosities of molten base are important in retarding rate of sedimentation of suspended high density drug particles during solidification in the moulds.

10. In addition to this, a fatty base should have acid value below 0.2.

11. Saponification value should be between 200 and 245.

12. Iodine value should be less than 7.

13. It should have only a small time interval after melting and before solidification starts.

CLASSIFICATION OF SUPPOSITORY BASES

Based on their physical characteristics, suppository bases are classified into three main categories-

a) Fatty or oleaginous bases

b) Water soluble or water miscible bases

c) Miscellaneous bases

A) FATTY OR OLEAGINOUS BASES :

These are the most widely used bases, as cocoa butter falls in this category. Apart from Cocoa butter, this class consists of other fatty or oleaginous materials, like hydrogenated fatty acids of vegetable oils and compounds of glycerin with high molecular weight fatty acids.

Cocoa butter (Theobroma oil) : It is a fat obtained from roasted seeds of *Theobroma Cacao*. It is a yellowish-white solid at room temperature, having a faint chocolate-like odour. It is a triglyceride, primarily of oleopalmistearin and oleodistearin. Its melting range is 30-36ºC, i.e., it melts at body temperature and yet remains solid at room temperature. Its Iodine value is between 34 and 38 and its acid value is not higher than 4.

Because of the high unsaturated triglyceride content, cocoa butter shows marked polymorphism. It exists in four different crystalline forms, which have different melting points and different rates of drug release.

Cocoa butter exists in four different crystalline states-

1. The α-form which melts at 24°C, is obtained by stirring liquefied cocoa butter to 0°C .
2. The β¹-form melts between 28 and 31°C and is obtained by stirring liquefied cocoa butter at 28-31°C.
3. The β-form is a stable form, melts between 34 and 35°C and is obtained due to conversion of the metastable β'-form, accompanied with volume contraction.
4. The γ-form, melts at 18°C. It is obtained by pouring cool (20°C) cocoa butter, before it solidifies, into a container, which is cooled to deep-freeze temperature.

Table 7.2: Types of Cocoa butter polymorphs

Polymorph	Melting range	How the polymorph is formed
α (Metastable)	24°C	Sudden cooling to 0°C
β' (Metastable)	28-31°C	Stirring at 28-31°C
β	34-35°C	Conversion of β'-form to this stable form
γ	18°C	Pouring cool liquefied cocoa butter (20°C) into a deep-frozen container.

When cocoa butter is hastily or carelessly melted at a temperature which is much higher than the minimum required temperature, and then rapidly chilled, low melting polymorphs are formed. As seen from Table 7.2, only β-form melts between 34 and 35°C. The formation of various forms of cocoa butter depends on the degree of heating, degree of cooling and conditions during processing. Prolonged heating above the critical temperature produces unstable crystals having lowered melting points. The unstable crystals revert to the stable β-form upon storage at higher temperatures, which usually takes 1-4 days.

Formation of unstable forms may be avoided by following means-

1. Addition of small amounts of stable crystals to molten cocoa butter accelerates conversion of unstable form to stable form.
2. Tempering the solidified melt at 28-32°C for long periods causes a quick change from unstable to stable form.
3. Incomplete melting of the mass prevents formation of the unstable form.

The instability of cocoa butter during heating, coupled with its property to adhere to moulds during solidification, cause considerable difficulties in the manufacturing processes.

Cocoa butter solidifies at a temperature 12-13°C below its melting point. It can be kept in fluid state at comparatively low temperatures because of this property, during its processing.

Cocoa butter can take up less amounts of water due to absence of emulsifiers.

Addition of emulsifiers, such as Tween-61® (5-10 per cent), increases water absorption. It also improves suspension of insoluble drugs. Adding materials such as silica or aluminium monostearate, which yield the mass thixotropic, also improves suspension stability.

Some drugs cause lowering in melting point of cocoa butter. Wax and Spermaceti were commonly used to correct this. Nowadays, many semisynthetic or completely synthetic bases, with higher melting ranges, have substituted cocoa butter, e.g. Adeps solidus. Table compares some properties of such semisynthetic bases with cocoa butter.

Table 7.3: Some properties of fatty suppository bases

Base	Melting range	Hydroxyl no.	Iodine no.
Cocoa butter	31 – 34	0	34-38
Adeps Solidus	33 – 37.5	< 5-30	< 3
Hydrokote	25	33.6 – 36.3 -	< 4
Suppocire AIML	34.5 – 35.5	20-30	< 2

Cocoa Butter Substitutes

Fatty suppository bases are prepared from a variety of materials of synthetic or natural origin, e.g. esterification, hydrogenation and fractionation of vegetable oils, such as coconut or palm kernel oils. Hydrogenation of corn oil reduces unsaturation and increases percentage of solid triglycerides. Lower melting triglycerides are then removed by solvent extraction. This product is referred to as "hard butter".

Inter-esterification is a common method of producing fatty suppository bases. In this process, coconut oil, palm kernel oil and/or palm oil refined, deodorised hydrogenated and then are finally inter-esterified to create narrow melting triglycerides.

Another common method uses re-esterification. The oils are split into fatty acids and glycerin by treating with high pressure steam. Glycerin is removed. The mixture now consists of C_6-C_{18} chain free fatty acids. The readily rancidified fatty acids, viz., caproic, caprylic and capric acids, are removed by fractional vacuum distillation. The remaining fatty acids are hydrogenated to harden them and to lower iodine value and then are re-esterified with excess of glycerin to form mixtures of mono, di and tri glycerides. The re-esterification is controlled to modify the melting range, good mould release, smoothness and viscosity.

A large number of suppository bases prepared in this way are available. The suppository base should have following characteristics-
1. Narrow interval between melting and solidification points.
2. High melting range in order to incorporate low melting drugs.
3. If the incorporated solids increase the viscosity of melted suppository, then smaller melting ranges are preferable.

4. Low iodine value and acid value to ensure longer shelf-life.

B) WATER SOLUBLE / HYDROPHILIC SUPPOSITORY BASES :

i) Glycerin Suppositories –

USP XX describes a formula for glycerin suppository which contains glycerin, sodium stearate and water. USP XX also gives an unofficial formula for glycerinated gelatin suppository.

Glycerinated gelatin suppositories do not melt, but dissolve in body fluids. The dissolution time may be manipulated by varying the percentage of the ingredients. These bases are hygroscopic and support microbial growth. Moisture resistant packaging and addition of preservative is needed to overcome these problems respectively.

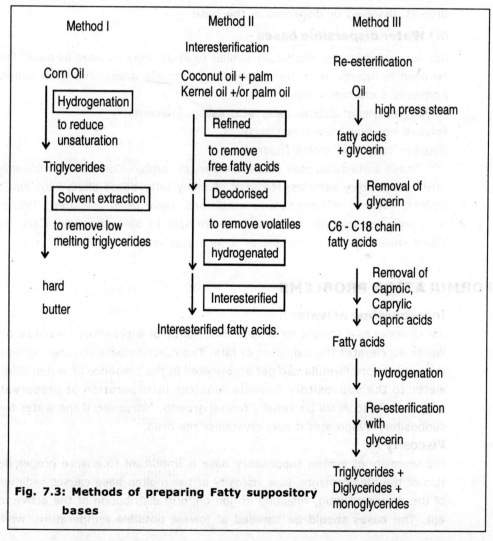

Fig. 7.3: Methods of preparing Fatty suppository bases

ii) Polyethylene Glycol Suppositories –

Polyethylene glycols have the general formula- $HOCH_2$ $(H_2COCH_2)_n$ CH_2OH. They are available as liquids (mol. wt. 200-600) and waxy solids (mol. wt. above 1000). Appropriate combinations of PEGs may be effectively used as suppository bases due to the wide range of melting points and solubilities of the PEGs. Varying degrees of heat stability and dissolution rates may be manipulated by altering the proportion. These bases are stable to hydrolysis and microbial attack and are physiologically inert.

The bases are free of water and have to be dipped in water prior to insertion. This avoids the possible irritation of mucous membranes by their drawing water from the mucosa.

PEG suppositories may be prepared by moulding or cold compression. The drug is dissolved or dispersed in the base.

iii) Water dispersible bases –

Non-ionic surfactants, chemically similar to PEGs, may be used as base. They can be used to incorporate water-soluble or oil-soluble drugs. The most widely used non-ionic surfactants are-

Polyoxy ethylene sorbitan fatty acid esters (Tweens).

Polyoxy ethylene stearates (Myrj).

Sorbitan fatty acid esters (Spans).

These surfactants may be used alone, in combination or in combination with other suppository vehicles. Mixtures of many fatty bases along with emulsifying agents, capable of forming w/o emulsions, have been prepared. These bases hold aqueous solutions or water and are said to be hydrophilic. Care must be taken while using a surfactant as it increases drug absorption.

FORMULATION PROBLEMS

Incorporation of water :

Use of water as a solvent for drug in formulation of suppository should be avoided. Water accelerates the oxidation of fats. The reaction between the ingredients of the suppository formula can get accelerated in the presence of water. Addition of water to the suppository formula requires incorporation of preservatives / antioxidants to avoid bacterial / fungal growth. Moreover, if the water from the suppository evaporates it may crystallise the drug.

Viscosity :

The viscosity of molten suppository base is important to ensure proper distribution of the medicaments. Low viscosity of the molten base causes sedimentation of the dispersed drug, resulting in non-uniform distribution of the active ingredient. The bases should be handled at lowest possible temperature, while processing, to avoid this problem. Addition of 2 per cent aluminium monostearate increases the viscosity and avoids sedimentation. Viscosity modifiers (cetyl / stearyl alcohol / stearic acid) may also be added.

Brittleness :

Some suppository bases have a tendency to crack, particularly, if they are chilled rapidly, e.g. synthetic fatty bases, bases containing high percentage of stearates and bases having high degree of hydrogenation. This problem may be overcome by the use of surfactants, which impart plasticity, and by cooling the suppository mass slowly.

Density :

The volume of suppository base is fixed. The weight of the suppository, therefore, depends on the density of the base. The weight of the suppository can be determined by knowing the volume of the mould and the density of the base. The active ingredient can then be added in such amounts that the exact quantity is present in each suppository.

Volume Contraction :

The molten suppository mass often contracts after cooling in the mould. This affects in following two ways:

1. Contraction ensures quick release from the mould, as the mass pulls away from the mould walls. This eliminates the use of mould-releasing or lubricating agents.

2. Due to contraction, a hole might form at the open end. This leads to decrease in weight and imperfect appearance. This can be avoided by pouring the mass at a temperature above its congealing temperature, into a warm mould. Sometimes the mould is overfilled and the excess mass, containing the hole, is scraped off.

Addition of lubricants and mould-release agents-

In some types of suppository bases, which do not undergo volume contraction, a strong tendency to adhere to the moulds is observed. This may be overcome by the use of mould-release or lubricating agents. Mineral oil, aqueous solution of sodium lauryl sulphate, silicones and alcohol are few examples of mould-releasing agents. The inside of the moulds may be coated with Teflon to avoid adhesion.

Use of antioxidants :

The high percentage of fats in the suppositories makes them liable to auto-oxidation and rancidity. High percentage of unsaturated fatty acids in the base makes it more prone to developing rancidity.

This problem may be overcome by the use of antioxidants. Some effective antioxidants are: m- or p- diphenols. Tocopherols, gossypol in cotton seed oil, sesamol in sesame oil, propyl gallate, Butylated Hydroxy Anisole (BHA) and Butylated Hydroxy Toluene (BHT).

PREPARATION OF SUPPOSITORIES

Suppositories are prepared by three methods-
    i)   Pour moulding from a melt
    ii) Compression
    iii) Hand Rolling and shaping

POUR MOULDING FROM A MELT :

The steps involved in pour moulding are indicated in the chart. Cocoa butter, Glycerinated gelatin, polyethylene glycol and most other bases, are suitable to be prepared by pour moulding.

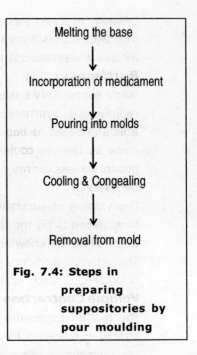

Fig. 7.4: Steps in preparing suppositories by pour moulding

Individual plastic moulds may be obtained to form a single suppository. Industrial moulds produce hundreds of suppositories in a single batch. Moulds commonly used in community pharmacy produce 6 or 12 suppositories. Moulds are commonly made from stainless steel, aluminium, brass or plastic.

Moulds may need lubrication prior to filling, to facilitate easy removal. The bases that undergo large volume contraction seldom need lubricants. The lubricants may be applied by wiping, brushing or spraying.

The weight of suppositories produced, using the same mould, varies with the density of the base. Addition of a medicament also alters the density. It is therefore essential to calibrate the mould with a usual suppository base (cocoa butter), so as to prepare a suppository containing uniform content of the active ingredient. The suppositories containing the base alone are first prepared. The total weight and average weight of each suppository is recorded. The suppositories are carefully melted in a calibrated beaker. The volume of the melt is determined for the total number as well as for the average weight of one suppository.

While preparing the medicated suppositories extemporaneously, the pharmacist needs to calculate the amount of base needed. By subtracting the volume of the drug form, the volume of the mould, the volume of the base required can be calculated. The volume may be converted to weight from the density of the material.

If the volume of the suppository mould is 15 ml and collective volume of the drug and other substances to be added is 5.8 ml, required volume of cocoa butter is 9.2 ml. Density of cocoa butter is 0.86 g/ml. Therefore, 9.2 x 0.86 = 7.9 gm of cocoa butter will be needed.

Another method of determining the amount of base in the preparation of medicated suppositories involves, dissolving or mixing the drug in a small portion of base, insufficient to fill one mould, adding melted base to the cavity to fill it completely, allowing the suppository to cool and congeal, removing and weighing the suppository, and subtracting the weight of the active ingredient from the total weight of the suppository to get the required weight of the base weighed.

The base is melted using least possible heat. Drug is incorporated into a portion of melted base. This is then stirred into the remaining base which has been allowed to cool almost to its congealing point. Volatile materials, if any, should be incorporated at this point with constant stirring.

The moulds are equilibrated to room temperature and the melt is carefully poured. The melt should be continuously stirred to avoid setting of suspended substances. The pouring should be performed just above the congealing point to avoid setting. To ensure completely filled mould on congealing, excess melt is poured and the excess is scraped off after congealing. The mould is usually refrigerated to hasten cooling. The suppositories are carefully removed after bringing the mould back to room temperature.

Automatic Moulding Machine

All the operations of moulding can be performed by a fully automatic moulding machine having an output of 3500-6000 suppositories per hour.

In the moulding machine, a cold turntable holds radially arranged moulds. A hopper maintained at constant temperature, holds the mass which is being stirred continuously. The lubricated moulds are filled to an excess. After solidification of the mass, the excess material is scraped off and collected for reuse. The solidified suppositories are ejected at ejecting stations, where the moulds are opened and suppositories are pushed out by steel rods. Air jets are used to blow loose particles out of the moulds.

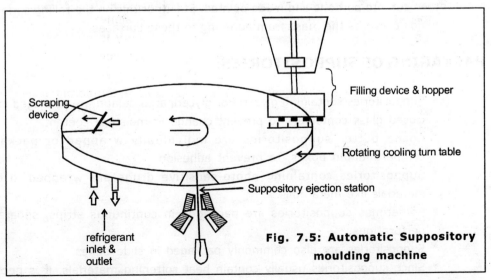

Fig. 7.5: Automatic Suppository moulding machine

Another type of moulding machine performs all the operations included in the rotary machine, but here the individual moulds are carried on a track through a cooling funnel where ejection and scrape-off takes place.

COMPRESSION MOULDING

Cold compression method of making suppositories makes more elegant suppositories. The cold grated base and the other ingredients are mixed thoroughly. The friction in the mixing process slightly softens the material. Softening can also be facilitated by using warm mixing kettles. In the suppository compression machine, a hand turned wheel pushes a piston against a suppository mass contained in a cylinder. This forces the mass out of the other end, into a die or a mould. When the die is filled, the movable endplate at the back of the die is removed. Upon application of additional pressure, the formed suppositories are ejected.

Compression moulding is particularly suitable for making suppositories containing heat-labile substances. Also, there is no likelihood of the suspended solids settling during moulding; hence this method is particularly suitable for suppositories containing high amounts of solids.

There are certain limitations as to shapes of suppositories that can be made by this method. It requires a compression moulding machine and hence is a little expensive.

HAND ROLLING AND SHAPING

This is the oldest and an historic method of making suppositories. A well blended suppository base containing the active ingredient is rolled into the desired shape. The active ingredients are finely powdered or dissolved in a small amount of water or wool fat for the ease of incorporation. The mass is then rolled into a cylindrical rod, which is then cut into portions and made pointed. Starch or talc on the rolling surfaces and hands prevents the mass from adhering to these surfaces.

PACKAGING OF SUPPOSITORIES:

* Suppositories containing glycerin or glycerinated gelatin are packaged in tightly closed glass containers to prevent change in moisture content.
* Cocoa butter suppositories are individually wrapped or packaged in compartmented boxes, to prevent adhesion.
* Suppositories containing photo-sensitive drugs are wrapped in opaque materials like metal foils.
* Sometimes suppositories are packaged in continuous strips, separated by perforations.
* Suppositories are also commonly packaged in slide boxes.
* Since suppositories usually contain heat softening materials, it is necessary

to store them in a cool place, or sometimes in refrigerators. Cocoa butter suppositories should be stored below 30ºC, glycerinated gelatin suppositories at 20-25ºC and polyethylene glycol suppositories at room temperature.

* High humidity in storage space can make the suppository spongy because of water absorption; whereas, excessive dryness can make the suppositories brittle.

QUALITY CONTROL OF SUPPOSITORIES :

Quality Control procedures listed in the US Pharmacopoeia for manufactured suppositories include identification, assay and, in some cases, water content, residual solvent, dissolution and content uniformity.

Identification :

Identification tests are commonly used for the identification and confirmation of official articles.

Assay :

Assay and test procedures are used to determine compliance with the pharmacopoeial standards of identity, strength, quality and purity. Chromatographic methods are commonly used for detection and quantisation.

Dissolution :

Dissolution testing is used to determine compliance with the dissolution requirements, if present in the individual monographs. The test measures the rate and extent of a drug dissolving in a defined medium, under defined conditions.

Water :

As many pharmacopoeial articles are either hydrates or contain water in adsorbed form, the determination of water content may be important in demonstrating compliance with Pharmacopoeial standards. Three methods are commonly used- titrimetric method, azeotropic method and gravimetric method.

Content uniformity :

Content uniformity is required in some monographs to ensure the consistency of dosage units. These dosage units should have drug substance content within a narrow range of the claim made on the label. Weight variation and content uniformity testing involving groups and individual dosage units are used.

Residual solvents :

For pharmacopoeial purposes, these are defined as organic volatile chemicals that are used or produced in the manufacture of drug substances or excipients, or in the preparation of drug products.

Suppository Quality Control includes physical and chemical aspects of the product. Physical analysis includes visual examination (physical appearance), uniformity of weight, uniformity of texture, melting point, liquefaction time, melting and solidification time and mechanical strength. Chemical testing includes dissolution testing.

Visual examination :

Colour and the surface characteristics of the suppository are assessed. It is important to ensure the absence of fissuring, pitting, fat blooming, exudation, sedimentation and the migration of the active ingredients.

Surface condition :

Brilliance, dullness, mottling, cracks, dark regions, axial cavities, bursts, air bubbles, holes, etc., should be checked.

Colour :

The intensity, nature and homogeneity of the colour should be verified.

Odour : A change in the odour may also be indicative of a degradation process.

Weight : Suppositories can be weighed on an automatic balance, obtaining the weight of ten suppositories. If the weight is found to be too small, probably the mould is being under-filled, or there are axial cavities or air bubbles caused by mechanical stirring. If the weight is found to be too high, probably the scraping has not been carried out properly. The weight may decrease during ageing, when the suppositories contain volatile substances, which evaporate through the packaging.

MELTING RANGE (MELTING POINT, MELTING ZONE) :-

Melting range is a more preferred term rather than melting point, as many suppository bases and medicated suppositories are mixtures and so do not have a precise

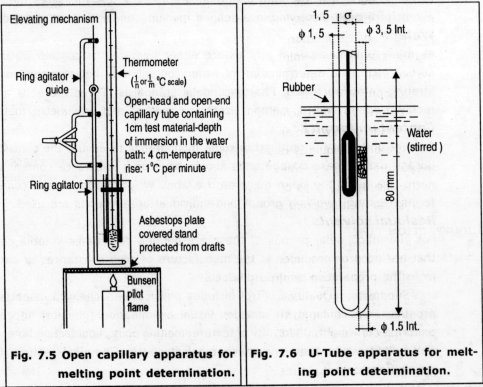

Elevating mechanism

Ring agitator guide

Thermometer ($\frac{1}{n}$ or $\frac{1}{m}$ °C scale)

Open-head and open-end capillary tube containing 1cm test material-depth of immersion in the water bath: 4 cm-temperature rise: 1°C per minute

Ring agitator

Asbestops plate covered stand protected from drafts

Bunsen pilot flame

Fig. 7.5 Open capillary apparatus for melting point determination.

1,5 σ
φ 1,5   φ 3, 5 Int.

Rubber

Water (stirred)

80 mm

φ 1.5 Int.

Fig. 7.6 U-Tube apparatus for melting point determination.

melting point. The release rate of the suppository is related to its melting point. A number of different techniques are used to study melting behaviour, including the open capillary tube, the U-tube, and the drop point methods (Figures 7.5, 7.6 and 7.7).

The methods used are similar in principle, but include different steps and techniques. In general, the equipment is set-up, the suppository dosage unit is placed in the apparatus, heat is applied and change in the system, such as melting or movement, is observed. In general, the melting point should be equal to or less than 37°C. The melting test consists of placing a suppository on the surface of water, thermostatically controlled at 37°C, and verifying the complete melting of the suppository in a few minutes.

Melting point determination

The use of a U-shaped capillary tube to determine melting point, provides precise information for excipient control and consistency in production for those suppositories containing soluble active principles. This method is not suitable when the suppositories have a high powder content, which prevents the fat from sliding inside the capillary tube, to give the end-point determination. The melting point can be determined by placing a small-diameter wire into the mould containing the suppository melt before the form solidifies. It is then immersed in water, and the temperature of the liquid is raised slowly (about 1°C every 2-3minutes), until the suppository slips off the wire. This is the melting point of the suppository.

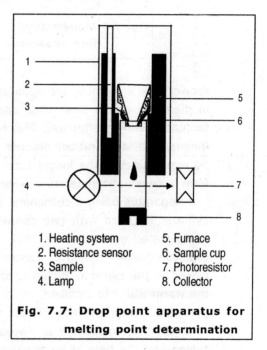

1. Heating system   5. Furnace
2. Resistance sensor   6. Sample cup
3. Sample   7. Photoresistor
4. Lamp   8. Collector

Fig. 7.7: Drop point apparatus for melting point determination

LIQUEFACTION TIME

Liquefaction testing provides information on the behaviour of a suppository when subjected to a maximum temperature of 37°C. The test commonly used is Krowczynski's method, which measures the time required for a suppository to liquefy under pressures similar to those found in the rectum (approximately 30 g), in the presence of water at 37°C. In general, liquefaction should take no longer than about 30 minutes. Two example set-ups are shown in Figures 7.8 and 7.9

Numerous techniques have been developed and used over the years. In

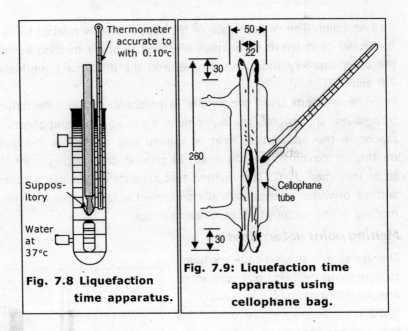

Fig. 7.8 Liquefaction time apparatus.

Fig. 7.9: Liquefaction time apparatus using cellophane bag.

Krowczynski's method, the apparatus consists of a glass tube, with a reduction in diameter at the base. One end is blocked with a small rubber stopper to facilitate cleaning after use. This tube and a thermometer are held in place, by means of a large rubber stopper with two holes, inside a longer tube with a 50 mm diameter. The longer tube has lateral tubes to allow the water, at 37°C, from a constant-temperature water bath to circulate.

Apparatus using a cellophane bag (Fig. 7.9) consists of a glass cylinder. The cylinder is fitted with two connections through which water, maintained at 37°C, can circulate. A cellulose dialyser tubing is moistened, opened and placed in the cylinder. Tubing is attached to allow the warm water to circulate, maintaining the temperature. When the appropriate temperature is reached, the suppository is placed in the dialysis tubing and the time of liquefaction measured.

SUPPOSITORY PENETRATION TEST

A suppository penetration test can be used to determine the temperature at which the suppository becomes sufficiently soft for a penetrating rod to drop through its length. The apparatus used is shown in Fig. 7.10.

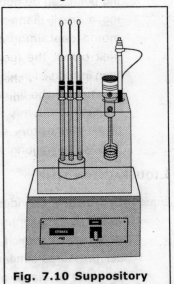

Fig. 7.10 Suppository penetration apparatus.

The temperature is adjusted to that required for the test, generally about 37°C. The suppository is placed in the device and the penetration rod gently moved into place. The device holding the suppository and penetration rod is lowered into the constant temperature bath and a stopwatch is started. When the penetration rod drops through the softened suppository, the time is recorded.

MELTING AND SOLIDIFICATION TIME

There is a relationship between melting and solidification that is important to characterise. The release of the active ingredient from the vehicle is related to the melting point of the vehicle and the solubility of the drug in the vehicle. Suppositories undergo phase change thrice during their "life". First, they are melted and then solidified; upon administration, they are again melted. An understanding of these factors and their relationships is critical for evaluating the bioavailability of the final suppository formulation. Higher the melting point, later the drug effects appear. If melting point is too high, the drug effects do not appear, leading to different results. These are obtained using different methods. Various methods are available to measure them. In one of the methods, liquid is shaken in an evacuated flask until turbid. Then the temperature, at which a transitory rise in temperature occurs during cooling, is noted.

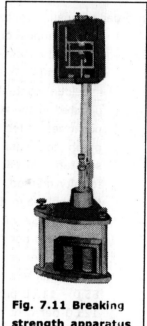

MECHANICAL STRENGTH/CRUSHING TEST

Suppositories can be classified as brittle or elastic by evaluating the mechanical force required to break them. Tests measure the mass (in kilograms) that a suppository can bear without breaking. A good result is one that shows at least 1.8-2 kg pressure. The laboratory set-up is shown in Fig. 7.11.

The suppository is positioned in an upright position and increasing weights are placed on it until it loses its structure and collapses. The purpose of the test is to verify that the suppository can be transported under normal conditions

Fig. 7.11 Breaking strength apparatus

DISSOLUTION TEST

One of the most important quality control tools available for *in vitro* assessment is dissolution testing. Dissolution testing is often required for suppositories to test for hardening and polymorphic transitions of active ingredients and suppository bases. Melting, deformation and dispersion in the dissolution medium often poses problems in dissolution testing of suppositories. Dissolution testing methods include the paddle method, basket method and membrane diffusion method. In order to control the variation in the ratio of mass to medium interface, various means have been used, including a wire mesh basket, or a membrane, to separate the sample chamber from the reservoir. Samples sealed in dialysis tubing, or natural membranes, may also be studied. Flow cell apparatus, which holds the sample in place with cotton, wire screening or glass beads, can also be used.

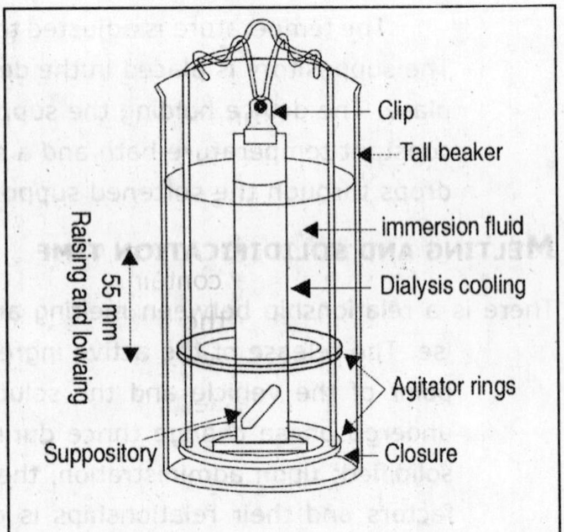

Fig. 7.12: Dissolution testing using membrane/ dialysis diffusion method

CONTENT UNIFORMITY TESTING

In order to ensure content uniformity, individual suppositories must be analysed to provide information on dose-to-dose uniformity. Testing is based on the assay of the individual content of drug substance(s) in a number of individual dosage units to determine whether the individual content is within the limits set. Ten units are assayed individually, as directed in the Assay in the individual monograph. The USP 30 criteria for suppositories states the following: Unless otherwise specified in the individual monograph, the requirements for dosage uniformity are met if the amount of the drug substance in each of the 10 dosage units as determined from the Content Uniformity method, lies within the range of 85.0-115.0 percent to 115.0 per cent of the label claim if the Relative standard deviation (RSD). If 1 unit is outside the range of 85.0 of 115.0 per cent of label claim, and no unit is outside the range of 75.0-125.0 per cent of label claim, or if the relative standard deviation is greater than 6.0 per cent,or if both conditions prevail, 20 additional units are tested. The requirements are met if not more than1 unit of the 30 is outside the range of 85.0 - 115.0 per cent of label claim, and no unit is outside the range of 75.0 - 125.0 per cent of label claim and the RSD of the 30 dosage units does not exceed 7.8 per cent.

AGEING TESTS

Changes over time may alter the physical and/or chemical properties of a suppository. Melting point fluctuations, for example, may occur either as a result of polymorphic changes in the excipient, or as a result of evaporation of a volatile medicament or because of physical or chemical reactions between medicaments or excipients. Some problems associated with ageing include the following:

- An odour may emanate from suppositories with vegetable extracts due to fungal contamination.
- Suppositories containing some dye may discolour due to oxidation of the dyes.
- The shape of some suppositories may be altered during storage at incorrect temperatures.
- Suppositories containing vegetable extracts or caffeine base may exhibit whitening on the surface.
- Suppositories containing camphor, menthol, or other volatile substances that may be lost due to vaporisation over time, may lose weight during storage.
- Other ageing phenomena, such as hardening, softening, blooming, mottling, and cracking may occur over time, depending upon the composition of the suppositories and storage conditions.

INDEX